2024

ADVANCES IN MOLECULAR PATHOLOGY

EDITOR-IN-CHIEF

Ahmad N. Abou Tayoun, PhD, FACMG

SECTION EDITORS

Stefan Rentas, PhD, FACMG

Jeremiah Karrs, DO

Erin Graf, PhD, D(ABMM)

Ann M. Moyer, MD, PhD

Nephi Walton, MD, MS, FACMG, FAMIA

Hunter Best, PhD, FACMG

ELSEVIER

Publishing Director, Medical Reference: Dolores Meloni
Editor: Taylor Hayes
Developmental Editor: Malvika Shah

Reprints: For copies of 100 or more of articles in this publication, please contact the Commercial Reprints Department, Elsevier Inc., 360 Park Avenue South, New York, NY 10010-1710. Tel: 212-633-3874; Fax: 212-633-3820; E-mail: reprints@elsevier.com.

Printed in the United States of America.

Editorial Office:
Elsevier, Inc.
1600 John F. Kennedy Blvd,
Suite 1800
Philadelphia, PA 19103-2899

International Standard Serial Number: 2589-4080
International Standard Book Number: 13: 978-0-443-31612-8

ADVANCES IN MOLECULAR PATHOLOGY

CONTRIBUTORS

AHMAD N. ABOU TAYOUN, PhD, FACMG
Director, Al Jalila Genomics Center, Al Jalila Children's Specialty Hospital, DUBAI, Associate Professor of Genetics, Mohammed Bin Rashid University, Dubai, UAE

ERICA F. ANDERSEN, PhD, FACMG
Section Chief, Cytogenetics and Genomic Microarray, ARUP Laboratories, Associate Professor, Department of Pathology, University of Utah School of Medicine, Salt Lake City, Utah, USA

MICHELE ANDERSON, DO
Fellow, Department of Pathology, Virginia Commonwealth University, Richmond, Virginia, USA

ALISON D. ARCHIBALD, PhD
Associate Professor, Department of Paediatrics, The University of Melbourne, Victorian Clinical Genetics Service, The Roal Children's Hospital, Group Leader, Reproductive Genetic Screening, Genomics in Society, Murdoch, Children's Research Institute, Parkville, Victoria, Australia

VAHID AZIMI, MD
Instructor, Division of Laboratory and Genomic Medicine, Pathology and Immunology, Washington University School of Medicine, St Louis, Missouri, USA

BRIANNA M. BEMBENEK, BA
Department of Pathology, Carver College of Medicine, University of Iowa, Iowa City, Iowa, USA; PhD Candidate, Mayo Clinic Graduate School of Biomedical Sciences, Mayo Clinic, Rochester, Minnesota, USA

HUNTER BEST, PhD, FACMG
Professor, Department of Pathology, University of Utah School of Medicine, Salt Lake City, UT; Medical Director, Molecular Genetics & Genomics, ARUP Laboratories, Salt Lake City, UT, USA

TIFFANY F. BOUGHTWOOD, MBA
Managing Director Australian Genomics, Genomics Health Alliances, Murdoch Children's Research Institute, Parkville, Victoria, Australia

SOMA ROY CHAKRABORTY, MD
Dartmouth Hitchcock Medical Center, Lebanon, New Hampshire, USA

SRIKAR CHAMALA, PhD
Director, Center for Pathology Informatics and Data Science, Children's Hospital Los Angeles, Department of Pathology, University of Southern California, Associate Professor of Clinical Pathology, USC Keck School of Medicine, Los Angeles, California, USA

KRISTY R. CROOKS, PhD
Associate Professor, Department of Pathology, University of Colorado Anschutz Medical Campus, Aurora, Colorado, USA

MARTIN B. DELATYCKI, MBBS, FRACP, PhD
Professor and Co-Director (Bruce Lefroy Centre for Genetic Health Research), Department of Paediatrics, The University of Melbourne, Victorian Clinical Genetics Service, Bruce Lefroy Centre, Murdoch Children's Research Institute, Parkville, Victoria, Australia

ROBERT H. DOLIN, MD
Senior Informaticist, Elimu Informatics, El Cerrito, California, USA

REBEKAH E. DUMM, PhD
Assistant Professor, Division of Laboratory and Genomic Medicine, Pathology and Immunology, Washington University School of Medicine, St Louis, Missouri, USA

MAKENZIE L. FULMER, PhD
Assistant Professor, Department of Pathology, University of Utah School of Medicine, ARUP Laboratories, Salt Lake City, Utah, USA

ERIC GOOLD, MD
Neuropathology Fellow, Department of Pathology, University of Utah, ARUP Laboratories, Salt Lake City, Utah, USA

BRET S.E. HEALE, PhD
Senior Consultant, Humanized Health Consulting, Salt Lake City, Utah, USA

RAJESWARI JAYAKUMAR, MD
Assistant Professor, Department of Pathology, Virginia Commonwealth University, Richmond, Virginia, USA

YUAN JI, PhD, DABCP, FACMG
Associate Professor, Department of Pathology, University of Utah School of Medicine, ARUP Laboratories, Salt Lake City, Utah, USA

JEREMIAH KARRS, DO
Hematopathologist, Pathology, Dartmouth Hitchcock Medical Center, Lebanon, New Hampshire, USA

PRABHJOT KAUR, MD
Director, Hematology Laboratory, Dartmouth Hitchcock Medical Center, Lebanon, New Hampshire, USA

WAHAB A. KHAN, PhD
Assistant Director (Molecular/Cytogenetics), Dartmouth Hitchcock Medical Center, Lebanon, New Hampshire, USA

EDWIN P. KIRK, MBBS, PhD
Professor, Centre for Clinical Genetics, Sydney Children's Hospital, Randwick, NSW Health Pathology Randwick Genomics Laboratory, School of Clinical Medicine, University of New South Wales, Randwick, New South Wales, Australia

NIGEL G. LAING, PhD
Emeritus Professor, Department of Diagnostic Genomics, Centre for Medical Research, University of Western Australia, Group Leader, Preventive Genetics Group, PathWest Laboratory Medicine, Nedlands, Western Australia, Australia

CARLO R. LARGIADÈR, PhD
Associate Professor, Vice Director, Department of Clinical Chemistry, Inselspital, Bern University Hospital, University of Bern, Bern, Switzerland

REYNOLD C. LY, PhD
Department of Research, Institute for Genomic Medicine, Clinical laboratory Director, Nationwide Children's Hospital, Columbus, Ohio, USA

VALARIE McMURTRY, MD, PhD
Assistant Professor, Department of Pathology, University of Utah, ARUP Laboratories, Salt Lake City, Utah, USA

RADHA NAGARAJAN, PhD
Information Services Department, Children's Hospital of Orange County, Orange, California, USA

JOHN M. O'SHEA, PhD
Laboratory Genetics and Genomics Fellow, Department of Pathology, University of Utah School of Medicine, ARUP Laboratories, Salt Lake City, Utah, USA

IFEYINWA E. OBIORAH, MD, PhD
Assistant Professor, Department of Pathology, Division of Hematopathology, University of Virginia Health, Charlottesville, Virginia, USA

STEVEN M. OFFER, PhD
Associate Professor, Department of Pathology, Carver College of Medicine, University of Iowa, Iowa City, Iowa, USA; Assistant Professor, Mayo Clinic Graduate School of Biomedical Sciences, Mayo Clinic, Rochester, Minnesota, USA

LUCILLA PIZZO, MS, PhD
Assistant Professor, Department of Pathology, University of Utah School of Medicine, ARUP Laboratories, Salt Lake City, Utah, USA

EVAN RAPS, MD
Assistant Professor, Department of Pathology, University of Utah, ARUP Laboratories, Salt Lake City, Utah, USA

SUSAN E. REALEGENO, PhD, D(ABMM)
Scientific Director, Quest Diagnostics, Infectious Disease Department, San Juan Capistrano, California, USA

MEGHAN W. STAROLIS, PhD, HCLD(ABB)
Senior Science Director, Infectious Disease, Quest Diagnostics, Molecular Infectious Disease Department, Chantilly, Virginia, USA

MARWAN K. TAYEH, PhD, FACMG
Associate Professor, Division of Diagnostic Genetics and Genomics, Department of Medical and Molecular Genetics, Director, Indiana University Genetic Testing Laboratories, Indiana University School of Medicine, Indianapolis, Indiana, USA

ERIN TUTTY, MGenCouns
PhD Candidate, Department of Paediatrics, Genomics in Society, Murdoch Children's Research Institute, The University of Melbourne, Parkville, Victoria, Australia

DEREK WALTON, JD
Walton Legal PLLC, Murray, Utah, USA

NEPHI WALTON, MD, MS, FACMG, FAMIA
Program Director, National Human Genome Research Institute, Bethesda, Maryland, USA

CHEN WANG, PhD, FAMIA
Associate Professor of Biomedical Informatics, Mayo Clinic, Rochester, Minnesota, USA

STEPHEN J. WICKS, PhD
Associate Professor, Department of Pathology, University of Colorado Anschutz Medical Campus, Aurora, Colorado, USA

JONATHAN WILCOCK, MD
Fellow, Department of Pathology, Division of Hematopathology, University of Virginia Health, Charlottesville, Virginia, USA

CONTENTS

VOLUME 7 • 2024

Education of Future Pharmacogenomics Laboratory Directors, *33*

By Reynold C. Ly, Marwan K. Tayeh, and Yuan Ji

Pharmacogenomic testing is increasingly performed in clinical laboratories for various hospital disciplines such as oncology, cardiology, and psychiatry. Thus, there is a need for more clinical laboratory directors to be proficient in clinical pharmacogenomic testing. However, there are limited opportunities and exposure to clinical pharmacogenomic testing in training programs. This article provides guidance to training programs or others not familiar with clinical pharmacogenomics on key points to consider for education in this testing.

Considerations in Clinical Laboratory Development of Pharmacogenomic Testing, *43*

By Stephen J. Wicks and Kristy R. Crooks

Personalized and precision medicine initiatives increasingly incorporate pharmacogenomic testing in efforts to improve health outcomes and reduce costs. During test development, laboratories should consider population-specific allele frequencies, the star allele nomenclature system, multigene-drug interactions, and non-pharmacogenomic clinical implications associated with pharmacogenes. Furthermore, the responsible integration of pharmacogenomic information into routine clinical practice requires providing provider and patient education, standardizing testing protocols, addressing reimbursement, and overcoming systemic barriers to equitable utility of pharmacogenomic information across populations.

Hematopathology

Advances in Structural Variant Detection in Hematolymphoid Malignancies: Optical Genome Mapping, *53*

By Soma Roy Chakraborty, Wahab A. Khan, Prabhjot Kaur, and Jeremiah Karrs

Optical genome mapping (OGM) is a new genome-wide technology that simplifies lab workflow by revealing both structural genomic changes and copy number variants in a single assay. This review comprehensively describes the OGM technique, outlining its unique strengths and weaknesses compared to standard-of-care techniques for hematologic malignancies. This review also explains how the OGM technique has the potential to transform front-line testing for various hematologic malignancies, including acute myeloid leukemia, myelodysplastic syndromes, acute lymphoblastic leukemia, multiple myeloma, and chronic lymphocytic leukemia.

Recent Advances in the Molecular Pathogenesis and Diagnosis of Chronic Myelomonocytic Leukemia, *63*

By Michele Anderson and Rajeswari Jayakumar

Purpose of Review: Chronic myelomonocytic leukemia (CMML) is a clonal hematopoietic malignancy defined by both proliferative and dysplastic features, monocytosis and a predilection for leukemic transformation. CMML is a poorly understood neoplasm with an overall dismal prognosis, and minimal treatment options. This review aims to summarize the diagnostic features in the updated World Health Organization 5th Edition, molecular findings in CMML, and current prognostic models, as well as provide recommendations for future studies.

Molecular Profiling of Small Mature B Cell Lymphomas; New Insights on Diagnosis and Treatment, *77*

By Jonathan Wilcock and Ifeyinwa E. Obiorah

A confident diagnosis of distinct small B cell lymphomas can be made in the majority of cases based on morphology and immunophenotypic studies. Further analysis with cytogenetic and fluorescence in situ hybridization testing is performed in certain cases. In the absence of helpful translocations, next-generation sequencing or copy number variation may follow to look for specific alterations, especially in the presence of therapy resistance. Notably, molecular results should not be interpreted in isolation but in the context of clinicopathological findings. Precise molecular features of each patient are helpful in the risk stratification and subsequent treatment of any patient.

Infectious Disease

Advances in Self-collection/Self-testing for Sexually Transmitted Infections and Implications for Health Equity, *89*

By Meghan W. Starolis and Susan E. Realegeno

The ability for a patient to collect their own sample for testing (self-collection) is critical for telehealth services, direct-to-consumer testing, and over-the counter testing. An assay can have specific claims from the Food and Drug Administration for self-collection, which will indicate if the sample can be collected in a health care setting (observed vs unobserved) or can be self-collected outside of a health care setting (ie, at home). Although there can be significant regulatory hurdles, expansion of self-collection can have positive implications for health equity by increasing access to testing as well as lowering barriers related to social stigmas and discomfort when seeking sexually transmitted infection testing in traditional health care settings.

Implementation, Optimization, and Stewardship of Advanced Molecular Testing for Infectious Diseases, *99*

By Vahid Azimi and Rebekah E. Dumm

Advanced molecular testing for infectious diseases is complex and results can be strongly influenced by testing methodology, specimen selection and patient population. Given their technical expertise and knowledge of laboratory workflows, clinical laboratories are well-suited to coordinate diagnostic stewardship efforts. In this review, the authors define the scope of published diagnostic stewardship for molecular infectious disease testing and review the reported impact of stewardship interventions with a focus on multiplex molecular panels for syndromic testing and sequencing-based assays.

Informatics

Genomics Clinical Decision Support with Fast Healthcare Interoperability Resources Genomics Operations, *113*

By Robert H. Dolin, Bret S.E. Heale, and Srikar Chamala

Next-generation sequencing can identify thousands to millions of variants, whose clinical significance can change over time as our knowledge evolves. To manage such a large volume of dynamic and complex data, new models of genomics-EHR integration are needed. FHIR Genomics Operations encapsulate data complexity, enable dynamic variant annotation, and offer an approach for driving advanced CDS that leverages a person's entire genome. Coupled with the tremendous growth and adoption of FHIR along with the growing adoption of SMART-on-FHIR and CDS Hooks, Operations are poised as a novel enabler of genomics-EHR integration to drive next generation advances in precision care.

Is Picture Archiving and Communication System a Model for Genomics?, *123*

By Srikar Chamala, Robert H. Dolin, and Nephi Walton

Integrating genomic data into electronic health records (EHRs) presents significant challenges due to the voluminous and complex nature of genomic data, differences between bioinformatics and EHR data standards, and the rapid evolution of knowledge that quickly outdated variant annotations. To manage this large and dynamic data volume, institutions are exploring the use of a genomic archiving and communication system (GACS) This study aims to analyze the picture archiving and communication system (PACS) model to identify insights that could enhance the development of GACS-based strategies, comparing various aspects such as workflow, data standards, EHR viewing, and storage in a "vendor neutral archive".

Fast Healthcare Interoperability Resource Genomics and Polygenic Risk Scores, *131*

By Bret S.E. Heale

Health Level 7's (HL7) Fast Healthcare Interoperability Resource (FHIR) is a critical clinically used standard in health care data exchange, with a flexible model that provides strong syntactic reliability and delivers semantic interoperability. Clinical polygenic risk scoring features were collected and used to populate an example in FHIR. A critical feature is the genetic similarity between a patient and the underlying population used to develop the score. The example delivers computable representation, including ancestry adjustment and genetic similarity measures, demonstrating that FHIR can communicate polygenic risk. FHIR's flexibility allows the representation to evolve as clinical polygenic risk reporting evolves.

Artificial Intelligence Applications in Genomics, *145*

By Radha Nagarajan, Chen Wang, Derek Walton, and Nephi Walton

Several factors have contributed to the rapid growth of genomic data, including the significant reduction in high-throughput sequencing costs, the availability of scalable and affordable cloud computing infrastructure for efficient storage and processing, increased knowledge of genomic variation leading to clinical utility for diagnosis, and the broader adoption and awareness of genomics, particularly through recreational genomics In this article, we will explore the current applications and technologies of artificial intelligence in genomics, examine its role in clinical settings, and discuss the challenges that must be addressed to further advance its integration and impact.

Hot Topics

A Concise Overview of Circulating Tumor DNA Detection for Solid Tumors, *155*

By Eric Goold, Evan Raps, and Valarie McMurtry

Detection of circulating tumor DNA (ctDNA) of solid tumors presents several challenges. There can be very low amounts of tumor DNA within plasma leading stochastic sampling bias or detection below the noise level of an assay resulting in false negatives. False positives can result from clonal hematopoiesis or sequencing errors. ctDNA detection methods can be classified by technique, such as amplicon-based sequencing, hybridization capture-based sequencing, and whole genome sequencing, and whether these technologies use a patient's a priori tumor information for personalized or tumor-informed panels. This review provides a brief overview of challenges faced by the field, current ctDNA methodology in solid tumors, and explores the current roll of ctDNA in non-small cell lung cancer and breast cancer.

Structural variants (SVs), including unbalanced copy-number variants as well as balanced rearrangements, play a crucial role in human genetic conditions. Polymerase chain reaction-free short-read whole-genome sequencing promises improved resolution of copy number and potentially balanced SVs along with routine single-nucleotide variant detection in the clinical setting. The identification of SVs using next-generation sequencing relies on distinctive read patterns or "signatures" diagnostic of different SV types. While multiple algorithms have been developed for SV identification, no single method consistently performs best across different SV types and sizes.

Next-generation sequencing has revolutionized the ability to interrogate the human genome and diagnose individuals with genetic disorders. Short-read sequencing offers high-throughput and read accuracy but has reduced capacity to detect structural variation and highly complex regions of the genome. Long-read sequencing has an improved ability to identify structural variation and complex, repetitive regions in the genome. Currently, short-read sequencing technologies are more widely used in clinical testing compared to long-read sequencing.

Advances in Molecular Pathology 7 (2024) xvii
ADVANCES IN MOLECULAR PATHOLOGY

Preface

Molecular Pathology: Another Year of Innovation

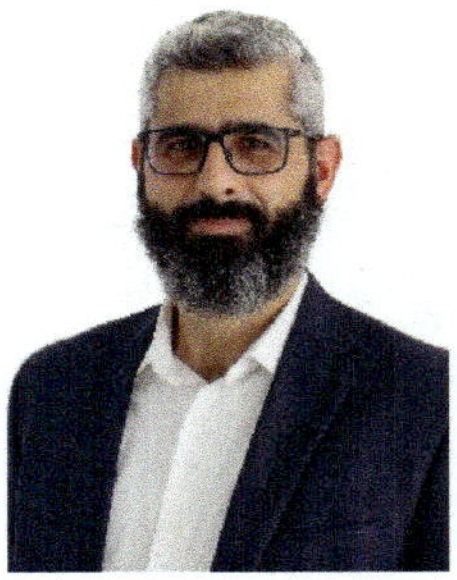

Ahmad N. Abou Tayoun, PhD, FACMG
Editor

It is an immense honor to take on the chief editor role from my mentor and colleague, Greg Tsongalis, the founding editor of this journal, the content of which we have all been enjoying over the past 6 years. Building on Greg's efforts over the years, and specifically the spectacular team of section editors he brought together, I am delighted to present the *seventh issue* of *Advances in Molecular Pathology*.

This issue reflects the *impressive* strides made in our field to improve patient care. It includes articles *illustrating* the application of molecular *approaches for diagnosing a diverse range of disorders, spanning* genetic diseases, hematologic malignancies, infectious diseases, pharmacogenomics, and solid tumors, and provides state-of-the-art overviews of recent topics, such as reproductive genetic carrier screening, structural variant detection, circulating tumor DNA, and the evolving sequencing technologies. Pertinent to the growing need for improved informatics tools to harness the large data sets routinely being generated in Molecular Pathology labs *amid rapid advances in emerging technologies*, this year we dedicate an "Informatics" section, which covers data analytics topics, such as artificial intelligence and the integration of genomics into electronic health records, among others.

I am immensely grateful to those friends and colleagues who once again agreed to become section editors and authors of the fantastic articles presented here.

Happy reading!

DISCLOSURES

The author has no conflicts of interest to disclose.

Ahmad N. Abou Tayoun, PhD, FACMG
Al Jalila Genomics Center
Al Jalila Children's Specialty Hospital

Genetics Department
Mohammed Bin Rashid University
Dubai, UAE

E-mail address: Ahmad.Tayoun@dubaihealth.ae

https://doi.org/10.1016/j.yamp.2024.08.002
2589-4080/24/

Genetics

Advances in Molecular Pathology 7 (2024) 1–14
ADVANCES IN MOLECULAR PATHOLOGY

Toward Accessible Reproductive Genetic Carrier Screening

Considerations for Implementation at Scale

Erin Tutty, MGenCouns[a,b], Alison D. Archibald, PhD[a,b,c], Tiffany F. Boughtwood, MBA[d,e], Edwin P. Kirk, MBBS, PhD[f,g,h], Nigel G. Laing, PhD[i,j,k], Martin B. Delatycki, MBBS, FRACP, PhD[b,c,l,*]

[a]Genomics in Society, Murdoch Children's Research Institute, Parkville, Victoria 3052, Australia; [b]Department of Paediatrics, The University of Melbourne, Parkville, Victoria 3052, Australia; [c]Victorian Clinical Genetics Service, The Roal Children's Hospital, Parkville, Victoria 3052, Australia; [d]Australian Genomics, Parkville, Victoria 3052, Australia; [e]Genomics Health Alliances, Murdoch Children's Research Institute, Parkville, Victoria 3052, Australia; [f]Centre for Clinical Genetics, Sydney Children's Hospital, Randwick, New South Wales 2031, Australia; [g]NSW Health Pathology Randwick Genomics Laboratory, Randwick, New South Wales 2031, Australia; [h]School of Clinical Medicine, University of New South Wales, Randwick, New South Wales 6009, Australia; [i]PathWest Laboratory Medicine, Department of Diagnostic Genomics, Nedlands, Western Australia 6009, Australia; [j]Centre for Medical Research, University of Western Australia, Nedlands, Western Australia 6009, Australia; [k]Harry Perkins Institute of Medical Research, Nedlands, Western Australia 6009, Australia; [l]Bruce Lefroy Centre, Murdoch Children's Research Institute, Parkville, Victoria 3052, Australia

KEYWORDS

• Reproductive genetic carrier screening • Preconception • Prenatal • Next generation sequencing • Implementation • Psychosocial

KEY POINTS

- Reproductive genetic carrier screening (RGCS) provides reproductive partners information about their chance of having children with severe, childhood onset genetic conditions.
- The advent of massive parallel sequencing meant that RGCS is available for hundreds of genes ("expanded" panels) to all people planning a pregnancy or in early pregnancy.
- The primary goal of RGCS is to promote reproductive autonomy; this can be achieved through carefully considered gene selection and variant reporting and access to genetic counseling.
- A couple-based approach, whereby reproductive couples are screened concurrently and receive a combined result (low or increased chance), provides information most useful for reproductive planning and most feasible at population scale.
- People generally do use results for reproductive planning, although reproductive decision-making after receipt of an increased chance result is psychosocially complex.

INTRODUCTION

Approximately 1% to 2% of reproductive couples (ie, the two genetic contributors to a pregnancy) have an "increased chance" of having children with autosomal recessive (AR) or X-linked (XL) conditions [1]. This figure is greater among consanguineous couples [2]. Most people with an increased chance are unaware of their carrier status until the birth of a child with the condition. Reproductive genetic carrier screening (RGCS) provides this information before or in early pregnancy.

RGCS was initially available for a limited number of conditions and offered to people from ancestral groups

*Corresponding author. Victorian Clinical Genetics Service, The Royal Children's Hospital, 4th Floor, 50 Flemington Road, Parkville, Victoria 3052, Australia. *E-mail address:* martin.delatycki@vcgs.org.au

https://doi.org/10.1016/j.yamp.2024.06.001 www.advancesinmolecularpathology.com
2589-4080/24/

with high carrier frequencies or those with a family history of the condition [2,3]. As genes were identified as the cause of AR and XL conditions, population-level screening became possible [2]. These programs demonstrated high levels of acceptability and feasibility [4,5] and also highlighted that using a priori risk alone, as an indicator for offering screening, underidentifies people with an increased chance [6]. The advent of massively parallel sequencing means it is now possible to screen hundreds of genes simultaneously [2]. This is sometimes described as "expanded" carrier screening. Professional bodies globally recommend that RGCS be offered to all people before or in early pregnancy [7–9].

GOALS OF REPRODUCTIVE GENETIC CARRIER SCREENING

RGCS aims to support reproductive autonomy: a person's ability to reproduce in a way that aligns with their goals and beliefs [10–12]. With RGCS, reproductive autonomy can be supported by providing information useful for reproductive planning ("reproductive utility") and ensuring people have access to support and resources needed to make informed reproductive decisions.

RGCS can be offered when forming a relationship (eg, the Dor Yeshorim premarital screening program for people of Jewish ancestry [2]), preconception or prenatally. Preconception RGCS is more ideal than prenatal RGCS, as it enables people with an increased chance to consider all available reproductive options. Options include using in vitro fertilization (IVF) with preimplantation genetic testing for monogenic disorders (PGT-M), prenatal diagnosis (PND) with or without termination for an affected pregnancy (TOP), not having (more) children, using donor gametes, adopting/fostering children, or using the information to plan and prepare to have a child with the genetic condition. When pregnant, people only have the options of PND with or without TOP, or not testing during pregnancy.

It is important to acknowledge that in supporting reproductive autonomy, the prevalence of some genetic conditions in the community will be reduced [10]. Prevention has been a specified aim of some ancestry-based screening programs, particularly in communities in which genetic conditions have significant disease burdens [12]. At a population level, however, prevention is not usually considered an ethically appropriate goal of RGCS [12]. Nevertheless, a person's desire to avoid a serious genetic condition in their children is a primary motivating factor in the decision to have RGCS [13,14].

IMPLEMENTING REPRODUCTIVE GENETIC CARRIER SCREENING

There is considerable variation in how RGCS is implemented worldwide, reflecting social, cultural, and political differences [3]. Very few nations have government-funded population-level screening for more than one or a few genes (Fig. 1) [3,15–17]. More commonly, RGCS is available on a user-pays basis through commercial providers with limited regulatory oversight [18]. Uncoordinated approaches to RGCS can risk inequity of access and increase demands on health systems. Thus, consideration is now being directed toward how to deliver RGCS effectively and appropriately at population scale [19]. This article will provide an overview of the current landscape of RGCS and will summarize learnings that can be used to promote the ethical and equitable implementation of RGCS now and into the future.

PRE-TEST CONSIDERATIONS

Societal Acceptability

Societal acceptability is critical to the successful implementation of RGCS. Studies in several nations have demonstrated positive attitudes toward RGCS among the public and those offered RGCS [20–23]. Some people may support the availability of RGCS for others even if they would not choose it for themselves [24]. People with a personal or family history of a genetic condition are also mostly supportive of RGCS, particularly if offered before conception [25–28], but there is some concern about it contributing to a less inclusive society [10,26]. Collaboration with patient groups can ensure RGCS is implemented in a socially acceptable manner.

Uptake is one measure of societal acceptability, though uptake rates are not necessarily indicative of autonomous choice. For example, the "quasi-mandatory" approach to hemoglobinopathy screening in Cyprus has high uptake but has raised questions about social pressure to participate [29]. With greater awareness and accessibility, there is potential for people to perceive RGCS as routine, or feel obligated to accept the offer, even if it does not align with their values [10]. Nevertheless, a systematic review noted that interest in RGCS when offered hypothetically is typically higher than observed uptake [30]. The same review identified considerable variation in uptake, ranging from 8% to 50% [30]. These findings may be explained by the intention–behavior gap, whereby external and internal factors (eg, the cost of RGCS or the timing

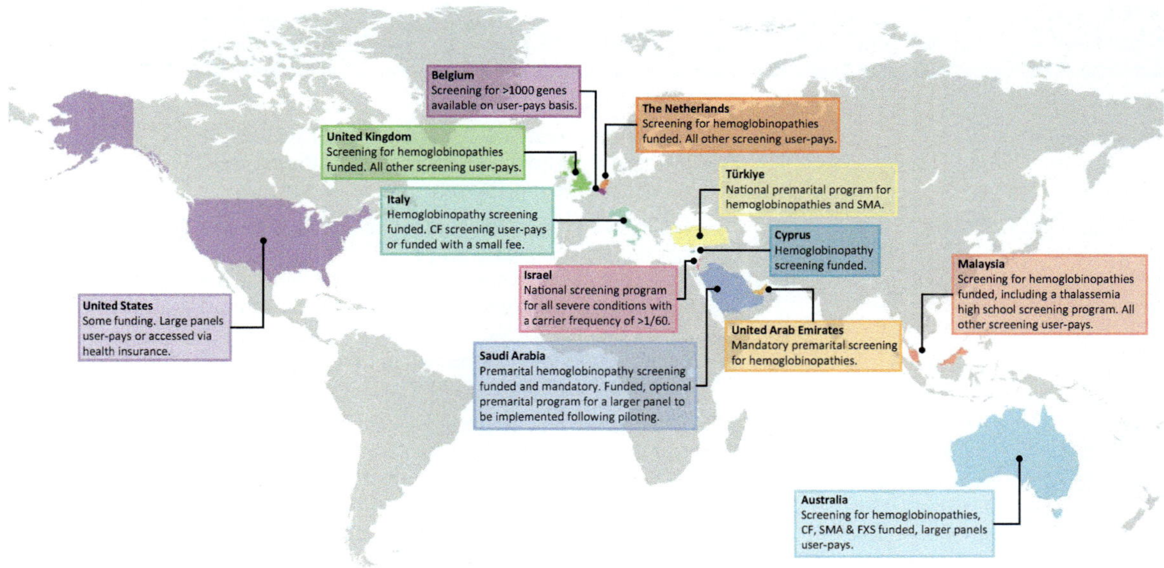

FIG. 1 Implementation of reproductive genetic carrier screening in selection locations. CF, cystic fibrosis; SMA, spinal muscular atrophy; FXS, fragile X syndrome. Note: Select locations used to illustrate examples of coordinated approaches to reproductive genetic carrier screening for the general population. [3,15-17] Not representative of all screening programs worldwide. Reproductive genetic carrier screening is also available through commercial providers in many countries.

of the offer) serve as barriers to completing a behavior [30].

Equity of Access

Most RGCS is accessed outside of specialized genetic centers, meaning the role of non-genetic health care providers (HCPs) in offering screening is crucial. Offers of RGCS are often ad hoc due to a range of infrastructural factors. Additional factors may also serve as barriers to participation, compounding inequity of access (Table 1).

The Australian Reproductive Genetic Carrier Screening Project ("Mackenzie's Mission") specifically addressed many barriers to accessing RGCS. It provides an RGCS model that can serve as an example of how health systems may increase equity of access in their jurisdictions (Box 1) [19].

Informed Decision-Making

An important measure of RGCS program feasibility and acceptability is whether people make informed decisions to participate [44]. Across three European population-based studies, greater than 70% of participants were assessed as having made an informed choice about RGCS [14,22,45]. Those who had RGCS reported minimal decisional conflict [22,46] and regret about their choice [40]. People who were offered RGCS as part of clinical care, rather than within a research study, have reported that decisions about screening were made quickly with limited deliberation [47]. Further, those who receive an increased chance result have expressed feeling unprepared for the result [47].

Reasons given to accept or decline RGCS are described in Table 2. Misconceptions about the relevance of RGCS highlight the importance of pre-test education being provided alongside the offer of RGCS [23]. However, as demand for RGCS increases, in-person modes of pre-test education may not be practical. Instead, multimedia tools such as decision aids can be used to facilitate decision-making about RGCS at population scale [43].

Multimedia tools can also ensure pre-test information is standardized, balanced, and appropriate to the target population [43]. Approaches for developing these tools and raising awareness of them in the community need further consideration. As technologies advance, pre-test education becomes increasingly complex, particularly with respect to communicating information about the conditions screened [48]. Consent approaches describing the screening process, the implications of results and the limitations of the test, may be most practical for large gene panels [7].

TABLE 1
Barriers to Accessing Reproductive Genetic Carrier Screening

Domain	Barriers
Infrastructure	• Health care systems not prioritizing RGCS [31,32] • Without a coordinated approach to offering RGCS and managing results, HCPs may be reluctant to engage [31]
HCP knowledge, skills, and prioritization	• HCPs have reported limited awareness of and/or engagement with current RGCS guidelines [31,33] • The complexity of genetic information, and a lack of familiarity with the conditions screened, deters some HCPs from ordering RGCS for their patients [31,33] • HCPs report challenges remembering to offer RGCS or prioritizing offering RGCS [33]
Cost	• The cost of RGCS is a significant barrier to equity of access • Uptake of commercially available RGCS in Australia was highest among people living in high socioeconomic areas [34]. Government funded RGCS for cystic fibrosis, spinal muscular atrophy, and fragile X syndrome became available in Australia 2023, but larger panels remain user-pays • In the United States, health insurance coverage may limit access to RGCS. Carlotti et al. [35] noted that lack of insurance coverage prevented male individuals from undergoing screening after their female reproductive partner was identified as a carrier of an AR condition
Logistical issues	• Questions have been raised about how best to facilitate access to RGCS for people living in regional and remote areas [33] and other locations with limited access to health care services. Similar issues may arise regarding access to post-result genetic counseling and reproductive options • Other logistical factors, such as the time required to organize RGCS and an aversion to blood tests can serve as barriers [36]
Lack of cultural and linguistic inclusivity	• People may experience barriers to engaging with RGCS if information and support is unavailable in their preferred language [37] • Discrimination resulting in mistrust of the genetics profession and/or the health care system can also deter people from accessing RGCS [38]
Timeliness	• The timeliness of the offer and/or result disclosure have been identified as important considerations for RGCS [39] • While undergoing RGCS before pregnancy may be ideal, preconception health care is under accessed [32]. Further, not all pregnancies are planned and those not planning a pregnancy are unlikely to access preconception health care. Self-funding RGCS may also be less of a priority before conception than during pregnancy • Late presentation for prenatal care may also serve as a barrier to RGCS access; HCPs may view offering RGCS as a low priority and patients may decline due to low perceived utility of results • Turnaround time for results may also limit the utility of results. In a preliminary evaluation of preconception RGCS in Belgium, mean turnaround time was 39 wk [40]. During this time, some couples became pregnant [40]

(*continued on next page*)

TABLE 1
(*continued*)

Domain	Barriers
Availability of reproductive options	• Availability of reproductive interventions can also limit the utility of results and, therefore, serve as a barrier to accessing RGCS • Termination of pregnancy is legal and funded in jurisdictions such as Australia, Cyprus, Israel, Italy, the Netherlands, and the United Kingdom (with the exception of Northern Ireland) [3]. By contrast, in some jurisdictions, such as Malaysia, Saudi Arabia, Northern Ireland, and parts of the United States, access to termination of pregnancy is either prohibited or restricted [3] • The availability of funded IVF with PGT-M also varies [3]. In Israel, for example, IVF with PGT-M for 2 children is funded through National Health Insurance. In most nations, however, IVF with PGT-M is either partially funded or user-pays [3]

Abbreviations: HCP, health care provider; IVF with PGT-M, in vitro fertilization with preimplantation genetic testing for monogenic disorders; RGCS, reproductive genetic carrier screening.

TEST CONSIDERATIONS

Gene Selection

Many hundreds of genes are candidates for inclusion in RGCS, and there are no agreed upon gene selection criteria. As a result, there is marked variation in what is available. Wang and colleagues [55] identified 2205 genes screened across 22 providers, with panels ranging in size from 44 to 2054 genes. Notably, only 15 genes were common across all panels [55]. A robust gene selection method is, therefore, needed to ensure that results have as much reproductive utility as possible [56–58].

The American College of Medical Genetics (ACMG) developed a tier-based approach to gene selection, informed primarily by carrier frequency. The "tier 3" list, consisting of 113 genes associated with conditions with a carrier frequency of at least 1 out of 200 [7], is recommended for everyone in the absence of a priori risk. The justification for this approach is that rare conditions may lack sufficient evidence to promote informed reproductive decision-making. However, there are limitations to this approach, as evidenced by the fact that the ACMG gene list excludes many well-known, severe conditions [59].

Screening for severe, childhood-onset conditions offers the greatest reproductive utility. The concept of "severity" is subjective, however [58,60], and the inclusion of a gene on a panel may be perceived as placing a judgment on the quality-of-life of those with the associated condition (Box 2) [57]. How best to define severity remains in question, although biomedical approaches to classifying condition severity have been developed [61]. Applying one such classification system to 176 genes commonly found on commercial RGCS panels, Arjunan and colleagues [62] found that 79% of genes were associated with severe/profound conditions, 20% with moderate conditions, and 1% with mild conditions. Challenges arise when a gene is associated with a spectrum of phenotypic severity (Box 3), a common phenomenon occurring for many genes.

People have expressed interest in screening for less severe conditions, even if the information would not alter their reproductive plans [27,65,68]. In the NextGen preconception study, conditions were categorized as lifespan-limiting, serious, mild, unpredictable, and adult-onset [68]. All participants received results about lifespan-limiting conditions, and although the remaining categories were optional, 93% chose to receive all results [68]. Providing this level of choice may be challenging in a population-level screening program [69], as it would increase the complexity of pre-test education provision and laboratory processes [68].

The availability of treatment to modify disease trajectory is also an important consideration in gene selection, particularly as gene therapies and other treatments for rare diseases evolve [70]. There may be overlap between genes included on RGCS panels and newborn screening, but this is not to suggest that one should replace the other. In Mackenzie's Mission, several genes associated with treatable conditions were screened on the basis that the treatment has significant burdens, or that diagnosis prior to newborn screening is of benefit (eg, methylmalonic acidemia) [57].

Further considerations in gene selection include technical capabilities of the test to identify variants,

BOX 1
Implementing Accessible Reproductive Genetic Carrier Screening in Australia

Mackenzie's Mission designed, implemented, and evaluated an accessible model of RGCS in Australia [19]. When the project was launched in 2019, access to RGCS in the general population was on a user-pays basis. Recognizing the inequity of access to RGCS, the Australian Government funded the Mackenzie's Mission research project through the Medical Research Future Fund. The project was designed to test ways to reduce or remove many common barriers to accessing RGCS.

- RGCS was provided free-of-charge to all participating reproductive couples.
- RGCS education was delivered to recruiting HCPs prior to them inviting their patients to take part in the study. HCPs noted the importance of flexibility in the timing and mode (eg, online or face-to-face) of the education [41].
- Theory-led interventions were trialed to increase HCP confidence in, and prioritization of, offering RGCS to patients [42].
- Recruiting HCPs were selected to ensure a diverse sample of participants. This included HCPs working in preconception and prenatal settings, in metropolitan, regional, remote, and very remote locations and across all socioeconomic areas.
- People could take part in the study either in preconception or in the first trimester of pregnancy.
- Participants enrolled in the study (and consented to RGCS) via an online portal. The portal included pre-test education and an optional decision-aid [43]. Participants could also contact a study genetic counselor for more information and support if required.
- To support the enrollment of participants who used a language other than English, enrollment was available via a translated version of the portal (Arabic and Simplified Chinese, the most common languages spoken other than English in Australia) or assisted by a study genetic counselor and an interpreter.
- The study team engaged with Aboriginal Community Controlled Health Organizations to develop culturally safe enrollment materials for First Nations people. This was done in consultation with a specifically formed study Indigenous Advisory Committee.
- A portal comprising inclusive language was developed to facilitate enrollment of people using known gamete donors to conceive.
- Genetic sample collection kits were posted to participants. Cheek swab samples were collected at home and returned to the laboratory by mail. This reduced time and travel requirements, particularly for participants living in regional and remote/very remote locations.
- Low chance results were accessible online, via the portal, with a copy of the result sent to the recruiting HCP. A low chance fact sheet was also provided, and there was an option to speak with a study genetic counselor for more information if needed.
- Increased chance results were managed by study genetic counselors. One cycle of IVF with PGT-M was funded by the study for couples who received an increased chance result.

Abbreviations: HCP, health care provider; IVF with PGT-M, in vitro fertilization with preimplantation genetic testing for monogenic disorders; RGCS, reproductive genetic carrier screening.

potential health implications for heterozygotes, and community values [57]. It is clear that gene selection is complex and associated with a myriad of ethical considerations.

Laboratory Processes

Most RGCS is now performed using sequencing methods (targeted gene panels or exome/genome sequencing) with separate assays required for *SMN1* and *FMR1*. Orthogonal methods such as multiplex ligation-dependent probe amplification may also be used to validate copy number variants detected in a subset of genes (eg, *DMD*). Sequencing is considered more effective than targeted genotyping for population-level RGCS, although variants associated with mild phenotypes and variants of uncertain significance (VUS) will be identified (although not necessarily reported) [9].

The responsible implementation of RGCS requires results to have high clinical validity [44]. This can be achieved by only reporting pathogenic (P) and likely pathogenic (LP) variants in the genes screened [7]. Providing as much information as possible regarding the predicted phenotype associated with the variant/variant combination is critical [57], considering that people are likely to make reproductive decisions based on the information. Box 4 describes an approach to reporting *FMR1* premutations that maximizes the reproductive utility of results. VUS are not generally reported

TABLE 2
Reasons Given to Accept or Decline the Offer of Reproductive Genetic Carrier Screening

Reasons Given for Accepting RGCS	Reasons Given for Declining RGCS
• To learn the chance of having children with a serious genetic condition [49–51] • To avoid a serious genetic condition in offspring [13,14,23,52] • To prevent suffering for future child(ren) and the family [20,23,52] • To be prepared for the birth of a child with the condition and/or put a plan in place to manage the condition after birth [14,23,51,53] • To be able to make informed reproductive decisions [51,53] • To avoid feeling regret about declining [14,23,49,54] • To receive peace-of-mind from a low chance result [13,51,53]	• Perceiving RGCS as irrelevant due to a lack of family history of genetic conditions [20,23] • A low perceived likelihood of having an increased chance of having children with a genetic condition [23,49] • An increased chance result would not alter reproductive plans [13,23,49,51,53] • Feeling that having RGCS would cause worry and/or anxiety [23,49,50,53] • A concern that RGCS could medicalize pregnancy [13,53] • Personal lack of interest or lack of interest from the reproductive partner [21,36]

Abbreviation: RGCS, reproductive genetic carrier screening.

in RGCS. Nevertheless, the ACMG recommends that laboratories should consider reporting VUS if consent for this has been provided before test [7]. Reporting VUS introduces ambiguity into RGCS results that has the potential to cause significant harm [71].

Restricting reporting to variants/variant combinations expected to result in severe forms of a condition can reduce uncertainty. Not all laboratories follow the same reporting practices [74] however, and some providers do issue increased chance results for attenuated and purely biochemical phenotypes [58]. Fehlberg and colleagues [75] noted the important role of the Mackenzie's Mission multidisciplinary Variant Review Committee in promoting consistent reporting practices across the 3 laboratories in the study. Further, it is not always possible to accurately predict the outcome of a variant/variant combination. As noted in Box 3, genetic counseling is essential in helping people navigate reproductive decision-making in situations where potentially ambiguous results are reported.

BOX 2
Severity Case Study A: GJB2

The inclusion of genes associated with nonsyndromic hearing loss (eg, *GJB2)* on screening panels is the subject of ethical debate. According to a classification system developed by Lazarin and colleagues, *GJB2*-related nonsyndromic hearing loss is of "moderate" severity [61]. Members of the D/deaf[a] community challenge the notion that hearing loss is a serious condition, however [63]. Those who identify as culturally deaf also typically reject medical inventions to aid hearing and consider deafness to be an identity rather than a disability [63]. Freeman and colleagues [64] interviewed hearing adults of deaf children and D/d adults to capture perspectives on gene selection for RGCS. Participants agreed that severity is an appropriate criterion to guide gene selection but did not consider deafness to meet this criterion [64]. Many were concerned that including hearing loss-related genes on screening panels may devalue the lives of those who are D/deaf [64]. Similar concerns have been raised in other studies [63]. For this reason, genes associated with nonsyndromic hearing loss were not included on the Mackenzie's Mission gene panel [63]. Freeman and colleagues [65] also examined views of this study cohort on screening for hearing loss-related genes. Of 655 participants, 63% felt that deafness is a serious condition, although 72% did not consider it to be a disability [65]. Most supported RGCS for deafness and just over a third of participants would use an increased chance result for deafness to change their reproductive plans [65]. This case study highlights the subjective nature of severity as well as the ethical considerations in gene selection.

[a] Uppercase D refers to cultural Deafness and lowercase d refers to noncultural deafness.

BOX 3
Severity Case Study B: GBA1

This case study demonstrates the complex genetic counseling and psychosocial scenario created by issuing increased chance results for conditions with variable severity. Gaucher disease is a lysosomal storage disorder caused by variants in the *GBA1* gene. Gaucher disease type 1 is the most common form of the condition and demonstrates considerable phenotypic variability; some individuals with biallelic *GBA1* variants are asymptomatic throughout life while others experience serious health issues and require enzyme replacement therapy in childhood. The inclusion of *GBA1* on screening panels is, therefore, controversial [66]. Zuckerman and colleagues [66] examined reproductive outcomes of couples identified as having an increased chance for Gaucher disease type 1 in Israel. A small number of couples pregnant with a fetus expected to have mild or moderate disease had a termination of pregnancy (two out of 13 and two out of three, respectively) [66]. In a qualitative follow-up study, Zuckerman and colleagues [67] found that many participants pursued screening on the recommendation of their HCP and received limited pre-test education. Consequently, participants were unprepared for the ambiguity of their increased chance result [67]. Notably, several participants expressed regret about the decision to have a termination of pregnancy [67]. Participants with an increased chance for mild disease (N = 101) also had some regret about the decision to have screening but 64% still felt that screening for Gaucher disease type 1 should be available [67]. The authors offered two explanations for this finding. First, post-result genetic counseling may have increased couples' sense of reproductive empowerment [67]. Second, normative beliefs about screening have led to generally positive attitudes and high screening uptake in Israel [67]. Ultimately, Zuckerman and colleagues [67] concluded that many of the potential harms associated with screening for genes such as *GBA1* can be allayed by access to high-quality post-result genetic counseling and medical advice.

It is important that gene selection and laboratory processes are continually reviewed and updated as technologies and knowledge evolve (Box 5) [57]. An unsolved challenge is how to address variant reinterpretation [9]. An acceptable and feasible approach to reanalysis has not yet been adequately addressed or trialed [59].

Sequential or Simultaneous Approach

RGCS has typically been implemented using a sequential approach. In this approach, one reproductive partner (often the female individual) undergoes RGCS first and, if identified as a carrier of an AR condition, screening is offered to the other partner. There are several limitations with the sequential approach. For

BOX 4
FMR1 Screening with AGG Interrupt Testing

Fragile X syndrome is a neurodevelopmental disorder caused by trinucleotide repeat expansion in the *FMR1* gene. The *FMR1* gene, located on the X chromosome, contains a repeated segment of 3 nucleotides, CGG, within the 5′ untranslated region. CGG repeats ranging from 6 to 54 are not associated with an increased chance of fragile X syndrome in offspring. An allele size of over 200 CGG repeats triggers hypermethylation of the *FMR1* promoter and subsequent gene silencing. This is known as a "full mutation." Carriers of fragile X syndrome have an allele size from 55 to 200 repeats (known as a "premutation"). The premutation allele demonstrates instability on transmission, whereby the premutation can expand into a full mutation when transmitted from mother to child. The chance of expansion is dependent on repeat size. A premutation with 65 to 69 repeats has approximately 5% chance of expansion to full mutation while a premutation with 100 to 200 repeats has a greater than 95% chance of expansion to full mutation [72]. The presence of one or more AGG nucleotide sequences interspersed within CGG repeats can confer allele stability when the premutation range is between 55 and 69 repeats [73]. One or more AGG repeats in an allele with 55 to 64 CGG repeats, or two or more AGG repeats in an allele with 65 to 69 CGG repeats, can reduce the chance of expansion to full mutation to close to zero [73]. Reporting premutations that are unlikely to expand to a full mutation can cause unnecessary anxiety and may lead to the use of unneeded reproductive interventions. Approximately 77% of premutation carriers identified through screening in the general population have between 55 and 69 CGG repeats [6]. Thus, incorporating AGG testing into *FMR1* screening protocols can provide more accurate reproductive risk information, minimizes harms, and reduces the number of increased chance results requiring detailed genetic counseling [6].

BOX 5
Digenic Inheritance

To date, RGCS has been performed for monogenic conditions. There is an increasing recognition of the importance of digenic and oligogenic inheritance in human genetic disease and growing databases (digenic disease database [DiDA] and oligogenic diseases database [OLIDA]) of suggested digenic or oligogenic gene combinations created [76,77]. However, the feasibility of RGCS for digenic or oligogenic conditions must be considered. As for monogenic conditions, RGCS for digenic/oligogenic conditions should be reserved for serious conditions with sufficiently strong evidence of genotype–phenotype correlation. Proposed ACMG-like guidelines [78] for digenic/oligogenic conditions include the necessity for sufficiently robust genetic and functional evidence of the association between the gene variant combination and the phenotype [79]. Genetic evidence requires a large family, or multiple families, with only affected individuals having the gene variant combination and individuals with variants in only one of the genes not having the phenotype. Similarly, functional evidence requires in vivo or in vitro data that the variant combination produces the phenotype while variants in individual genes do not. Four-point scales were developed for both genetic and functional evidences: 0, absent; 1, weak; 2, moderate; and 3, strong. Applying the scales to the greater than 900 gene combinations in OLIDA, only 3 digenic combinations scored 3 for both genetic and functional evidences: *MFN2/GDAP1* in Charcot-Marie-Tooth disease, *SLC3A1/SLC7A9* in cystinuria and *MuRF1/MuRF2* in hypertrophic cardiomyopathy [77]. A recent definitive example of digenic inheritance is variants in *TTN* and the XL gene *SRPK3* causing an early onset, slowly progressive myopathy [80]. Thirty-three people with myopathy (31 male and two female individuals [both female individuals showed skewed X-inactivation]) were identified in 25 families. Only individuals with variants in both *TTN* and *SRPK3* were affected. Multiple unaffected male individuals had only *SRPK3* or *TTN* variants. In functional analyses, only doubly mutant *SPRK3/TTN* zebrafish had a myopathy, singly mutant *SRPK3* or *TTN* zebrafish did not. To provide RGCS for digenic conditions, variant curators would have to identify variants in specific gene pairs, rather than in the same autosomal gene or an XL gene as for monogenic diseases. This could be done, expanding RGCS to non-Mendelian conditions.

Abbreviations: ACMG, American College of Medical Genetics; RGCS, reproductive genetic carrier screening.

example, a meta-analysis found that rates of partner testing range from 42% to 77% in the United States [81]. Heightened anxiety while waiting for partner results is also well documented [82]. In a simultaneous approach, the reproductive couple is screened together, engaging both partners in screening simultaneously and expediting the process for those screened prenatally [32,83]. Results can be reported individually or as a combined reported (low or increased chance for the couple). Advantages and disadvantages to individual and combined ("couple-based") reporting are described in Table 3.

As gene panels increase in size, so too does the likelihood that an individual will be a carrier of one or more conditions. Simultaneous screening with combined reporting is, therefore, most practical at population scale [75]. Combined reporting also offers the greatest reproductive utility and has been positively received by potential and actual users [13,83].

POST-RESULT CONSIDERATIONS

Reproductive Decision-Making

It is essential that people feel empowered to make reproductive decisions that align with their values. Genetic counselors can promote reproductive empowerment by practicing "nondirectiveness," a technique that involves providing balanced information and support for patient decisions regardless of the choice made. Studies demonstrate that reproductive decision-making is complex and associated with individual and societal factors [85].

Perceived severity is highly influential in people's reproductive choices [85]. In one study, 32 out of 42 (76%) couples with an increased chance for a profound/severe condition chose to act on the information [86]. Wang and colleagues [56] found that as RGCS panels increase in size, the percentage use of reproductive interventions decreases. This finding could reflect that larger panels may include a greater number of genes associated with moderate or treatable conditions.

The timing of receiving results may also influence the use of reproductive interventions. In a study of three gene RGCS, 81% of people pregnant at receipt of their increased chance had PND, and 86% of those with an affected pregnancy opted for TOP [6]. These figures are higher than reported by Ghiossi and colleagues [86] and Johansen Taber and colleagues [87] for panels that comprised 86 and 176 genes, respectively. For example, Johansen Taber and colleagues [87] reported

TABLE 3
Advantages and Disadvantages of Approaches to Result Reporting

	Advantages	Disadvantages
Individual results	• Carrier status can be shared with relatives[a] • Increased self-knowledge [82]	• Potential negative psychological responses to individual carrier status [82] • High workforce demands. Lynch et al. [84] reported that the median time taken to counsel an individual about carrier status is 64 minutes • Individual carrier status for AR conditions offers no reproductive utility
Combined results	• Provides the opportunity to report variant combinations with the greatest likelihood of a severe phenotype [57] • Reduces burdens on the health system, including laboratory and genetic counseling services [44,83]	• Does not address the needs of people whose reproductive partner is unavailable (eg, those using an anonymous gamete donor) or unwilling to have RGCS • Results cannot be used with a new reproductive partner without returning to the provider for rescreening and/or rematching of stored genomic data [83]

[a] Facilitation of cascade testing has traditionally been cited as an important outcome of learning one's individual carrier status. This becomes less of an issue if reproductive screening carrier screening is offered freely at population scale where reproductive-aged relatives can access couple-based screening for themselves [45].

that 37% of pregnant couples at increased chance had PND and 40% of those with an affected pregnancy opted for TOP. Recent studies suggest a preference for IVF with PGT-M over PND with TOP when RGCS is accessed preconception [86–88]. Use, or intended use, of IVF with PGT-M (59%–100%) in these studies may reflect the fact that a high proportion of participants were already pursuing IVF [85]. Those already pursuing IVF may also be more likely to consider PGT-M for mild and moderate conditions [85].

Societal factors may mean that TOP or IVF with PGT-M is not acceptable or accessible. The cost of IVF with PGT-M can also be prohibitive, and there are few health systems that provide financial assistance. The physical and emotional impacts of undertaking a reproductive intervention should also not be overlooked [11,85].

Psychosocial Implications

Most studies have shown that RGCS can be delivered at a population scale with minimal psychosocial consequences for those who receive low chance results [14,46,89]. Given that many people embark on RGCS expecting to receive a reassuring result [13,51,53], it is not surprising that anxiety is minimal and decision satisfaction is high [40,89]. Receipt of a low chance result is also associated with increased reproductive empowerment [39,46].

Conversely, receiving an increased chance result is a psychosocially significant event. Common reactions include shock and anxiety, particularly if disclosed during pregnancy [47]. Those screened preconception may also express grief over the loss of an expected reproductive journey [39]. There is, however, evidence to indicate that with time, people find value in their increased chance result given the reproductive autonomy it provides [47]. Studies also highlight the value of genetic counseling in addressing the psychological impacts of receiving an increased chance result [47]. Further research is needed to explore how genetic counseling can address the long-term psychological impacts of increased chance results.

SUMMARY

The advent of massively parallel sequencing means it is now possible to offer RGCS for hundreds of genes. This review offers insights into how to support the implementation of RGCS in an acceptable and feasible way. Multimedia decision support tools can be used to facilitate informed decision-making at scale [43]. People are more likely to alter their reproductive plans based on an increased chance for a serious genetic condition, thus a robust approach to gene selection, focusing on genes expected to result in severe, childhood-onset conditions, is critical [57]. Reproductive decision-making is nevertheless psychosocially complex and associated with individual and societal factors [85].

Consistent themes in this review are the importance of genetic counseling and system capacity [48]. Growth in the genetic counselor workforce has not kept pace with demand for RGCS, however, meaning genetic counselors are in limited supply. Health technology assessment and addressing data management issues are also needed. Further, cost is a universal barrier to accessing RGCS [3]. Continued engagement in these issues from health systems and professional bodies will promote the responsible implementation of RGCS into the future.

CLINICS CARE POINTS

- Traditional models of pre-test counseling for RGCS are impractical at population scale; new service delivery models are needed to facilitate informed choice.
- Gene selection and variant reporting practices should aim to maximize the reproductive utility of results.
- Simultaneous screening with combined results provides information most useful for reproductive planning and makes the best use of limited laboratory and genetic counseling resources.
- Access to genetic counseling is essential to promote value-consistent reproductive decision-making and psychological adaptation to an increased chance result.

DISCLOSURE

E. Tutty is supported by an Australian Government Resarch Training Program Scholarship. A.D. Archibald and M.B. Delatycki are employed by VCGS, a not-for-profit provider of genetic testing. E.P. Kirk is employed by NSW Health Pathology, a service that provides a fee-for-service reproductive genetic carrier screening, and by Genea, a fertility company that refers patients for reproductive genetic carrier screening. N.G. Laing is employed by PathWest, a genetic testing provider. T.F. Boughtwood has nothing to disclose.

REFERENCES

[1] Ropers H-H. On the future of genetic risk assessment. J Community Genet 2012;3(3):229–36.

[2] Antonarakis SE. Carrier screening for recessive disorders. Nat Rev Genet 2019;20(9):549–61.

[3] Delatycki MB, Alkuraya F, Archibald A, et al. International perspectives on the implementation of reproductive carrier screening. Prenat Diagn 2020;40(3):301–10.

[4] Ioannou L, McClaren BJ, Massie J, et al. Population-based carrier screening for cystic fibrosis: a systematic review of 23 years of research. Genet Med 2014;16(3): 207–16.

[5] Hill MK, Archibald AD, Cohen J, et al. A systematic review of population screening for fragile X syndrome. Genet Med 2010;12(7):396–410.

[6] Archibald AD, Smith MJ, Burgess T, et al. Reproductive genetic carrier screening for cystic fibrosis, fragile X syndrome, and spinal muscular atrophy in Australia: outcomes of 12,000 tests. Genet Med 2018;20(5):513–23.

[7] Gregg AR, Aarabi M, Klugman S, et al. Screening for autosomal recessive and X-linked conditions during pregnancy and preconception: a practice resource of the American College of Medical Genetics and Genomics (ACMG). Genet Med 2021;23(10):1793–806.

[8] Genomics in general practice. (2018).

[9] Sagaser KG, Malinowski J, Westerfield L, et al. Expanded carrier screening for reproductive risk assessment: An evidence-based practice guideline from the National Society of Genetic Counselors. J Genet Counsel 2023; 32(3):540–57.

[10] Dive L, Newson AJ. Ethics of reproductive genetic carrier screening: From the clinic to the population. Publ Health Ethics 2021;14(2):202–17.

[11] van der Hout S, Dondorp W, de Wert G. The aims of expanded universal carrier screening: Autonomy, prevention, and responsible parenthood. Bioethics 2019;33(5):568–76.

[12] De Wert GMWR, Dondorp WJ, Knoppers BM. Preconception care and genetic risk: ethical issues. J Community Genet 2012;3(3):221–8.

[13] Schuurmans J, Birnie E, Ranchor AV, et al. GP-provided couple-based expanded preconception carrier screening in the Dutch general population: who accepts the test-offer and why? Eur J Hum Genet 2020;28(2):182–92.

[14] van Dijke I, Lakeman P, Sabiri N, et al. Couples' experiences with expanded carrier screening: evaluation of a university hospital screening offer. Eur J Hum Genet 2021;29(8):1252–8.

[15] Tan HY, Hussein N, Lee YK, et al. Adolescents' experiences and views of the national school-based thalassaemia screening programme in Malaysia: a qualitative study. J Community Genet 2023;14(4):361–9.

[16] Fidan C, Akdur R, Unver CN, et al. Carrier screening programs for rare diseases in developed countries and the case of Turkey: A systematic review. Intractable Rare Dis Res 2023;12(3):161–9.

[17] Belhoul KM, Abdulrahman M, Alraei RF. Hemoglobinopathy carrier prevalence in the United Arab Emirates: First Analysis of The Dubai Health Authority Premarital Screening Program Results. Hemoglobin 2013;37(4): 359–68.

[18] Borry P, Henneman L, Lakeman P, et al. Preconceptional genetic carrier testing and the commercial offer directly-to-consumers. Hum Reprod 2011;26(5):972–7.
[19] Archibald AD, McClaren BJ, Caruana J, et al. The Australian Reproductive Genetic Carrier Screening Project (Mackenzie's Mission): Design and Implementation. J Personalized Med 2022;12(11):1781.
[20] Zhang F, Tan J, Shao B, et al. Current attitudes and preconceptions towards expanded carrier screening in the Eastern Chinese reproductive-aged population. J Assist Reprod Genet 2021;38(3):697–707.
[21] Ong R, Howting DR, Alethea Christian H, et al. Measuring the impact of genetic knowledge on intentions and attitudes of the community towards expanded preconception carrier screening. J Med Genet 2018; 55(11):744–52.
[22] Van Steijvoort E, Peeters H, Vandecruys H, et al. Exploring informed choice in preconception reproductive genetic carrier screening by using a modified Multidimensional Measure of Informed Choice. Patient Educ Counsel 2022;105(11):3313–8.
[23] Nijmeijer SCM, Conijn T, Lakeman P, et al. Attitudes of the general population towards preconception expanded carrier screening for autosomal recessive disorders including inborn errors of metabolism. Mol Genet Metabol 2019;126(1):14–22.
[24] Pereira N, Wood M, Luong E, et al. Expanded genetic carrier screening in clinical practice: a current survey of patient impressions and attitudes. J Assist Reprod Genet 2019;36:709–16.
[25] Boardman FK, Clark C, Jungkurth E, et al. Social and cultural influences on genetic screening programme acceptability: A mixed-methods study of the views of adults, carriers, and family members living with thalassemia in the UK. J Genet Counsel 2020;29(6):1026–40.
[26] Woudstra AJ, van den Heuvel LM, van Vliet-Lachotzki EH, et al. Views of patients and parents of children with genetic disorders on population-based expanded carrier screening. Prenat Diagn 2022;42(9): 1201–10.
[27] Thomas LA, Lewis S, Massie J, et al. Which types of conditions should be included in reproductive genetic carrier screening? Views of parents of children with a genetic condition. Eur J Med Genet 2020;63(12):104075.
[28] Boardman FK, Young PJ, Warren O, et al. The role of experiential knowledge within attitudes towards genetic carrier screening: A comparison of people with and without experience of spinal muscular atrophy. Health Expect 2018;21(1):201–11.
[29] Hoedemaekers R, Have HT. Geneticization: the cyprus paradigm. J Med Philos 1998;23(3):274–87.
[30] Van Steijvoort E, Chokoshvili D, W Cannon J, et al. Interest in expanded carrier screening among individuals and couples in the general population: systematic review of the literature. Hum Reprod Update 2020;26(3):335–55.
[31] Holtkamp KCA, Vos EM, Rigter T, et al. Stakeholder perspectives on the implementation of genetic carrier screening in a changing landscape. BMC Health Serv Res 2017;17(1):146.
[32] Kraft SA, Duenas D, Wilfond BS, et al. The evolving landscape of expanded carrier screening: challenges and opportunities. Genet Med 2019;21(4):790–7.
[33] Best S, Long J, Theodorou T, et al. Health practitioners' perceptions of the barriers and enablers to the implementation of reproductive genetic carrier screening: A systematic review. Prenat Diagn 2021;41(6):708–19.
[34] Robson SJ, Caramins M, Saad M, et al. Socioeconomic status and uptake of reproductive carrier screening in Australia. Aust N Z J Obstet Gynaecol 2020;60(6):976–9.
[35] Carlotti K, Hines K, Weida J, et al. Perceived barriers to paternal expanded carrier screening following a positive maternal result: To screen or not to screen. J Genet Counsel 2021;30(2):470–7.
[36] Gilmore MJ, Schneider J, Davis JV, et al. Reasons for declining preconception expanded carrier screening using genome sequencing. J Genet Counsel 2017;26(5): 971–9.
[37] Gafni-Amsalem C, Aboleil-Zoubi O, Chervinsky E, et al. Educational tools support informed decision-making for genetic carrier screening in a heterogenic Israeli population. J Community Genet 2023. https://doi.org/10.1007/s12687-023-00694-4.
[38] Arjunan A, Darnes DR, Sagaser KG, et al. Addressing Reproductive Healthcare Disparities through Equitable Carrier Screening: Medical Racism and Genetic Discrimination in United States' History Highlights the Needs for Change in Obstetrical Genetics Care. Societies 2022; 12(2):33.
[39] Richardson E, McEwen A, Newton-John T, et al. Outcomes of importance to patients in reproductive genetic carrier screening: a qualitative study to inform a core outcome set. J Personalized Med 2022;12(8).
[40] Van Steijvoort E, Peeters H, Vandecruys H, et al. Experiences of nonpregnant couples after receiving reproductive genetic carrier screening results in Belgium. Eur J Hum Genet 2023;31(6):696–702.
[41] Best S, Long JC, Fehlberg Z, et al. The more you do it, the easier it gets: using behaviour change theory to support health care professionals offering reproductive genetic carrier screening. Eur J Hum Genet 2023;31(4):430–44.
[42] Best S, Long JC, Fehlberg Z, et al. Using a theory informed approach to design, execute, and evaluate implementation strategies to support offering reproductive genetic carrier screening in Australia. BMC Health Serv Res 2023;23(1):1276.
[43] King E, Halliday J, Archibald AD, et al. Development and use of the Australian reproductive genetic carrier screening decision aid. Eur J Hum Genet 2022;30(2): 194–202.
[44] Henneman L, Borry P, Chokoshvili D, et al. Responsible implementation of expanded carrier screening. Eur J Hum Genet 2016;24(6):e1–12.
[45] Schuurmans J, Birnie E, van den Heuvel LM, et al. Feasibility of couple-based expanded carrier screening offered

by general practitioners. Eur J Hum Genet 2019;27(5):691–700.
[46] Birnie E, Schuurmans J, Plantinga M, et al. Couple-based expanded carrier screening provided by general practitioners to couples in the Dutch general population: psychological outcomes and reproductive intentions. Genet Med 2021;23(9):1761–8.
[47] Beard CA, Amor DJ, Di Pietro L, et al. "I'm Healthy, It's Not Going To Be Me": Exploring experiences of carriers identified through a population reproductive genetic carrier screening panel in Australia. Am J Med Genet 2016;170(8):2052–9.
[48] Edwards S, Laing N. Genetic counselling needs for reproductive genetic carrier screening: a scoping review. J Personalized Med 2022;12(10):1699.
[49] Van Steijvoort E, Demuynck R, Peeters H, et al. Reasons affecting the uptake of reproductive genetic carrier screening among nonpregnant reproductive-aged women in Flanders (Belgium). J Genet Counsel 2022;31(5):1043–53.
[50] Cheng HYH, Wong GCY, Chan Y-KK, et al. Expanded carrier screening in chinese population – a survey on views and acceptance of pregnant and non-pregnant women. Front Genet 2020. https://doi.org/10.3389/fgene.2020.594091.
[51] Rabkina L, Swanson A, Aufox S, et al. What women want: General population perspectives and access to preconception expanded carrier screening. Prenat Diagn 2021;41(9):1057–65.
[52] Ragnar ME, Tydén T, Kihlbom U, et al. Swedish parents' interest in preconception genetic carrier screening. Ups J Med Sci 2016;121(4):289–94.
[53] Schneider JL, Goddard KAB, Davis J, et al. "Is It Worth Knowing?" Focus Group Participants' Perceived Utility of Genomic Preconception Carrier Screening. J Genet Counsel 2016;25(1):135–45.
[54] Van Steijvoort E, Cassou M, De Schutter C, et al. Exploring attitudes and experiences with reproductive genetic carrier screening among couples seeking medically assisted reproduction: a longitudinal survey study. J Assist Reprod Genet 2024. https://doi.org/10.1007/s10815-023-03010-8.
[55] Wang T, Scuffham P, Byrnes J, et al. An overview of reproductive carrier screening panels for autosomal recessive and/or X-linked conditions: How much do we know? Prenat Diagn 2023;43(11):1416–24.
[56] Wang T, Kiss D, McFadden K, et al. Clinical utility of reproductive carrier screening for preconception and pregnant couples for multiple genetic conditions: a systematic review and meta-analysis. Expert Rev Mol Diagn 2023;23(5):419–29.
[57] Kirk EP, Ong R, Boggs K, et al. Gene selection for the Australian Reproductive Genetic Carrier Screening Project ("Mackenzie's Mission"). Eur J Hum Genet 2021;29(1):79–87.
[58] Dive L, Archibald AD, Newson AJ. Ethical considerations in gene selection for reproductive carrier screening. Hum Genet 2022;141(5):1003–12.
[59] Righetti S, Dive L, Archibald AD, et al. Correspondence on "Screening for autosomal recessive and X-linked conditions during pregnancy and preconception: A practice resource of the American College of Medical Genetics and Genomics (ACMG)" by Gregg et al. Genet Med 2022;24(5):1158–61.
[60] Dive L, Archibald AD, Freeman L, et al. How should severity be understood in the context of reproductive genetic carrier screening? Bioethics 2023;37(4):359–66.
[61] Lazarin GA, Hawthorne F, Collins NS, et al. Systematic classification of disease severity for evaluation of expanded carrier screening panels. PLoS One 2014;9(12):e114391.
[62] Arjunan A, Bellerose H, Torres R, et al. Evaluation and classification of severity for 176 genes on an expanded carrier screening panel. Prenat Diagn 2020;40(10):1246–57.
[63] Freeman L, Righetti S, Delatycki MB, et al. The views of people with a lived experience of deafness and the general public regarding genetic testing for deafness in the reproductive setting: A systematic review. Genet Med 2022;24(9):1803–13.
[64] Freeman L, Bristowe L, Kirk EP, et al. Should genes for non-syndromic hearing loss be included in reproductive genetic carrier screening: Views of people with a personal or family experience of deafness. J Genet Counsel 2023;42(13).
[65] Freeman L, Delatycki MB, Leach Scully J, et al. Views of reproductive genetic carrier screening participants regarding screening for genes associated with non-syndromic hearing loss. Prenat Diagn 2022;42(13):1658–66.
[66] Zuckerman S, Lahad A, Shmueli A, et al. Carrier screening for Gaucher disease: lessons for low-penetrance, treatable diseases. JAMA 2007;298(11):1281–90.
[67] Zuckerman S, Lahad A, Zimran A, et al. Attitudes of couples identified through screening as carriers of Gaucher disease type 1. Clin Genet 2008;74(6):566–70.
[68] Wilfond BS, Kauffman TL, Jarvik GP, et al. Lessons learned from a study of genomics-based carrier screening for reproductive decision making. Health Aff 2018;37(5):809–16.
[69] Dive L, Holmes I, Newson AJ. Is it just for a screening program to give people all the information they want? Am J Bioeth 2023;23(7):34–42.
[70] Newson AJ, Dive L, Cini J, et al. Ethical aspects of the changing landscape for spinal muscular atrophy management in Australia. Aus J Gen Prac 2022;51(3):131–5.
[71] Silver J, Norton ME. Expanded carrier screening and the complexity of implementation. Obstet Gynecol 2021;137(2):345–50.
[72] Nolin SL, Brown WT, Glicksman A, et al. Expansion of the fragile X CGG repeat in females with premutation or intermediate alleles. Am J Med Genet 2003;72(2):454–64.
[73] Nolin SL, Glicksman A, Ersalesi N, et al. Fragile X full mutation expansions are inhibited by one or more AGG interruptions in premutation carriers. Genet Med 2015;17(5):358–64.

[74] Ramdaney A, Dunn DM, Weiss RB, et al. Beware the laboratory report: discrepancy in variant classification on reproductive carrier screening. Genet Med 2018;20(3): 374–5.

[75] Fehlberg Z, Best S, Long JC, et al. Scaling-up and future sustainability of a national reproductive genetic carrier screening program. NPJ Genom Med 2023;8(1):18.

[76] Gazzo AM, Daneels D, Cilia E, et al. DIDA: A curated and annotated digenic diseases database. Nucleic Acids Res 2016;44(D1):D900–7.

[77] Nachtegael C, Gravel B, Dillen A, et al. Scaling up oligogenic diseases research with OLIDA: the Oligogenic Diseases Database. Database 2022. https://doi.org/10.1093/database/baac023.

[78] Richards S, Aziz N, Bale S, et al. Standards and guidelines for the interpretation of sequence variants: a joint consensus recommendation of the American College of Medical Genetics and Genomics and the Association for Molecular Pathology. Genet Med 2015;17(5):405–24.

[79] Papadimitriou S, Gravel B, Nachtegael C, et al. Toward reporting standards for the pathogenicity of variant combinations involved in multilocus/oligogenic diseases. HGG Adv 2023;4(1):100165.

[80] Töpf A, Cox D, Zaharieva IT, et al. Digenic inheritance involving a muscle-specific protein kinase and the giant titin protein causes a skeletal muscle myopathy. Nat Genet 2024. https://doi.org/10.1038/s41588-023-01651-0.

[81] Ramdaney A, Lichten L, Propst L, et al. Expanded carrier screening in the United States: A systematic evidence review exploring client and provider experiences. J Genet Counsel 2022;31(4):937–48.

[82] Lewis C, Skirton H, Jones R. Can we make assumptions about the psychosocial impact of living as a carrier, based on studies assessing the effects of carrier testing? J Genet Counsel 2011;20(1):80–97.

[83] Plantinga M, Birnie E, Schuurmans J, et al. Expanded carrier screening for autosomal recessive conditions in health care: arguments for a couple-based approach and examination of couples' views. Prenat Diagn 2019; 39(5):369–78.

[84] Lynch FL, Himes P, Gilmore MJ, et al. Time costs for genetic counseling in preconception carrier screening with genome sequencing. J Genet Counsel 2018;27(4): 823–33.

[85] Cannon J, Van Steijvoort E, Borry P, et al. How does carrier status for recessive disorders influence reproductive decisions? A systematic review of the literature. Expert Rev Mol Diagn 2019;19(12):1117–29.

[86] Ghiossi CE, Goldberg JD, Haque IS, et al. Clinical utility of expanded carrier screening: reproductive behaviors of at-risk couples. J Genet Counsel 2018;27(3):616–25.

[87] Johansen Taber KA, Beauchamp KA, Lazarin GA, et al. Clinical utility of expanded carrier screening: results-guided actionability and outcomes. Obstet Gynecol Surv 2019;74(10):582–4.

[88] Capalbo A, Fabiani M, Caroselli S, et al. Clinical validity and utility of preconception expanded carrier screening for the management of reproductive genetic risk in IVF and general population. Hum Reprod 2021;36(7): 2050–61.

[89] Kraft SA, Schneider JL, Leo MC, et al. Patient actions and reactions after receiving negative results from expanded carrier screening. Clin Genet 2018;93(5):962–71.

Pharmacogenomics

Advances in Molecular Pathology 7 (2024) 15–32
ADVANCES IN MOLECULAR PATHOLOGY

Review of Neurologic and Developmental Conditions Associated with Pediatric Dihydropyrimidine Dehydrogenase Deficiency

Brianna M. Bembenek, BA[a,b], Carlo R. Largiadèr, PhD[c], Steven M. Offer, PhD[a,b,*]

[a]Department of Pathology, Carver College of Medicine, University of Iowa, 500 Newton Road, Iowa City, IA 52242, USA; [b]Mayo Clinic Graduate School of Biomedical Sciences, Mayo Clinic, 200 1st Street Southwest, Rochester, MN 55905, USA; [c]Department of Clinical Chemistry, Inselspital, Bern University Hospital, University of Bern, Freiburgstrasse / INO F, 3010 Bern, Switzerland

KEYWORDS

- Pediatric DPD deficiency • Dihydropyrimidine dehydrogenase • Disorders of pyrimidine catabolism
- Neurodevelopmental disorder

KEY POINTS

- Deficiency of the pyrimidine metabolism enzyme dihydropyrimidase dehydrogenase (DPD) is most commonly studied in the context of chemotherapy toxicity; however, DPD deficiency is also linked to a neurologic developmental disorder.
- While a variety of mechanisms potentially contribute to neurodevelopmental symptoms associated with pediatric DPD deficiency, dysregulated pathways have yet to be directed identified or studied in this context.
- A review of case studies has identified correlations between pediatric DPD deficiency and clinical presentation but has also highlighted an unexplained variability in symptom presentation.
- The biochemical similarities between pediatric DPD deficiency and deficiencies of other pyrimidine catabolism enzymes indicates that signaling pathways linked to the downstream metabolites β-alanine and β-aminoisobutyric acid are likely involved.

INTRODUCTION

Pediatric dihydropyrimidine dehydrogenase (DPD) deficiency is broadly defined as a neurologic developmental disorder accompanied by the detection of deleterious variation in the gene encoding DPD (*DPYD*) that results in reduced function of the encoded protein (DPD) for which no other explanation for the disorder can be identified. This condition has been reported to present with a variety of symptoms that range from mild-to-severe delay of motor and intellectual development. These symptoms are typically identified in early childhood and are accompanied by elevated levels of thymine and uracil [1], as well as reduced levels of N-carbamyl-β-alanine [2], N-carbamyl-β-aminoisobutyric acid [2], β-alanine [3], and β-aminoisobutyric acid (BAIBA) [4], in body fluids. Patients most commonly present with delayed cognitive and motor development and epilepsy, with delayed growth, microcephaly, facial dysmorphia, autism, hypotonia, and ocular abnormalities occurring less frequently [3,5–9].

Pediatric DPD deficiency differs from the more extensively studied general DPD deficiency, which

*Corresponding author, *E-mail address:* steven-offer@uiowa.edu

https://doi.org/10.1016/j.yamp.2024.07.005 www.advancesinmolecularpathology.com
2589-4080/24/

greatly increases the risk of chemotherapy-induced toxicity to the anticancer drug 5-fluorouracil (5-FU) or its prodrug form [10,11]. In chemotherapy-related DPD deficiency, subjects do not display any overt signs of the disorder until after administration of 5-FU for the treatment of cancer, which typically does not occur until later in life.

DPD is the initial and rate-defining enzyme for the catabolism of the pyrimidines uracil and thymine [12,13]. Uracil is reduced to 5,6-dihydrouracil and, subsequently, further metabolized by dihydropyrimidinase (DHP) and β-ureidopropionase (BUP) enzymes to β-alanine. Thymine follows a similar catabolism pathway and is ultimately converted to BAIBA [14] (Fig. 1). DPD also metabolizes pyrimidine analogs such as 5-FU [15], which explains the elevated rates of 5-FU toxicity in individuals with DPD deficiency. The most commonly studied deleterious *DPYD* variant is *DPYD**2A (c.1905 + 1G>A, IVS14 + 1G>A, rs3918290) [16], an intronic variant that results in the skipping of exon 14 [17,18] and production of inactive DPD [19,20]. Other well-studied variants associated with reduced DPD function leading to increased 5-FU toxicity risk include *DPYD**13 (c.1679 T>G, p.I560S, rs55886062), c.2846 A>T (p.D949 V, rs67376798), and c.1129-5923C>G (rs75017182) [21].

While these variants are well studied within the field of cancer pharmacology, there is less known regarding their role in pediatric DPD deficiency. The prevalence of pediatric DPD deficiency is extremely low, as not all individuals with *DPYD* genetic variation develop the corresponding neurologic and developmental symptoms [3,22,23]. It has been suggested that individuals who are homozygous for deleterious *DPYD* variations are more likely to develop the pediatric condition in comparison to heterozygous individuals [8]; however, no clear correlation between *DPYD* genotype and risk for pediatric DPD deficiency has been established [3,24].

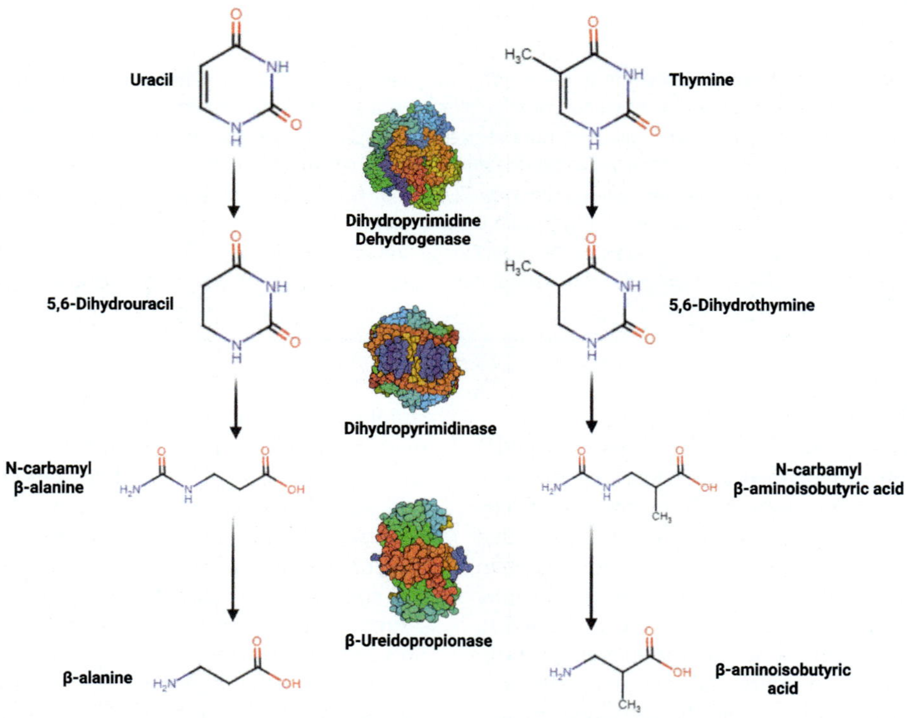

FIG. 1 Metabolites and enzymes involved in pyrimidine catabolism. Uracil and thymine follow a similar degradation pathway, where they are first reduced by DPD [141] into dihydrouracil and thymine, respectively. DHP [142] then catalyzes a hydrolytic ring opening to convert dihydrouracil to N-carbamyl β-alanine and dihydrothymine to N-carbamyl β-aminoisobutyric acid. In the final step of catabolism, BUP [143] performs a decarbamylation of N-carbamyl β-alanine and N-carbamyl β-aminoisobutyric acid to produce β-alanine and BAIBA, respectively. (Created with Biorender.com.)

PEDIATRIC DIHYDROPYRIMIDINE DEHYDROGENASE DEFICIENCY

Numerous published cases of pediatric DPD deficiency demonstrate the wide degree of symptom variability. Delayed motor and intellectual development, along with seizures, are the most frequently reported conditions [25] (Table 1). Vision-related symptoms, including microphthalmia, ptosis, nystagmus, microcornea, and ophthalmoplegia, are also commonly reported [3,8,26–28]. Newborns and infants with pediatric DPD deficiency tend to display respiratory defects and feeding difficulties, with symptoms generally decreasing in severity with age [29,30]. Patients are also likely to have autism spectrum disorder (ASD) and abnormal social behaviors, with many cases being co-diagnosed with autism [8,28,31].

Additional symptoms show greater variability between cases. For example, individuals with the same *DPYD* variant have presented with hypotonia [5,6,8,26, 27,32–35] or hypertonia [30,36–39]. Patients have been shown to develop macrocephaly [8] or microcephaly [5,24,29,34,36,40,41]. Some patients present with normal MRI, whereas others display decreased corpus callosum size, prominent sulcal spaces and ventricles, white and/or gray matter loss, T2-lesions, or cerebral atrophy [5,6,9,27,33,35,38].

Biochemically, patients consistently present with thymine-uraciluria with the presence of the abnormal metabolite 5-hydroxymethyluracil, which is formed via oxidation of thymine by ten-eleven translocation proteins [42]. Patients also display decreased or absent DPD activity, depending on the nature of their genetic variation(s) (Table 2). Patients with severe symptoms tend to carry homozygous or compound heterozygous deleterious genetic variants and/or large deletions of *DPYD*. The *DPYD**2A variant appears to be the most common documented genetic variant, consistent with the known high prevalence of this genetic variation in the population [16].

Within patients with other pediatric disorders, individuals with *DPYD* variants have been suggested to develop distinct symptoms. For example, a patient carrying variants in *DPYD* and *UBE3A* presented with the characteristic Angelman syndrome symptoms (linked to *UBE3A*), including paroxysm of laughter, hyperactivity, ataxia, microcephaly, and electroencephalogram (EEG) pattern of rhythmic frontal high amplitude 2 to 3 Hz, rhythmic high amplitude 4 to 6 Hz, and parieto-occipital 4 to 5 Hz spike waves. Additionally, the patient showed symptoms characteristic of pediatric DPD deficiency, including feeding difficulties, developmental impairment, hypotonia, microcephaly, poorly coordinated movements, delayed speech development, play behavior, and social skills, and T2-hyperintense lesions in occipital white matter [34]. Another patient with a *GLB1* variant (associated with GM1 gangliosidosis) displayed global hypomyelination and abnormal basal ganglia characteristic of gangliosidosis, while also presenting with global developmental delay, hypotonia, nystagmus, and status epilepticus with febrile seizures characteristic of pediatric DPD deficiency [27].

Pediatric DPD deficiency has also been linked to ASD in patients with and without genetic variation in known ASD-associated genes. Homozygosity for *DPYD**2A [3] and heterozygous *DPYD* exon 6 deletion (leading to hemizygosity of this region) [31] have been linked to ASD independent of any other known genetic risk factor. ASD has also been reported in patients with *DPYD* heterozygous deletions in conjunction with *PTCHD1* genetic variation [31], *PTPB2* deletion [31], or a combination of various *SNX7*, *MIR137*, and *LPPR5* heterozygous deletions [28]. Copy number variation (CNV) loss and gain of genes within the 1p21.3p21.2 region, including *DPYD*, have additionally been linked to the onset of intellectual disability, ASD, language disorders, seizures, and dysmorphic features [43]. Despite suggestive evidence linking *DPYD* to ASD, a clear correlation and mechanism have yet to be established.

DEFICIENCIES OF OTHER PYRIMIDINE CATABOLISM ENZYMES

Dihydropyrimidinase Deficiency

Genetic variants in other genes involved in pyrimidine catabolism have also been linked to similar pediatric conditions. Variants in *DPYS*, the gene-encoding DHP, which acts downstream of DPD [44], have been reported in patients with symptoms that are similar to those associated with pediatric DPD deficiency [45–53]. DHP deficiency is extremely rare. Only 31 cases have been reported in the literature to date [48], and the prevalence has been estimated to be 1 in 10,000 based on a study in Japan [54]. The symptoms of DHP deficiency are also highly variable and range from asymptomatic to severe neurodevelopmental delay, seizures, and gastrointestinal abnormalities [45–47,50,53]. Patients with microcephaly [46,47,53] and loss of white matter and cerebral atrophy on MRI [47,48,50–53] have been reported. Patients variably present with delayed growth, feeding problems, hypotonia, autism, dysmorphic features, ataxia, and optic disc pallor [47,53].

TABLE 1
Reported Genetic Variation in Pediatric Dihydropyrimidine Dehydrogenase Deficiency

Subject ID	*DPYD* Variation	Zygosity	References
1	Complete deletion	Homozygous	Mattia et al, [26] 1992
2	Unknown	Unknown	Henderson et al, [40] 1995
3	Unknown	Unknown	Jakobs et al, [41] 1991
4	c.1905 + 1G>A (rs3918290)	Homozygous	Au et al, [32] 2003
5	c.1340–3473_c.1524 + 10154del13812 (exon 12 deletion)	Homozygous	Van Kuilenburg et al, [8] 2009
6	c.1340–3473_c.1524 + 10154del13812 (exon 12 deletion)	Homozygous	Van Kuilenburg et al, [8] 2009
7	c.1340–3473_c.1524 + 10154del13812 (exon 12 deletion)	Homozygous	Van Kuilenburg et al, [8] 2009
8	c.1741_2058del (exon 14–16 deletion)	Homozygous	Van Kuilenburg et al, [8] 2009
9	c.299_302del, p.Phe100Serfs*15 (rs72549309)/Complete deletion	Compound heterozygous	Van Kuilenburg et al, [8] 2009
10	c.299_302del, p.Phe100Serfs*15 (rs72549309)	Homozygous	Vreken et al, [24] 1997
11	c.299_302del, p.Phe100Serfs*15 (rs72549309)	Homozygous	Vreken et al, [24] 1997
12	c.505_513del, p.Pro169_Ile171del	Homozygous	Van Kuilenburg et al, [30]2010
13	c.1905 + 1G>A (rs3918290)/c.187A>G, p.Lys63Glu (rs367619008)	Compound heterozygous	Weidensee et al, [25] 2011
14	c.1905 + 1G>A (rs3918290)	Homozygous	Fernandez-Salguero et al, [16] 1997
15	c.1905 + 1G>A (rs3918290)	Homozygous	Brussel et al, [33] 2006
16	c.2043–2058del, p.Lue682Ilefs*24 (rs773499329)	Homozygous	Ong et al, [27] 2012
17	c.1651 G>A, p.Ala551Thr (rs777425216)	Homozygous	Chen et al, [5] 2014
18	c.1651 G>A, p.Ala551Thr (rs777425216)	Homozygous	Chen et al, [5] 2014
19	c.257 C>T, p.Pro86Leu (rs568132506)	Homozygous	van Kuilenburg et al, [9]2019
20	c.85 T>C, p.Cys29Arg (rs1801265)[a]	Homozygous	Van Kuilenburg et al, [7] 1999
21	c.1905 + 1G>A (rs3918290)	Homozygous	Holopainen et al, [151] 1997
22	Unknown	Unknown	Wilcken et al, [39] 1985
23	c.1905 + 1G>A (rs3918290)	Homozygous	Christensen et al, [152] 1998
24	c.1905 + 1G>A (rs3918290)	Homozygous	Christensen et al, [152] 1998
25	c.1905 + 1G>A (rs3918290)	Homozygous	Christensen et al, [152] 1998
26	c.1905 + 1G>A (rs3918290)	Homozygous	Al-Sanna'a et al, [29] 2005
27	Unknown	Unknown	Berger et al, [36] 1984
28	Unknown	Unknown	Berger et al, [36] 1984
29	Unknown	Unknown	Berger et al, [36] 1984
30	Complete deletion	Homozygous	Dockery and Westhuyzen, [153] 1991
31	Complete deletion	Homozygous	Dockery and Westhuyzen, [153] 1991

(*continued on next page*)

TABLE 1
(*continued*)

Subject ID	*DPYD* Variation	Zygosity	References
32	Complete deletion	Homozygous	Tabata et al, [154] 1991
33	c.1905 + 1G>A (rs3918290)	Homozygous	Yau et al, [35] 2004
34	Unknown	Unknown	Brockstedt et al, [37] 1990
35	c.1905 + 1G>A (rs3918290)	Homozygous	Fiumara et al, [38] 2003
36	Unknown	Unknown	Enns et al, [6] 2004
37	Unknown	Unknown	Braakhekke et al, [23] 1987
38	Unknown	Unknown	Bakkeren et al, [155] 1984
39	Unknown	Unknown	Bakker et al, [156] 1994
40	c.2059–22T>G (rs747189276)	Homozygous	Fleger et al, [34] 2017
41	c.1905 + 1G>A (rs3918290)	Homozygous	Schmidt et al, [157] 2005
42	Unknown	Unknown	Schmidt et al, [157] 2005
43	c.1905 + 1G>A (rs3918290)	Homozygous	Van Kuilenburg et al, [3] 1999
44	c.1905 + 1G>A (rs3918290)	Homozygous	Van Kuilenburg et al, [3] 1999
45	c.703 C>T, p.Arg235Trp (rs1801266)	Heterozygous	Van Kuilenburg et al, [3] 1999

[a] Denotes an allele currently classified as "normal function."

Biochemically, DHP deficiency leads to moderately increased levels of uracil and thymine and severely increased levels of dihydrouracil and dihydrothymine in plasma, cerebrospinal fluid (CSF), and urine [45–48,53,54]. Affected individuals also show decreased levels of N-carbamyl-β-alanine [51], N-carbamyl-β-aminoisobutyric acid [51], β-alanine [52], and BAIBA [52]. Measures of DHP activity from liver biopsies show minimal-to-no DHP activity in patients with DHP deficiency [50]. Reported *DPYS* variants tend to localize to exons 1 and 5 to 9 [44,48,51–53].

The similarity in symptoms when comparing patients with pediatric DPD deficiency and severe forms of DHP deficiency may indicate that β-alanine and BAIBA play roles in brain development, as low levels of these compounds are correlated with delayed intellectual development. However, there are notable differences that have been reported between the 2 conditions. Patients with pediatric DPD deficiency are more likely to have motor deficits, hearing loss, and hepatomegaly and display a greater heterogeneity of symptoms, such as hypertonia/hypotonia and macrocephaly/microcephaly (see Table 1).

B-ureidopropionase Deficiency

Neurodevelopmental syndrome similar to those associated with pediatric DPD deficiency has been reported in patients with BUP deficiency. The prevalence of this disorder is estimated to be 1 in 6000 individuals based on a study in Japan [55]. Approximately 40 individuals with BUP deficiency have been described in the literature [56,57]. Patients with BUP deficiency display a variety of symptoms ranging from asymptomatic to severe developmental delay, hypotonia, dystonia, seizures, microcephaly, dysmorphic features, and language disorders [56–61]. Less commonly, gastrointestinal abnormalities have been reported [62,63]. One co-diagnosis of BUP deficiency and West syndrome was reported in a child with hypsarrhythmia on EEG [59]. Another patient was diagnosed with both BUP deficiency and a mitochondrial gene (*MT-TL1*) mutation [64]. The patient displayed common symptoms of BUP deficiency, including convulsions and delayed development, but also suffered from mitochondrial encephalomyopathy with lactic acidosis and stroke-like episodes (MELAS) syndrome-specific symptoms, including dizziness, hyperlactacidemia, and metabolic acidosis [64].

Biochemically, patients have elevated levels of N-carbamyl-β-alanine and N-carbamyl-β-aminoisobutyric acid in urine, plasma, and CSF, along with moderately elevated levels of dihydrouracil and dihydrothymine [55–58,61–65]. N-carbamyl β-amino acids can function as inhibitors of DHP, which may explain the moderately elevated dihydrouracil and dihydrothymine observed in

TABLE 2
Reported Symptoms of Pediatric Dihydropyrimidine Dehydrogenase Deficiency

Subject ID	Age in Report	Delayed Motor Development	Delayed Intellectual Development	Language Disorders	Macrocephaly	Microcephaly	Seizures	ASD	Hypertonia	Hypotonia	Dysmorphic Features	Eye Disorders	Abnormal MRI
1	2	+	+							+	+	+	
2	Neonatal					+					+		
3	Neonatal	+	+			+							
4	<1 mo						+			+			
5	8	+	+				+						
6	1	+	+	+		+	+	+		+			
7	1	+	+	+			+			+			
8	<5 mo	+	+							+	+		
9	3	+	+		+					+	+	+	
10	Unknown					+	+						
11	Unknown						+						
12	1.3	+	+				+		+				
13	8	+	+										
14	2	+	+										
15	1	+	+							+			+
16	1.6	+	+				+			+		+	+
17	11	+	+			+	+			+			+
18	6	+	+			+	+						+
19	12	+	+	+			+						+
20	3	+	+	+									
21	7						+						+
22	<2 mo					+			+				
23	8	+	+				+						
24	3.5	+	+										
25	<8 mo	+	+										
26	3					+			+		+		
27	4	+	+	+			+						
28	14		+				+						

29	1.25		+		+							
30	30		+		+							
31	30		+		+							
32	<8 mo	+	+			+						
33	<8 mo	+				+			+	+	+	+
34	2	+	+	+	+	+		+			+	+
35	3		+	+	+	+		+				+
36	2.6	+	+	+	+	+			+		+	+
37	6				+	+						
38	6				+	+						
39	2	+	+								+	
40	3.5	+	+	+	+				+			
41	3					+						
42	4	+	+	+		+						
43	7	+	+			+	+					
44	14	+									+	
45	6	+	+		+	+				+	+	+

Note: + indicates that a patient is reported as positive for a given symptom. An empty space indicates that the condition was not reported and/or not tested for.

patients with BUP deficiency [66]. Β-alanine and BAIBA levels tend to be moderately and severely decreased, respectively [60]. Measurements of BUP activity from liver biopsies are typically non-detectable [60]. The majority of *UPB1* genetic variation reported in the literature involves single nucleotide variants (SNVs) or splicing variants located within exons 1 to 4, exons 6 to 10, and introns 1, 7, and 8 [56,57,59,61,67]. There is a lack of correlation between the genotype and clinical presentation; however, patients with biallelic splicing variants tend to experience more severe neurologic symptoms compared to individuals with homozygous or compound heterozygous missense variants [60,63].

Patients with BUP deficiency tend to experience similar, but often more severe, neurodevelopmental symptoms compared to pediatric DPD deficiency. Because of these similarities, decreased levels of β-alanine and BAIBA are thought to be the primary cause of symptoms [68]. However, N-carbamyl-β-alanine has been shown to exert neurotoxic effects in vitro [69]. It is noted that patients with DPD and DHP deficiency have decreased levels of N-carbamyl-β-alanine, and BUP deficiency typically presents with only moderately elevated N-carbamyl-β-alanine levels in CSF [60]. Overall, this suggests that decreased β-alanine and BAIBA are more likely to contribute to neurodevelopmental symptoms in DPD, DHP, and BUP deficiencies.

POTENTIAL MECHANISMS OF ONSET

Pyrimidines in the Brain

The major pyrimidine present in the plasma is uridine [70]. Circulating uridine and cytidine are important for maintaining brain electrophysiological activity and carbohydrate and phospholipid content [71]. Limited de novo synthesis of pyrimidines occurs in the brain [72], indicating that pyrimidines in the brain are taken up from the plasma, typically in the form of uridine [73]. Uridine is the only pyrimidine able to cross the blood–brain barrier (BBB) in rats—cytidine and thymidine cannot [73]. Neurons and glial cells can also take up uridine from the extracellular space using equilibrative nucleoside transporters and concentrative nucleoside transporters [74]. Further, extracellular uridine levels increase based on the neural activity of a particular brain region after pharmacologically induced depolarization [75,76] or epilepsy [77], indicating that uridine transport may be affected by changes in signaling.

Within the central nervous system (CNS), pyrimidines can directly act as signaling molecules that can bind purinergic receptors [78] that are expressed on various neural cell types and promote a variety of neuroprotective functions, including $P2Y_2$, $P2Y_4$, $P2Y_6$, and $P2Y_{14}$ [79–82] (Fig. 2). Uridine nucleotides can additionally bind orphan G protein-coupled receptors (GPCRs), such as GPR17, which is activated by both uracil nucleotides and cysteinyl leukotrienes [83]. Typically, these molecules are released in areas of neuroinflammation, which show elevated levels of GPR17 expression, indicating that GPR17 may play a role in mediating the brain's inflammatory response [84]. GPR17 is also expressed on neural progenitor cells, especially in the adult brain in regions where neurogenesis can occur [83]. GPR17 is important for oligodendrocyte precursor cell (OPC) differentiation to oligodendrocytes, as it is typically co-expressed on OPCs with early oligodendrocyte markers [85,86]. In cases of acute and chronic stress, OPCs expressing GPR17 play a role in remyelination of the damaged area through differentiation to oligodendrocytes [86]. Up-regulation of GPR17 in neurons surrounding areas of damage is observed, which correlated with neuronal death, along with recruitment of active microglia [87–89].

Uridine also regulates neurotransmitter release within the brain. Specifically, uracil nucleotides can modulate gamma-aminobutyric acid (GABA) [90] and dopamine [91] release. Administration of oral uridine-5′-monophosphate was shown to increase dopamine [91] and acetylcholine (ACh) [92] release. Promotion of GABA release may be consistent with uridine's role as an antiepileptic agent, as it protects against seizures in animal models of epilepsy [93–95]. Uridine treatment competitively inhibits GABA binding to its receptors [90,96], allowing uridine to regulate inhibitory signaling via its activation of GABA receptors [90]. Alternative models suggest that elevated uridine levels increase the rate of RNA synthesis following seizures, which may contribute to uridine's action as an anticonvulsant [94].

β-alanine in the Brain

β-alanine is the resulting product of uracil catabolism and functions as a neurotransmitter within the CNS [97]. β-alanine is released following depolarization to decrease neural excitability [98]. β-alanine can be synthesized by 3 mechanisms in vivo: L-aspartate decarboxylation by gut microbes [99], as a byproduct of pyruvate conversion to L-alanine, and as the end product of uracil catabolism [100]. Neurons and glial cells cannot synthesize β-alanine via uracil catabolism since they lack BUP activity [101]. Instead, GABA transporters (GAT1-4) likely transport β-alanine across the BBB and into cells [102,103]. Cells can also uptake β-alanine from the synapse via a taurine/β-alanine transporter [104] dependent on the sodium-chloride gradient [105].

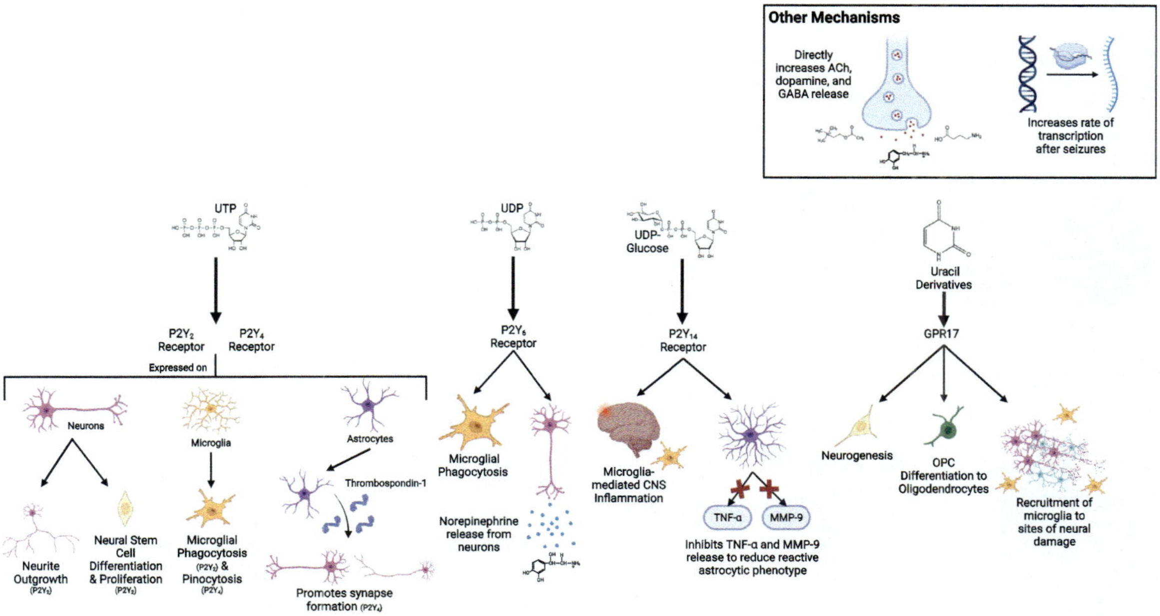

FIG. 2 Uracil effects in the CNS. Uracil derivatives, including uridine, uridine-5′-triphosphate (UTP), uridine diphosphate (UDP), and UDP-glucose, can bind to purinergic receptors ($P2Y_2$, $P2Y_4$, $P2Y_6$, and $P2Y_{14}$) and GPCRs. Binding of UTP to $P2Y_2$ receptors can promote neurite outgrowth, neural stem cell (NSC) differentiation and proliferation, and microglial phagocytosis. Activation of the $P2Y_4$ receptor can promote synapse formation via astrocytic release of thrombospondin-1 and microglial pinocytosis. UDP binding to the $P2Y_6$ receptor also promotes microglial phagocytosis and additionally stimulates the release of norepinephrine (NE) from neurons. $P2Y_{14}$ receptor activation mediates CNS inflammation via microglial activation and reduces the reactive astrocytic phenotype by inhibiting TNF-α and MMP-9 release from astrocytes. The orphan GPCR, GPR17, has been shown to play a role in neural progenitor differentiation to neurons, OPC differentiation to oligodendrocytes, and recruitment of microglia to areas of neural damage, as its expression is positively correlated with neuronal damage. Uracil derivatives can also directly promote the release of ACh, dopamine, and GABA from neurons and increase the RNA synthesis rate following seizure occurrence. (Created with Biorender.com.)

Within the CNS, β-alanine can act as an inhibitory neurotransmitter through multiple mechanisms: binding the GABA-A receptor, binding glycine strychnine-insensitive site on the N-methyl-D-aspartate (NMDA) excitatory glutamatergic receptor, binding glycine strychnine sensitive receptor site, and binding GAT protein for reuptake [106] (Fig. 3). When binding to the inhibitory GABA-A receptor, β-alanine can produce a similar response to GABA binding, indicating that β-alanine likely can hyperpolarize neurons within the CNS [107]. B-alanine also acts as an agonist of the glycine receptor, as its binding allows the chloride channel to open, resulting in neural hyperpolarization [108–110]. β-alanine binding to the glycine receptor elicits the same response as glycine binding, indicating that it is a full agonist of the receptor regulating neural excitation [111–113]. Further, β-alanine binding to the strychnine-insensitive glycine site of the excitatory NMDA receptor inhibits glycine binding and prevents NMDA receptor activation, decreasing neural excitability [114,115]. β-alanine can additionally prolong GABA presence within the synapse by inhibiting its reuptake by GAT-2, as β-alanine can competitively inhibit GABA transport via its own reuptake [102,103]. The increased GABA availability can suppress abnormal excitability and reduce epileptiform activity [3,116]. Further, β-alanine can regulate dopamine levels in the *nucleus accumbens* via its binding to the strychnine-sensitive glycine receptor [117].

Most β-alanine within the body is stored as carnosine, a dipeptide with L-histidine that is synthesized by carnosine synthase [118]. β-alanine is the limiting reagent in carnosine synthesis, as it is mainly obtained from uracil catabolism in the liver [119]. Carnosine can cross the BBB [120]; however, most carnosine present in the brain

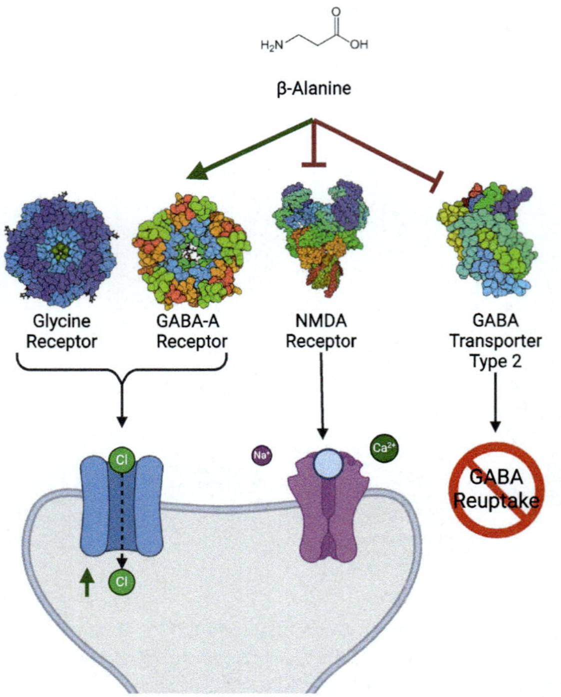

FIG. 3 β-alanine as an inhibitory neurotransmitter within the CNS. β-alanine is a known agonist of the inhibitory glycine [144] and GABA-A [145] ionotropic chloride channels, leading to neural hyperpolarization following β-alanine binding. Binding to the strychnine-insensitive glycine site of NMDA receptors [146] inhibits their activation and prevents Ca^{+2} influx into neurons, further inhibiting depolarization. β-alanine prolongs GABA presence within the synaptic space by utilizing GAT-2 [147] as a reuptake presence and competitively inhibiting GABA reuptake. (Created with Biorender.com.)

is produced through de novo synthesis [121]. While carnosine has been found to be synthesized in olfactory bulb neurons [122], in other brain regions, it is mostly located in mature astrocytes and oligodendrocytes [123,124]. Carnosine is likely synthesized by glial cells [119]; however, only oligodendrocytes have been shown to express carnosine-synthetase activity [123,125]. Interestingly, most carnosine is used by neurons and astrocytes [125]. Carnosine can also function as a neuroprotective molecule by inhibiting calcium uptake by the mitochondria [126], act as an antioxidant [121,126], reduce reductive oxygen species (ROS) production [127,128], modulate the brain immune response by increasing interleukin (IL)-1β release to suppress apoptosis [129,130], increase extracellular GABA [129], decrease extracellular glutamate [129], buffer pH during excitotoxicity [128], and chelate divalent cations, such as zinc and copper [131,132]. In animal models of epilepsy, intraperitoneal injections of carnosine can decrease the length of seizures and increase the time between seizures [120,133]. Reductions in carnosine, β-alanine, and histidine levels have also been observed in children with ASD [134].

β-aminoisobutyric Acid

BAIBA is the product of thymine catabolism. A minority of BAIBA (<10%) can also be produced via valine catabolism [135]. Impaired thymine catabolism decreases BAIBA levels in urine, plasma, and CSF [4]. BAIBA is classically known for its leptin-dependent metabolic affects, and BAIBA binding to GPR41 on white adipocytes stimulates leptin release [136] (Fig. 4). A recent study indicates that BAIBA can reduce hypothalamus inflammation via reversal of microglial activation [137]. BAIBA's neuroprotective role through the prevention of ROS-induced neurotoxicity [138] is a potential explanation for the elevated urine levels of 8-hydroxydeoxyguanosine in patients with pediatric DPD deficiency, an indicator of oxidative stress [60,139].

PROPOSED TREATMENT OPTIONS

Proposed treatments for pediatric DPD deficiency have focused on reversing the biochemical deficits through β-alanine and BAIBA supplementation. In one study, administration of β-alanine and BAIBA improved clinical symptoms in a patient with DPD deficiency suffering from arthrogryposis multiplex congenita [140] who initially presented with reduced fetal movement, arthrogryposis, feeding difficulties, and hypercapnia at birth. The patient's uracil and thymine excretion values were greatly elevated, with 1046 mmol/mol creatinine for uracil and 331 mmol/mol creatinine for thymine. DPD activity in peripheral blood mononuclear cells was undetectable, and the patient was found to be homozygous for *DPYD**2A. The patient's hypercapnia subsided following β-alanine supplementation at 5 weeks of age at a dose of 100 mg/kg bodyweight per day. At 9 months of age, BAIBA supplement was started (50 mg/kg bodyweight per day), which was found to improve feeding and increase muscle activity. The authors concluded that supplementation with β-alanine and BAIBA may be a sufficient therapeutic approach to improve the clinical symptoms of pediatric DPD deficiency [140].

However, β-alanine supplementation alone was insufficient to treat neurologic symptoms in BUP deficiency [68]. The patient presented with visual impairment, irritability, hypotonia, and dystonia from birth. At 28 months, β-alanine (174 mg/kg bodyweight per day) was administered for 1.5 years until the patient

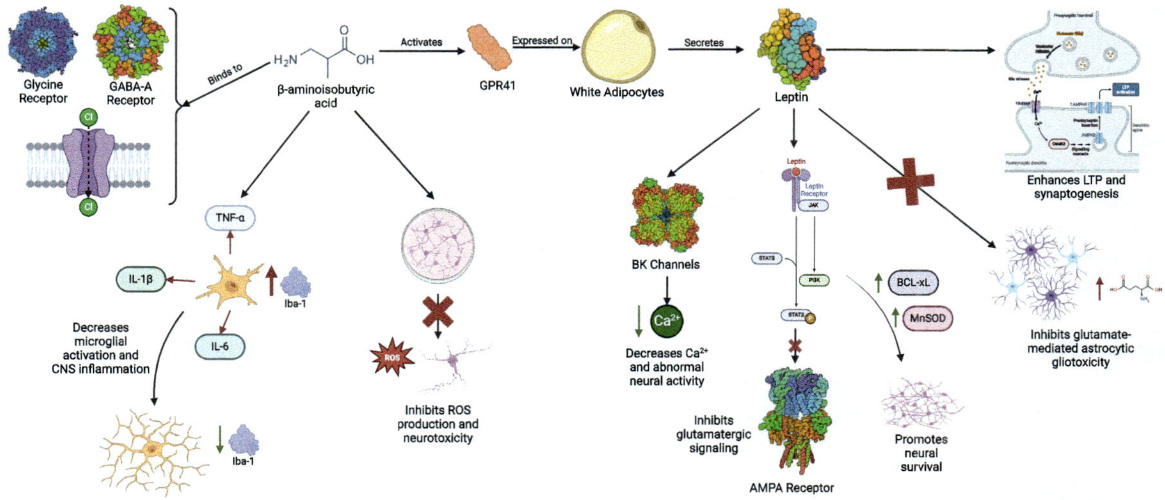

FIG. 4 Antiepileptic functions of BAIBA in the CNS. BAIBA can bind to and activate the inhibitory ionotropic glycine [144] and GABA-A receptors [145]. It additionally decreases the inflammatory phenotype of microglia, inhibits pro-inflammatory cytokine release, and also inhibits ROS production contributing to neurotoxicity. BAIBA can act via GPR41 receptors to promote leptin [148] secretion from white adipocytes, and leptin can have neuroprotective effects within the CNS. Leptin activates BK channels [149] to decrease neuronal excitability, inhibits AMPA receptor [150] activation and promotes neural survival via the JAK/PI3K signaling pathway, enhances synaptogenesis via CAMKII, and inhibits gliotoxicity that occurs due to high glutamate levels. (Created with Biorender.com.)

reached the age of 3.8 years. β-alanine supplementation increased head growth and reduced the severity of microcephaly during the first 2 years of life. Abnormal β-activity was shown to return to normal after 7 weeks of β-alanine supplementation. At 5 years of age, the patient still experienced severe dystonia, severe language deficits, impaired vision, delayed myelination, cerebral hypoplasia, and mild cerebral atrophy. Plasma β-alanine increased during supplementation but returned to the lower end of the normal range by the age of 2.9 years. β-alanine was slightly increased within CSF during treatment. The authors ultimately concluded that there was not sufficient clinical improvement [68].

SUMMARY AND OPPORTUNITIES FOR ADVANCEMENT

While there are a variety of mechanisms that could contribute to the onset of the neurodevelopmental symptoms in pediatric DPD deficiency, the potentially dysregulated pathways have yet to be directly investigated in this context. While case studies have established correlations between *DPYD* variants and the reported clinical presentations, the variability of symptoms that have been reported remains unexplained. The biochemical similarity between deficiencies of other pyrimidine catabolism enzymes, indicates that a lack of β-alanine and BAIBA likely contributes to neurologic dysfunction [60]. While treatment with both compounds alleviated symptoms in one patient [140] and β-alanine alone reduced microcephaly in another subject patient with BUP deficiency [68], further research is required to determine whether dietary supplementation is an appropriate treatment or whether there are other more suitable therapeutic targets.

CLINICS CARE POINTS

- Pediatric DPD deficiency is a neurodevelopmental disorder characterized by incomplete penetrance and variable expressivity associated with genetic variation in *DPYD*.
- This disorder is typically diagnosed biochemically by high uracil and thymine levels in patients' blood, urine, or cerebrospinal fluid and can be confirmed via sequencing of *DPYD* to test for genetic variants.
- There are no current therapeutic options for pediatric DPD deficiency and most treatments focus on alleviation of individual symptoms.

DISCLOSURE

The authors have nothing to disclose.

FUNDING

This work is supported by research grants from the DPD Deficiency Foundation (S.M. Offer, P.I.) and the Mayo Clinic Center for Individualized Medicine (S.M. Offer, P.I.; B.M. Bembenek, Co-I).

REFERENCES

[1] Micheli V, Camici M, Tozzi MG, et al. Neurological disorders of purine and pyrimidine metabolism. Curr Top Med Chem 2011;11(8):923–47. https://doi.org/10.2174/156802611795347645.

[2] van Gennip AH, Abeling NG, Vreken P, et al. Inborn errors of pyrimidine degradation: clinical, biochemical and molecular aspects. J Inherit Metab Dis 1997;20(2):203–13. https://doi.org/10.1023/a:1005356806329.

[3] Van Kuilenburg AB, Vreken P, Abeling NG, et al. Genotype and phenotype in patients with dihydropyrimidine dehydrogenase deficiency. Hum Genet 1999;104(1):1–9. https://doi.org/10.1007/pl00008711.

[4] Van Kuilenburg AB, Stroomer AE, Van Lenthe H, et al. New insights in dihydropyrimidine dehydrogenase deficiency: a pivotal role for beta-aminoisobutyric acid? Biochem J 2004;379(Pt 1):119–24. https://doi.org/10.1042/BJ20031463.

[5] Chen BC, Mohd Rawi R, Meinsma R, et al. Dihydropyrimidine dehydrogenase deficiency in two malaysian siblings with abnormal MRI findings. Mol Syndromol 2014;5(6):299–303. https://doi.org/10.1159/000366074.

[6] Enns GM, Barkovich AJ, van Kuilenburg AB, et al. Head imaging abnormalities in dihydropyrimidine dehydrogenase deficiency. J Inherit Metab Dis 2004;27(4):513–22. https://doi.org/10.1023/B:BOLI.0000037350.24142.d5.

[7] Van Kuilenburg AB, Vreken P, Riva D, et al. Clinical and biochemical abnormalities in a patient with dihydropyrimidine dehydrogenase deficiency due to homozygosity for the C29R mutation. J Inherit Metab Dis 1999;22(2):191–2. https://doi.org/10.1023/a:1005470524203.

[8] van Kuilenburg AB, Meijer J, Mul AN, et al. Analysis of severely affected patients with dihydropyrimidine dehydrogenase deficiency reveals large intragenic rearrangements of DPYD and a de novo interstitial deletion del(1)(p13.3p21.3). Hum Genet 2009;125(5–6):581–90. https://doi.org/10.1007/s00439-009-0653-6.

[9] van Kuilenburg ABP, Meijer J, Meinsma R, et al. Dihydropyrimidine Dehydrogenase Deficiency: Homozygosity for an Extremely Rare Variant in DPYD due to Uniparental Isodisomy of Chromosome 1. JIMD Rep 2019;45:65–9. https://doi.org/10.1007/8904_2018_138.

[10] Johnson MR, Diasio RB. Importance of dihydropyrimidine dehydrogenase (DPD) deficiency in patients exhibiting toxicity following treatment with 5-fluorouracil. Adv Enzyme Regul 2001;41:151–7. https://doi.org/10.1016/s0065-2571(00)00011-x.

[11] van Kuilenburg AB. Dihydropyrimidine dehydrogenase and the efficacy and toxicity of 5-fluorouracil. Eur J Cancer 2004;40(7):939–50. https://doi.org/10.1016/j.ejca.2003.12.004.

[12] Podschun B, Cook PF, Schnackerz KD. Kinetic mechanism of dihydropyrimidine dehydrogenase from pig liver. J Biol Chem 1990;265(22):12966–72.

[13] Porter DJ, Spector T. Dihydropyrimidine dehydrogenase. Kinetic mechanism for reduction of uracil by NADPH. J Biol Chem 1993;268(26):19321–7.

[14] Fink K, Cline RE, Henderson RB, et al. Metabolism of thymine (methyl-C14 or -2-C14) by rat liver in vitro. J Biol Chem 1956;221(1):425–33.

[15] Heggie GD, Sommadossi JP, Cross DS, et al. Clinical pharmacokinetics of 5-fluorouracil and its metabolites in plasma, urine, and bile. Cancer Res 1987;47(8):2203–6.

[16] Fernandez-Salguero PM, Sapone A, Wei X, et al. Lack of correlation between phenotype and genotype for the polymorphically expressed dihydropyrimidine dehydrogenase in a family of Pakistani origin. Pharmacogenetics 1997;7(2):161–3. https://doi.org/10.1097/00008571-199704000-00012.

[17] Van Kuilenburg AB, Vreken P, Beex LV, et al. Heterozygosity for a point mutation in an invariant splice donor site of dihydropyrimidine dehydrogenase and severe 5-fluorouracil related toxicity. Eur J Cancer 1997;33(13):2258–64. https://doi.org/10.1016/s0959-8049(97)00261-x.

[18] Wei X, McLeod HL, McMurrough J, et al. Molecular basis of the human dihydropyrimidine dehydrogenase deficiency and 5-fluorouracil toxicity. J Clin Invest 1996;98(3):610–5. https://doi.org/10.1172/JCI118830.

[19] Johnson MR, Hageboutros A, Wang K, et al. Life-threatening toxicity in a dihydropyrimidine dehydrogenase-deficient patient after treatment with topical 5-fluorouracil. Clin Cancer Res 1999;5(8):2006–11.

[20] Offer SM, Wegner NJ, Fossum C, et al. Phenotypic profiling of DPYD variations relevant to 5-fluorouracil sensitivity using real-time cellular analysis and in vitro measurement of enzyme activity. Cancer Res 2013;73(6):1958–68. https://doi.org/10.1158/0008-5472.CAN-12-3858.

[21] Amstutz U, Henricks LM, Offer SM, et al. Clinical Pharmacogenetics Implementation Consortium (CPIC) Guideline for Dihydropyrimidine Dehydrogenase Genotype and Fluoropyrimidine Dosing: 2017 Update. Clin Pharmacol Ther 2018;103(2):210–6. https://doi.org/10.1002/cpt.911.

[22] Page T. Metabolic approaches to the treatment of autism spectrum disorders. J Autism Dev Disord 2000;30(5):463–9. https://doi.org/10.1023/a:1005563926383.

[23] Braakhekke JP, Renier WO, Gabreels FJ, et al. Dihydropyrimidine dehydrogenase deficiency. Neurological

aspects. J Neurol Sci 1987;78(1):71–7. https://doi.org/10.1016/0022-510x(87)90079-7.

[24] Vreken P, Van Kuilenburg AB, Meinsma R, et al. Identification of a four-base deletion (delTCAT296-299) in the dihydropyrimidine dehydrogenase gene with variable clinical expression. Hum Genet 1997;100(2):263–5. https://doi.org/10.1007/s004390050502.

[25] Weidensee S, Goettig P, Bertone M, et al. A mild phenotype of dihydropyrimidine dehydrogenase deficiency and developmental retardation associated with a missense mutation affecting cofactor binding. Clin Biochem 2011;44(8–9):722–4. https://doi.org/10.1016/j.clinbiochem.2011.03.033.

[26] Mattia FR, Wardinsky TD, Tuttle DJ, et al. Interstitial deletion of the short arm of chromosome 1 (46XY, del(1)(p13p22.3)). Am J Med Genet 1992;44(5):551–4. https://doi.org/10.1002/ajmg.1320440503.

[27] Ong MT, Chow GC, Morton RE. Dual diagnosis of dihydropyrimidine dehydrogenase deficiency and GM(1) gangliosidosis. Pediatr Neurol 2012;46(3):178–81. https://doi.org/10.1016/j.pediatrneurol.2011.12.005.

[28] Willemsen MH, Valles A, Kirkels LA, et al. Chromosome 1p21.3 microdeletions comprising DPYD and MIR137 are associated with intellectual disability. J Med Genet 2011;48(12):810–8. https://doi.org/10.1136/jmedgenet-2011-100294.

[29] Al-Sanna'a NA, Van Kuilenburg AB, Atrak TM, et al. Dihydropyrimidine dehydrogenase deficiency presenting at birth. J Inherit Metab Dis 2005;28(5):793–6. https://doi.org/10.1007/s10545-005-4218-0.

[30] van Kuilenburg AB, Meijer J, Gokcay G, et al. Dihydropyrimidine dehydrogenase deficiency caused by a novel genomic deletion c.505_513del of DPYD. Nucleos Nucleot Nucleic Acids 2010;29(4–6):509–14. https://doi.org/10.1080/15257771003730227.

[31] Carter MT, Nikkel SM, Fernandez BA, et al. Hemizygous deletions on chromosome 1p21.3 involving the DPYD gene in individuals with autism spectrum disorder. Clin Genet 2011;80(5):435–43. https://doi.org/10.1111/j.1399-0004.2010.01578.x.

[32] Au KM, Lai CK, Yuen YP, et al. Diagnosis of dihydropyrimidine dehydrogenase deficiency in a neonate with thymine-uraciluria. Hong Kong Med J 2003;9(2):130–2.

[33] Brussel W, van Kuilenburg AB, Janssens PM. A neonate with recurrent vomiting and generalized hypotonia diagnosed with a deficiency of dihydropyrimidine dehydrogenase. Nucleos Nucleot Nucleic Acids 2006;25(9–11):1099–102. https://doi.org/10.1080/15257770600894063.

[34] Fleger M, Willomitzer J, Meinsma R, et al. Dihydropyrimidine Dehydrogenase Deficiency: Metabolic Disease or Biochemical Phenotype? JIMD Rep 2017;37:49–54. https://doi.org/10.1007/8904_2017_14.

[35] Yau EKC, Shek CC, Chan KY, et al. Dihydropyrimidine dehydrogenase deficiency: a baby boy with ocular abnormalities, neonatal seizure and global developmental delay. HK J Paediatr 2004;9:167–70.

[36] Berger R, Stoker-de Vries SA, Wadman SK, et al. Dihydropyrimidine dehydrogenase deficiency leading to thymine-uraciluria. An inborn error of pyrimidine metabolism. Clin Chim Acta 1984;141(2–3):227–34. https://doi.org/10.1016/0009-8981(84)90014-7.

[37] Brockstedt M, Jakobs C, Smit LM, et al. A new case of dihydropyrimidine dehydrogenase deficiency. J Inherit Metab Dis 1990;13(1):121–4. https://doi.org/10.1007/BF01799339.

[38] Fiumara A, van Kuilenburg AB, Caruso U, et al. Dihydropyrimidine dehydrogenase deficiency and acute neurological presentation. J Inherit Metab Dis 2003;26(4):407–9. https://doi.org/10.1023/a:1025123622821.

[39] Wilcken B, Hammond J, Berger R, et al. Dihydropyrimidine dehydrogenase deficiency–a further case. J Inherit Metab Dis 1985;8(Suppl 2):115–6. https://doi.org/10.1007/BF01811485.

[40] Henderson MJ, Jones S, Walker P, et al. Heterogeneity of symptomatology in two male siblings with thymine uraciluria. J Inherit Metab Dis 1995;18(1):85–6. https://doi.org/10.1007/BF00711383.

[41] Jakobs C, Stellaard F, Smit LM, et al. The first prenatal diagnosis of dihydropyrimidine dehydrogenase deficiency. Eur J Pediatr 1991;150(4):291. https://doi.org/10.1007/BF01955535.

[42] Pfaffeneder T, Spada F, Wagner M, et al. Tet oxidizes thymine to 5-hydroxymethyluracil in mouse embryonic stem cell DNA. Nat Chem Biol 2014;10(7):574–81. https://doi.org/10.1038/nchembio.1532.

[43] Brecevic L, Rincic M, Krsnik Z, et al. Association of new deletion/duplication region at chromosome 1p21 with intellectual disability, severe speech deficit and autism spectrum disorder-like behavior: an all-in approach to solving the DPYD enigma. Transl Neurosci 2015;6(1):59–86. https://doi.org/10.1515/tnsci-2015-0007.

[44] Hamajima N, Kouwaki M, Vreken P, et al. Dihydropyrimidinase deficiency: structural organization, chromosomal localization, and mutation analysis of the human dihydropyrimidinase gene. Am J Hum Genet 1998;63(3):717–26. https://doi.org/10.1086/302022.

[45] Duran M, Rovers P, de Bree PK, et al. Dihydropyrimidinuria: a new inborn error of pyrimidine metabolism. J Inherit Metab Dis 1991;14(3):367–70. https://doi.org/10.1007/BF01811705.

[46] Henderson MJ, Ward K, Simmonds HA, et al. Dihydropyrimidinase deficiency presenting in infancy with severe developmental delay. J Inherit Metab Dis 1993;16(3):574–6. https://doi.org/10.1007/BF00711685.

[47] Putman CW, Rotteveel JJ, Wevers RA, et al. Dihydropyrimidinase deficiency, a progressive neurological disorder? Neuropediatrics 1997;28(2):106–10. https://doi.org/10.1055/s-2007-973681.

[48] Nakajima Y, Meijer J, Dobritzsch D, et al. Dihydropyrimidinase deficiency in four East Asian patients due to novel and rare DPYS mutations affecting protein structural integrity and catalytic activity. Mol Genet Metab

2017;122(4):216–22. https://doi.org/10.1016/j.ymgme.2017.10.003.

[49] Ohba S, Kidouchi K, Sumi S, et al. Dihydropyrimidinuria: the first case in Japan. Adv Exp Med Biol 1994;370:383–6. https://doi.org/10.1007/978-1-4615-2584-4_83.

[50] van Gennip AH, de Abreu RA, van Lenthe H, et al. Dihydropyrimidinase deficiency: confirmation of the enzyme defect in dihydropyrimidinuria. J Inherit Metab Dis 1997;20(3):339–42. https://doi.org/10.1023/a:1005309423960.

[51] van Kuilenburg AB, Meijer J, Dobritzsch D, et al. Clinical, biochemical and genetic findings in two siblings with a dihydropyrimidinase deficiency. Mol Genet Metab 2007;91(2):157–64. https://doi.org/10.1016/j.ymgme.2007.02.008.

[52] van Kuilenburg AB, Stroomer AE, Bosch AM, et al. Beta-alanine and beta-aminoisobutyric acid levels in two siblings with dihydropyrimidinase deficiency. Nucleos Nucleot Nucleic Acids 2008;27(6):825–9. https://doi.org/10.1080/15257770802146445.

[53] van Kuilenburg AB, Dobritzsch D, Meijer J, et al. Dihydropyrimidinase deficiency: Phenotype, genotype and structural consequences in 17 patients. Biochim Biophys Acta 2010;1802(7–8):639–48. https://doi.org/10.1016/j.bbadis.2010.03.013.

[54] Sumi S, Imaeda M, Kidouchi K, et al. Population and family studies of dihydropyrimidinuria: prevalence, inheritance mode, and risk of fluorouracil toxicity. Am J Med Genet 1998;78(4):336–40. https://doi.org/10.1002/(sici)1096-8628(19980724)78:4<336::aid-ajmg6>3.0.co;2-j.

[55] Kuhara T, Ohse M, Inoue Y, et al. Five cases of beta-ureidopropionase deficiency detected by GC/MS analysis of urine metabolome. J Mass Spectrom 2009;44(2):214–21. https://doi.org/10.1002/jms.1500.

[56] Dobritzsch D, Meijer J, Meinsma R, et al. beta-Ureidopropionase deficiency due to novel and rare UPB1 mutations affecting pre-mRNA splicing and protein structural integrity and catalytic activity. Mol Genet Metab 2022;136(3):177–85. https://doi.org/10.1016/j.ymgme.2022.01.102.

[57] Fang Y, Cai C, Wang C, et al. Clinical and genetic analysis of 7 Chinese patients with beta-ureidopropionase deficiency. Medicine (Baltimore) 2019;98(1):e14021. https://doi.org/10.1097/MD.0000000000014021.

[58] Akiyama T, Shibata T, Yoshinaga H, et al. A Japanese case of beta-ureidopropionase deficiency with dysmorphic features. Brain Dev 2017;39(1):58–61. https://doi.org/10.1016/j.braindev.2016.08.001.

[59] Nakajima Y, Meijer J, Dobritzsch D, et al. Clinical, biochemical and molecular analysis of 13 Japanese patients with beta-ureidopropionase deficiency demonstrates high prevalence of the c.977G > A (p.R326Q) mutation [corrected]. J Inherit Metab Dis 2014;37(5):801–12. https://doi.org/10.1007/s10545-014-9682-y.

[60] van Kuilenburg AB, Meinsma R, Beke E, et al. beta-Ureidopropionase deficiency: an inborn error of pyrimidine degradation associated with neurological abnormalities. Hum Mol Genet 2004;13(22):2793–801. https://doi.org/10.1093/hmg/ddh303.

[61] van Kuilenburg AB, Dobritzsch D, Meijer J, et al. ss-ureidopropionase deficiency: phenotype, genotype and protein structural consequences in 16 patients. Biochim Biophys Acta 2012;1822(7):1096–108. https://doi.org/10.1016/j.bbadis.2012.04.001.

[62] Shu J, Lv X, Jiang S, et al. Genetic analysis of the UPB1 gene in two new Chinese families with beta-ureidopropionase deficiency and the carrier frequency of the mutation c.977G>A in Northern China. Childs Nerv Syst 2014;30(12):2109–14. https://doi.org/10.1007/s00381-014-2541-1.

[63] Yaplito-Lee J, Pitt J, Meijer J, et al. Beta-ureidopropionase deficiency presenting with congenital anomalies of the urogenital and colorectal systems. Mol Genet Metab 2008;93(2):190–4. https://doi.org/10.1016/j.ymgme.2007.09.009.

[64] Shu J, Zhi X, Chen J, et al. Case Report: A Case of beta-Ureidopropionase Deficiency Complicated With MELAS Syndrome Caused by UPB1 Variant and Mitochondrial Gene Variant. Front Pediatr 2022;10:838341. https://doi.org/10.3389/fped.2022.838341.

[65] Ohse M, Matsuo M, Ishida A, et al. Screening and diagnosis of beta-ureidopropionase deficiency by gas chromatographic/mass spectrometric analysis of urine. J Mass Spectrom 2002;37(9):954–62. https://doi.org/10.1002/jms.354.

[66] Kikugawa M, Kaneko M, Fujimoto-Sakata S, et al. Purification, characterization and inhibition of dihydropyrimidinase from rat liver. Eur J Biochem 1994;219(1–2):393–9. https://doi.org/10.1111/j.1432-1033.1994.tb19951.x.

[67] van Kuilenburg AB, Meinsma R, Assman B, et al. Genetic analysis of the first 4 patients with beta-ureidopropionase deficiency. Nucleos Nucleot Nucleic Acids 2006;25(9–11):1093–8. https://doi.org/10.1080/15257770600956870.

[68] Assmann B, Gohlich G, Baethmann M, et al. Clinical findings and a therapeutic trial in the first patient with beta-ureidopropionase deficiency. Neuropediatrics 2006;37(1):20–5. https://doi.org/10.1055/s-2006-923933.

[69] Kolker S, Okun JG, Horster F, et al. 3-Ureidopropionate contributes to the neuropathology of 3-ureidopropionase deficiency and severe propionic aciduria: a hypothesis. J Neurosci Res 2001;66(4):666–73. https://doi.org/10.1002/jnr.10012.

[70] Cansev M. Uridine and cytidine in the brain: their transport and utilization. Brain Res Rev 2006;52(2):389–97. https://doi.org/10.1016/j.brainresrev.2006.05.001.

[71] Geiger A, Yamasaki S. Cytidine and uridine requirement of the brain. J Neurochem 1956;1(2):93–100. https://doi.org/10.1111/j.1471-4159.1956.tb12059.x.

[72] Bourget PA, Tremblay GC. Pyrimidine biosynthesis in rat brain. J Neurochem 1972;19(7):1617–24. https://doi.org/10.1111/j.1471-4159.1972.tb06207.x.

[73] Cornford EM, Oldendorf WH. Independent blood-brain barrier transport systems for nucleic acid precursors. Biochim Biophys Acta 1975;394(2):211–9. https://doi.org/10.1016/0005-2736(75)90259-x.

[74] Lu H, Chen C, Klaassen C. Tissue distribution of concentrative and equilibrative nucleoside transporters in male and female rats and mice. Drug Metab Dispos 2004;32(12):1455–61. https://doi.org/10.1124/dmd.104.001123.

[75] Dobolyi A, Szikra T, Kekesi AK, et al. Uridine is released by depolarization and inhibits unit activity in the rat hippocampus. Neuroreport 1999;10(14):3049–53. https://doi.org/10.1097/00001756-199909290-00032.

[76] Dobolyi A, Reichart A, Szikra T, et al. Sustained depolarisation induces changes in the extracellular concentrations of purine and pyrimidine nucleosides in the rat thalamus. Neurochem Int 2000;37(1):71–9. https://doi.org/10.1016/s0197-0186(99)00162-x.

[77] Slezia A, Kekesi AK, Szikra T, et al. Uridine release during aminopyridine-induced epilepsy. Neurobiol Dis 2004;16(3):490–9. https://doi.org/10.1016/j.nbd.2004.02.011.

[78] Jacobson KA, Paoletta S, Katritch V, et al. Nucleotides Acting at P2Y Receptors: Connecting Structure and Function. Mol Pharmacol 2015;88(2):220–30. https://doi.org/10.1124/mol.114.095711.

[79] Li HQ, Chen C, Dou Y, et al. P2Y4 receptor-mediated pinocytosis contributes to amyloid beta-induced self-uptake by microglia. Mol Cell Biol 2013;33(21):4282–93. https://doi.org/10.1128/MCB.00544-13.

[80] Miras-Portugal MT, Queipo MJ, Gil-Redondo JC, et al. P2 receptor interaction and signalling cascades in neuroprotection. Brain Res Bull 2019;151:74–83. https://doi.org/10.1016/j.brainresbull.2018.12.012.

[81] Moore DJ, Murdock PR, Watson JM, et al. GPR105, a novel Gi/o-coupled UDP-glucose receptor expressed on brain glia and peripheral immune cells, is regulated by immunologic challenge: possible role in neuroimmune function. Brain Res Mol Brain Res 2003;118(1–2):10–23. https://doi.org/10.1016/s0169-328x(03)00330-9.

[82] Koizumi S, Shigemoto-Mogami Y, Nasu-Tada K, et al. UDP acting at P2Y6 receptors is a mediator of microglial phagocytosis. Nature 2007;446(7139):1091–5. https://doi.org/10.1038/nature05704.

[83] Lecca D, Trincavelli ML, Gelosa P, et al. The recently identified P2Y-like receptor GPR17 is a sensor of brain damage and a new target for brain repair. PLoS One 2008;3(10):e3579. https://doi.org/10.1371/journal.pone.0003579.

[84] Fumagalli M, Lecca D, Abbracchio MP. CNS remyelination as a novel reparative approach to neurodegenerative diseases: The roles of purinergic signaling and the P2Y-like receptor GPR17. Neuropharmacology 2016;104:82–93. https://doi.org/10.1016/j.neuropharm.2015.10.005.

[85] Fratangeli A, Parmigiani E, Fumagalli M, et al. The regulated expression, intracellular trafficking, and membrane recycling of the P2Y-like receptor GPR17 in Oli-neu oligodendroglial cells. J Biol Chem 2013;288(7):5241–56. https://doi.org/10.1074/jbc.M112.404996.

[86] Fumagalli M, Daniele S, Lecca D, et al. Phenotypic changes, signaling pathway, and functional correlates of GPR17-expressing neural precursor cells during oligodendrocyte differentiation. J Biol Chem 2011;286(12):10593–604. https://doi.org/10.1074/jbc.M110.162867.

[87] Fumagalli M, Lecca D, Abbracchio MP. Role of purinergic signalling in neuro-immune cells and adult neural progenitors. Front Biosci (Landmark Ed) 2011;16(6):2326–41. https://doi.org/10.2741/3856.

[88] Ceruti S, Villa G, Genovese T, et al. The P2Y-like receptor GPR17 as a sensor of damage and a new potential target in spinal cord injury. Brain 2009;132:2206–18. https://doi.org/10.1093/brain/awp147.

[89] Zhao B, Zhao CZ, Zhang XY, et al. The new P2Y-like receptor G protein-coupled receptor 17 mediates acute neuronal injury and late microgliosis after focal cerebral ischemia in rats. Neuroscience 2012;202:42–57. https://doi.org/10.1016/j.neuroscience.2011.11.066.

[90] Guarneri P, Guarneri R, La Bella V, et al. Interaction between uridine and GABA-mediated inhibitory transmission: studies in vivo and in vitro. Epilepsia Nov-Dec 1985;26(6):666–71. https://doi.org/10.1111/j.1528-1157.1985.tb05709.x.

[91] Wang L, Pooler AM, Albrecht MA, et al. Dietary uridine-5′-monophosphate supplementation increases potassium-evoked dopamine release and promotes neurite outgrowth in aged rats. J Mol Neurosci 2005;27(1):137–45. https://doi.org/10.1385/JMN:27:1:137.

[92] Wang L, Albrecht MA, Wurtman RJ. Dietary supplementation with uridine-5′-monophosphate (UMP), a membrane phosphatide precursor, increases acetylcholine level and release in striatum of aged rat. Brain Res 2007;1133(1):42–8. https://doi.org/10.1016/j.brainres.2006.11.048.

[93] Roberts CA. Anticonvulsant effects of uridine: comparative analysis of metrazol and penicillin induced foci. Brain Res 1973;55(2):291–308. https://doi.org/10.1016/0006-8993(73)90296-5.

[94] Roberts CA, Kreisman NR, Waltman M. Uridine anticonvulsant effects: selective control of nucleoside incorporation in experimental epilepsy. Epilepsia 1974;15(4):479–500. https://doi.org/10.1111/j.1528-1157.1974.tb04023.x.

[95] Zhao Q, Marolewski A, Rusche JR, et al. Effects of uridine in models of epileptogenesis and seizures. Epilepsy Res 2006;70(1):73–82. https://doi.org/10.1016/j.eplepsyres.2006.03.003.

[96] Guarneri P, Guarneri R, Mocciaro C, et al. Interaction of uridine with GABA binding sites in cerebellar membranes of the rat. Neurochem Res 1983;8(12):1537–45. https://doi.org/10.1007/BF00964155.

[97] DeFeudis FV, Martin del Rio R. Is beta-alanine an inhibitory neurotransmitter? Gen Pharmacol 1977;8(3):177–80. https://doi.org/10.1016/0306-3623(77)90046-5.

[98] Mathers DA, Grewal A, Wang YH. Beta-alanine induced ion channels in the membrane of cultured spinal cord neurons. Neurosci Lett 1990;108(1–2):127–31. https://doi.org/10.1016/0304-3940(90)90718-o.

[99] Cronan JE Jr. Beta-alanine synthesis in Escherichia coli. J Bacteriol 1980;141(3):1291–7. https://doi.org/10.1128/jb.141.3.1291-1297.1980.

[100] Hayaishi O, Nishizuka Y, Tatibana M, et al. Enzymatic studies on the metabolism of beta-alanine. J Biol Chem 1961;236:781–90.

[101] Minard FN, Grant DS. 5,6-dihydrouracil: its occurrence and metabolism in rat brain. Biochim Biophys Acta 1970;209(1):255–7. https://doi.org/10.1016/0005-2787(70)90682-9.

[102] Tamura S, Nelson H, Tamura A, et al. Short external loops as potential substrate binding site of gamma-aminobutyric acid transporters. J Biol Chem 1995; 270(48):28712–5. https://doi.org/10.1074/jbc.270.48.28712.

[103] Borden LA. Gaba transporter heterogeneity: Pharmacology and cellular localization. Neurochem Int 1996; 29(4):335–56. https://doi.org/10.1016/0197-0186(95)00158-1.

[104] Liu QR, Lopez-Corcuera B, Nelson H, et al. Cloning and expression of a cDNA encoding the transporter of taurine and beta-alanine in mouse brain. Proc Natl Acad Sci U S A 1992;89(24):12145–9. https://doi.org/10.1073/pnas.89.24.12145.

[105] Zafra F, Aragon MC, Valdivieso F, et al. beta-Alanine transport into plasma membrane vesicles derived from rat brain synaptosomes. Neurochem Res 1984;9(5): 695–707. https://doi.org/10.1007/BF00964516.

[106] Williams M, Risley EA, Totaro JA. Interactions of taurine and beta-alanine with central nervous system neurotransmitter receptors. Life Sci 1980;26(7):557–60. https://doi.org/10.1016/0024-3205(80)90319-7.

[107] Horikoshi T, Asanuma A, Yanagisawa K, et al. Taurine and beta-alanine act on both GABA and glycine receptors in Xenopus oocyte injected with mouse brain messenger RNA. Brain Res 1988;464(2):97–105. https://doi.org/10.1016/0169-328x(88)90002-2.

[108] Laube B, Langosch D, Betz H, et al. Hyperekplexia mutations of the glycine receptor unmask the inhibitory subsite for beta-amino-acids. Neuroreport 1995;6(6): 897–900. https://doi.org/10.1097/00001756-199504190-00018.

[109] Rajendra S, Lynch JW, Pierce KD, et al. Mutation of an arginine residue in the human glycine receptor transforms beta-alanine and taurine from agonists into competitive antagonists. Neuron 1995;14(1):169–75. https://doi.org/10.1016/0896-6273(95)90251-1.

[110] Tremblay N, Warren R, Dykes RW. The effects of strychnine on neurons in cat somatosensory cortex and its interaction with the inhibitory amino acids, glycine, taurine and beta-alanine. Neuroscience 1988;26(3):745–62. https://doi.org/10.1016/0306-4522(88)90096-6.

[111] Choquet D, Korn H. Does beta-alanine activate more than one chloride channel associated receptor? Neurosci Lett 1988;84(3):329–34. https://doi.org/10.1016/0304-3940(88)90530-7.

[112] Boehm S, Harvey RJ, von Holst A, et al. Glycine receptors in cultured chick sympathetic neurons are excitatory and trigger neurotransmitter release. J Physiol 1997;504(Pt 3):683–94. https://doi.org/10.1111/j.1469-7793.1997.683bd.x.

[113] Krishtal OA, Osipchuk Yu V, Vrublevsky SV. Properties of glycine-activated conductances in rat brain neurones. Neurosci Lett 1988;84(3):271–6. https://doi.org/10.1016/0304-3940(88)90519-8.

[114] Ogita K, Suzuki T, Yoneda Y. Strychnine-insensitive binding of [3H]glycine to synaptic membranes in rat brain, treated with Triton X-100. Neuropharmacology 1989;28(11):1263–70. https://doi.org/10.1016/0028-3908(89)90220-7.

[115] Pullan LM, Powel RJ. Comparison of binding at strychnine-sensitive (inhibitory glycine receptor) and strychnine-insensitive (N-methyl-D-aspartate receptor) glycine binding sites. Neurosci Lett 1992;148(1–2):199–201. https://doi.org/10.1016/0304-3940(92)90838-x.

[116] Pfeiffer M, Draguhn A, Meierkord H, et al. Effects of gamma-aminobutyric acid (GABA) agonists and GABA uptake inhibitors on pharmacosensitive and pharmacoresistant epileptiform activity in vitro. Br J Pharmacol 1996;119(3):569–77. https://doi.org/10.1111/j.1476-5381.1996.tb15710.x.

[117] Ericson M, Clarke RB, Chau P, et al. beta-Alanine elevates dopamine levels in the rat nucleus accumbens: antagonism by strychnine. Amino Acids 2010;38(4): 1051–5. https://doi.org/10.1007/s00726-009-0313-0.

[118] Kalyankar GD, Meister A. Enzymatic synthesis of carnosine and related beta-alanyl and gamma-aminobutyryl peptides. J Biol Chem 1959;234:3210–8.

[119] Bauer K, Hallermayer K, Salnikow J, et al. Biosynthesis of carnosine and related peptides by glial cells in primary culture. J Biol Chem 1982;257(7):3593–7.

[120] Jin CL, Yang LX, Wu XH, et al. Effects of carnosine on amygdaloid-kindled seizures in Sprague-Dawley rats. Neuroscience 2005;135(3):939–47. https://doi.org/10.1016/j.neuroscience.2005.06.066.

[121] Berezhnoy DS, Stvolinsky SL, Lopachev AV, et al. Carnosine as an effective neuroprotector in brain pathology and potential neuromodulator in normal conditions. Amino Acids 2019;51(1):139–50. https://doi.org/10.1007/s00726-018-2667-7.

[122] Biffo S, Grillo M, Margolis FL. Cellular localization of carnosine-like and anserine-like immunoreactivities in rodent and avian central nervous system. Neuroscience 1990;35(3):637–51. https://doi.org/10.1016/0306-4522(90)90335-2.

[123] DeMarchis S, Melcangi RC, Modena C, et al. Identification of the glial cell types containing carnosine-related peptides

in the rat brain. Neurosci Lett 1997;237(1):37–40. https://doi.org/10.1016/S0304-3940(97)00800-8.

[124] De Marchis S, Modena C, Peretto P, et al. Carnosine-related dipeptides in neurons and glia. Biochemistry (Mosc) 2000;65(7):824–33.

[125] Hoffmann AM, Bakardjiev A, Bauer K. Carnosine-synthesis in cultures of rat glial cells is restricted to oligodendrocytes and carnosine uptake to astrocytes. Neurosci Lett 1996;215(1):29–32. https://doi.org/10.1016/s0304-3940(96)12937-2.

[126] Bae ON, Majid A. Role of histidine/histamine in carnosine-induced neuroprotection during ischemic brain damage. Brain Res 2013;1527:246–54. https://doi.org/10.1016/j.brainres.2013.07.004.

[127] Boldyrev AA, Johnson P, Wei Y, et al. Carnosine and taurine protect rat cerebellar granular cells from free radical damage. Neurosci Lett 1999;263(2–3):169–72. https://doi.org/10.1016/s0304-3940(99)00150-0.

[128] Lopachev AV, Lopacheva OM, Abaimov DA, et al. Neuroprotective Effect of Carnosine on Primary Culture of Rat Cerebellar Cells under Oxidative Stress. Biochemistry (Mosc) 2016;81(5):511–20. https://doi.org/10.1134/S0006297916050084.

[129] Ouyang L, Tian Y, Bao Y, et al. Carnosine decreased neuronal cell death through targeting glutamate system and astrocyte mitochondrial bioenergetics in cultured neuron/astrocyte exposed to OGD/recovery. Brain Res Bull 2016;124:76–84. https://doi.org/10.1016/j.brainresbull.2016.03.019.

[130] Tan KM, Candlish JK. Carnosine and anserine as modulators of neutrophil function. Clin Lab Haematol 1998;20(4):239–44. https://doi.org/10.1046/j.1365-2257.1998.00123.x.

[131] Horning MS, Blakemore LJ, Trombley PQ. Endogenous mechanisms of neuroprotection: role of zinc, copper, and carnosine. Brain Res 2000;852(1):56–61. https://doi.org/10.1016/s0006-8993(99)02215-5.

[132] Trombley PQ, Horning MS, Blakemore LJ. Carnosine modulates zinc and copper effects on amino acid receptors and synaptic transmission. Neuroreport 1998;9(15):3503–7. https://doi.org/10.1097/00001756-199810260-00031.

[133] Kozan R, Sefil F, Bagirici F. Anticonvulsant effect of carnosine on penicillin-induced epileptiform activity in rats. Brain Res 2008;1239:249–55. https://doi.org/10.1016/j.brainres.2008.08.019.

[134] Ming X, Stein TP, Barnes V, et al. Metabolic perturbance in autism spectrum disorders: a metabolomics study. J Proteome Res 2012;11(12):5856–62. https://doi.org/10.1021/pr300910n.

[135] van Gennip AH, Kamerling JP, de Bree PK, et al. Linear relationship between the R- and S-enantiomers of a beta-aminoisobutyric acid in human urine. Clin Chim Acta 1981;116(3):261–7. https://doi.org/10.1016/0009-8981(81)90045-0.

[136] Begriche K, Massart J, Abbey-Toby A, et al. Beta-aminoisobutyric acid prevents diet-induced obesity in mice with partial leptin deficiency. Obesity (Silver Spring) 2008;16(9):2053–67. https://doi.org/10.1038/oby.2008.337.

[137] Park BS, Tu TH, Lee H, et al. Beta-Aminoisobutyric Acid Inhibits Hypothalamic Inflammation by Reversing Microglia Activation. Cells 2019;8(12). https://doi.org/10.3390/cells8121609.

[138] Minato T, Nakamura N, Saiki T, et al. beta-Aminoisobutyric acid, L-BAIBA, protects PC12 cells from hydrogen peroxide-induced oxidative stress and apoptosis via activation of the AMPK and PI3K/Akt pathway. IBRO Neurosci Rep 2022;12:65–72. https://doi.org/10.1016/j.ibneur.2021.12.001.

[139] van Kuilenburg AB, Stroomer AE, Abeling NG, et al. A pivotal role for beta-aminoisobutyric acid and oxidative stress in dihydropyrimidine dehydrogenase deficiency? Nucleos Nucleot Nucleic Acids 2006;25(9–11):1103–6. https://doi.org/10.1080/15257770600894097.

[140] Schweitzer-Krantz S, Van Kuilenburg AB, van Gennip AH, et al. Dihydropyrimidine dehydrogenase deficiency and arthrogryposis multiplex congenita: clinical improvement under substitution of beta-alanine and beta-aminoisobutyric acid. J Inhert Metab Dis 2002;25(Suppl 1):155.

[141] Dobritzsch D, Ricagno S, Schneider G, et al. Crystal structure of the productive ternary complex of dihydropyrimidine dehydrogenase with NADPH and 5-iodouracil. Implications for mechanism of inhibition and electron transfer. J Biol Chem 2002;277(15):13155–66. https://doi.org/10.1074/jbc.M111877200.

[142] M. Wellin, T. Karlberg, J. Andersson, et al., Human dihydropyrimidinase structure summary. In: research collaboratory for structural bioinformatics (RCSB) protein data bank. 2008. Available at: https://www.rcsb.org/structure/2VR2. Accessed March 3, 2024.

[143] Maurer D, Lohkamp B, Krumpel M, et al. Crystal structure and pH-dependent allosteric regulation of human beta-ureidopropionase, an enzyme involved in anticancer drug metabolism. Biochem J 2018;475(14):2395–416. https://doi.org/10.1042/BCJ20180222.

[144] Kumar A, Basak S, Rao S, et al. Mechanisms of activation and desensitization of full-length glycine receptor in lipid nanodiscs. Nat Commun 2020;11(1):3752. https://doi.org/10.1038/s41467-020-17364-5.

[145] Phulera S, Zhu H, Yu J, et al. Cryo-EM structure of the benzodiazepine-sensitive alpha1beta1gamma2S tri-heteromeric GABA(A) receptor in complex with GABA. Elife 2018;7. https://doi.org/10.7554/eLife.39383.

[146] Chou TH, Tajima N, Romero-Hernandez A, et al. Structural Basis of Functional Transitions in Mammalian NMDA Receptors. Cell 2020;182(2):357–371 e13. https://doi.org/10.1016/j.cell.2020.05.052.

[147] Motiwala Z, Aduri NG, Shaye H, et al. Structural basis of GABA reuptake inhibition. Nature 2022;606(7915):820–6. https://doi.org/10.1038/s41586-022-04814-x.

[148] Zhang F, Basinski MB, Beals JM, et al. Crystal structure of the obese protein leptin-E100. Nature 1997;387(6629):206–9. https://doi.org/10.1038/387206a0.

[149] Tao X, Zhao C, MacKinnon R. Membrane protein isolation and structure determination in cell-derived membrane vesicles. Proc Natl Acad Sci U S A 2023;120(18). https://doi.org/10.1073/pnas.2302325120:e2302325120.

[150] Herguedas B, Garcia-Nafria J, Cais O, et al. Structure and organization of heteromeric AMPA-type glutamate receptors. Science 2016;352(6285):aad3873. https://doi.org/10.1126/science.aad3873.

[151] Holopainen I, Pulkki K, Heinonen OJ, et al. Partial epilepsy in a girl with a symptom-free sister: first two Finnish patients with dihydropyrimidine dehydrogenase deficiency. J Inherit Metab Dis 1997;20(5):719–20. https://doi.org/10.1023/a:1005399131620.

[152] Christensen E, Cezanne I, Kjaergaard S, et al. Clinical variability in three Danish patients with dihydropyrimidine dehydrogenase deficiency all homozygous for the same mutation. J Inherit Metab Dis 1998;21(3):272–5. https://doi.org/10.1023/a:1005328424310.

[153] Dockery H, Van der Westhuzyen J. Monosomy of 1p13.3-22.3 in twins. Clin Genet 1991;39(3):223–7. https://doi.org/10.1111/j.1399-0004.1991.tb03016.x.

[154] Tabata H, Sone K, Kobayashi T, et al. Short arm deletion of chromosome 1: del(1)(p13.3p22.3) in a female infant with an extreme tetralogy of Fallot. Clin Genet 1991;39(2):132–5. https://doi.org/10.1111/j.1399-0004.1991.tb02999.x.

[155] Bakkeren JA, De Abreu RA, Sengers RC, et al. Elevated urine, blood and cerebrospinal fluid levels of uracil and thymine in a child with dihydrothymine dehydrogenase deficiency. Clin Chim Acta 1984;140(3):247–56. https://doi.org/10.1016/0009-8981(84)90206-7.

[156] Bakker HD, Rubio Gozalbo ME, van Gennip AH. Dihydropyrimidine dehydrogenase deficiency presenting with psychomotor retardation and ocular abnormalities. J Inherit Metab Dis 1994;17(5):640–1. https://doi.org/10.1007/BF00711611.

[157] Schmidt C, Hofmann U, Kohlmuller D, et al. Comprehensive analysis of pyrimidine metabolism in 450 children with unspecific neurological symptoms using high-pressure liquid chromatography-electrospray ionization tandem mass spectometry. J Inherit Metab Dis 2005;28:1109–22. https://doi.org/10.1007/s10545-005-0133-7.

Advances in Molecular Pathology 7 (2024) 33–41
ADVANCES IN MOLECULAR PATHOLOGY

Education of Future Pharmacogenomics Laboratory Directors

Reynold C. Ly, PhD[a,*], Marwan K. Tayeh, PhD[b], Yuan Ji, PhD[c]
[a]Department of Research, Institute for Genomic Medicine, Nationwide Children's Hospital, 575 Children's Crossroad, Columbus, OH 43215, USA; [b]Indiana University Genetic Testing Laboratories, Division of Diagnostic Genetics and Genomics, Department of Medical and Molecular Genetics, Indiana University School of Medicine, 975 West Walnut Street, IB350, Indianapolis, IN 46202, USA; [c]ARUP Laboratories, Department of Pathology, University of Utah School of Medicine, Mail Code 115, 500 Chipeta Way, Salt Lake City, UT 84108, USA

KEYWORDS

- Pharmacogenomics • Pharmacogenomics education • Germline pharmacogenomic testing
- Targeted genotyping • Next-generation sequencing • Star-allele nomenclature • Single nucleotide polymorphism
- Copy number variation

KEY POINTS

- Currently, there are limited exposure and training in pharmacogenomics among fellowship training programs that vary depending on the expertise of training faculty and program directors.
- Pharmacogenomic testing is increasingly offered by genetic testing or pathology laboratories, which necessitates the need for laboratory directors who are educated and proficient in pharmacogenomics.
- Given the variability in exposure to pharmacogenomics during fellowship training, the authors propose key skills, education, and important pharmacogenomic resources that should be incorporated into education of trainees and others learning clinical pharmacogenomic laboratory testing.

INTRODUCTION

Pharmacogenomics (PGx) is the study of inherited or acquired genetic differences in drug response phenotypes including drug efficacy and adverse drug reactions [1]. The goal of clinical PGx is to find the right drug at the right dose at the right time for the right patient. Over the last decade, germline testing for PGx indications has been increasingly used for patient care in various hospital disciplines. As clinical PGx testing continues to be adopted and utilized, there will be an increased need for clinical laboratory directors to be trained and familiar with clinical PGx testing. Currently, there are few training programs that offer exposure to this testing. This article highlights key points that should be considered for trainees or laboratory directors who are not familiar with clinical PGx, including differences between PGx and hereditary genetics, current training options, educational materials, and other related resources, and points to consider for training future PGx laboratory directors.

DIFFERENCES BETWEEN PHARMACOGENOMICS AND HEREDITARY GENETICS

Hereditary genetics focuses on identifying rare genetic variants in disease-causing genes with following different modes of inheritance such as autosomal dominant and/or recessive inheritance. PGx has several key differences. The following section will review these

*Corresponding author, *E-mail address:* reynold.ly@nationwidechildrens.org

https://doi.org/10.1016/j.yamp.2024.06.003
www.advancesinmolecularpathology.com
2589-4080/24/

differences including the focus of PGx on pharmacokinetic (PK) and pharmacodynamic (PD) genes, phenotype, inheritance, and allele frequency as well as star (*) allele nomenclature, haplotype calling, diplotype assignment, and copy number variation.

Focus on Pharmacokinetic and Pharmacodynamic Genes

Current clinical PGx testing mostly focuses on genetic variants in genes encoding components of PK pathways, such as drug-metabolizing enzymes and transporters, and PD pathways including proteins involved in the drug's mechanism of action, such as drug receptors. Most tested PGx genes include those encoding the cytochrome p450 enzymes that are primarily responsible for the metabolism of many drugs, such as clopidogrel, simvastatin, warfarin, sertraline, and tacrolimus. The cytochrome P450 enzymes are primarily expressed in the liver and 75% to 80% of commonly used drugs are metabolized by enzymes encoded by *CYP2C9*, *CYP2C19*, *CYP2D6*, and *CYP3A4/5* [2]. PGx is unique where the impact of a genetic variant can be different from drug to drug, depending on whether the drug is an active drug or a prodrug that requires metabolism for its downstream effect. In addition, transporters interact with drugs to move them across epithelial membranes or tissues, such as the clinically relevant OAT1B1 protein, encoded by *SLCO1B1*, that is responsible for hepatic uptake of simvastatin into hepatocytes. Loss-of-function variants in *SLCO1B1* result in decreased hepatic uptake of simvastatin and are associated with an increased risk for drug-induced myopathy [3,4].

Furthermore, PGx also includes PD pharmacogenes such as the *HLA* genes. For instance, patients with human immunodeficiency virus and the *HLA-B*57:01* allele are at a significantly increased risk for hypersensitivity reactions including severe, life-threatening Steven-Johnson syndrome or toxic epidermal necrolysis when treated with abacavir [5]. Additionally, individuals with deleterious variants in *RYR1* or *CACN1AS* are at increased risk for malignant hyperthermia from halogenated volatile anesthetic agents or depolarizing muscle relaxants [6].

Phenotype, Inheritance, and Pharmacogenomics Allele Frequency

Clinical PGx uses genotype-guided prediction of a patient's phenotype using metabolizer status, especially for tests performed on genes encoding drug-metabolizing enzymes. There are 5 Clinical Pharmacogenomics Implementation Consortium (CPIC)-approved metabolizer status terms used in clinical PGx test reports including poor, intermediate, normal, rapid, and ultrarapid metabolizers [7]. Metabolizer status is determined based on functional status assigned to both alleles in an individual such as no function or decreased function [8]. Some genes like *CYP2D6* and *DPYD* use an activity score system as part of the genotype-to-phenotype translation to determine metabolizer phenotype. Briefly, each allele is assigned an activity value, and the sum of both alleles is used to determine the metabolizer phenotype [7,9,10]. Because both alleles can influence metabolizer status, the mode of inheritance for PGx alleles in genes encoding drug-metabolizing enzymes and transporters is generally considered autosomal codominant.

With hereditary genetics, most disease-causing variants are rare, while clinically relevant PGx variants in CYP genes such as *CYP2D6* are common and can vary among populations. For instance, the *CYP2D6*4* allele has been observed in the European population at a 19% allele frequency, while only at a frequency of 3% to 5% among those of African ancestry. In contrast, *CYP2D6*29* is commonly observed in populations of African ancestry (9%–12%), but at a frequency of less than 0.5% in Europeans. The Pharmacogenomics Knowledge Base (PharmGKB) has standardized and defined biogeographical ancestry groups with allele frequency data available [11]. It is critical to consider the frequency of PGx alleles by ancestry to ensure appropriate alleles are included for testing of the target patient population(s) to avoid exclusion of a key allele that could lead to "inaccurate" genotyping and impact phenotype assignment and ultimately affect patients' drug treatment and care [12,13]. In addition to common PGx alleles, rare variants in PGx genes can also influence drug response in CYP450 enzymes and other drug-metabolizing enzymes [14–16]. As PGx testing transitions from targeted testing of common variants to sequencing-based platforms, these rare variants will also need to be considered along with common PGx alleles although they might not be assigned a star allele. This will be further discussed in the upcoming section "Understanding the Strengths and Limitations of Targeted Testing and Sequencing Approaches."

Star Allele Nomenclature

Clinical PGx star (*) allele nomenclature usually focuses on defining haplotypes for certain pharmacogenes that are composed of one or more, often multiple, single nucleotide variants (SNVs) or small insertions/deletions that are typically less than 50 nucleotides. The legacy PGx nomenclature system designates combinations of sequence variants (ie, haplotype) by star (*) alleles, where **1* is assigned when none of the targeted variants tested for are detected (an exception is *NAT2* for which the default no variant assignment is **4* allele) [7]. A new numerical star allele number is assigned for novel haplotypes as they are chronologically discovered. Although the star (*) allele nomenclature system is widely used among early adopters of clinical PGx tests, it is important to recognize both the legacy nomenclature and the standard genomic nomenclature, such as the Human Genome Variation Society system, which is especially important when PGx is performed on a sequencing-based platform. When clinical laboratories assign star (*) alleles and diplotypes based on the observed genotypes, they should follow the standard star allele definitions as cataloged by the Pharmacogene Variation Consortium (PharmVar; www.pharmvar.org). Laboratories may use external resources provided by PGx reporting software vendors to help with haplotype calling, diplotype assignment, and result interpretation/reporting but should ensure standard nomenclature and translations are included in the reports.

Haplotype Calling, Diplotype Assignment, and Copy Number Variation

Although numerous variants may be present on a given star (*) allele, those that are known to impact function are designated by PharmVar as "core" variants. The core variants are typically the functionally causal variants or variant(s) in tight linkage disequilibrium with functional variants and usually are selected as analytical targets for clinical PGx testing [7,17]. For example, *CYP2D6*4* is defined by the c.506-1G>A splice site variant (rs3892097, NM_000106.6) as the core allele. There are currently more than 30 defined *CYP2D6*4* suballeles listed by PharmVar (https://www.pharmvar.org/gene/CYP2D6, last accessed on April 13, 2024). All suballeles listed under a star (*) number are assumed to be functionally equivalent.

Unlike hereditary genetics, pharmacogenomic analysis requires the identification of haplotypes followed by diplotype assignment to determine metabolizer phenotype. Haplotypes are first identified by testing for "core variants" associated with their given star (*) allele. For certain PGx genes such as *CYP2D6*, haplotype calling can be challenging as there are over 150 known haplotypes or star alleles. In this case, there are multiple "core" variants or star alleles that are examined before determining the diplotype. Briefly, diplotype refers to the pair of haplotypes, where one haplotype is maternally inherited and the other is paternally inherited. An individual typically has 2 haplotypes unless there is a gene deletion or duplication. The diplotype is typically reported on the clinical PGx test report along with metabolizer phenotype.

Additionally, some pharmacogenes are affected by structural variants or copy number variants (CNVs), including gene deletions, duplications, multiplications, and gene rearrangements. For *CYP2D6*, a comprehensive summary of these CNVs is provided by the structural variation document on the PharmVar *CYP2D6* gene page (https://www.pharmvar.org/gene/CYP2D6). PharmVar provides nomenclature for the highly polymorphic human *CYP2D6* gene locus, where CNVs are described by adding a multiplication sign (x) and the number of gene copies after the affected allele. If the copy number is known, duplications/multiplications are recommended to be reported as x2, x3, and so forth [18,19].

It is important to note that for PGx testing, there is a residual risk that the individual has a rare genotype, depending on how comprehensive a test is. In a genotyping assay, if none of the tested variants were detected, a default **1* is assigned, despite that there is a residual risk that the individual has a rare non-**1* genotype. Such residual risk is dependent on the number of alleles tested and allele frequencies. For example, the defining variants for the normal function *CYP2D6*2* allele are c.886C>T (p.Arg296Cys, rs16947, NM_000106.6) and c.1457G>C (p.Ser486Thr, rs1135840, NM_000106.6) [18]. However, these 2 variants also occur on other alleles such as *CYP2D6*8*, **11*, **12*, **17*, **29*, and many others, in addition to the unique core SNVs on each allele. If a given test fails to capture these additional core SNVs, it will result in a *CYP2D6*2* default assignment and misclassification of a nonfunctional allele as a normal function allele, leading to an inaccurate phenotype prediction [7]. Hence, it is important to consider such issues when developing a PGx test.

CURRENT TRAINING OPTIONS FOR CLINICAL LABORATORY DIRECTORS

The Milestones defined by Accreditation Council for Graduate Medical Education (ACGME) is a framework to assess a trainee or fellow's development in key knowledge areas or skills for competency required for a specialty or subspecialty. The same framework is shared by ACGME programs for different specialty training and arranged into levels from novice to expert in each of the 6 defined ACGME Competencies (Patient Care, Medical Knowledge, Professionalism, Interpersonal and Communication Skills, Practice-based Learning and Improvement, and Systems-based Practice).

Laboratory Genetics and Genomics (LGG) Fellowship Programs are one of the major sources of training laboratory directors for clinical laboratories that offer genetic testing utilizing molecular genetics, cytogenetics, and next-generation sequencing. At present, there are 38 ACGME-accredited LGG Programs (https://apps.acgme.org/ads/Public/Programs/Search, last accessed on April 13, 2024). Although the ACGME-accredited training length for the LGG Fellowship Program is 2 years, the LGG training length can vary between programs and is usually 2 to 3 years. All ACGME-accredited LGG programs are required to use the default ACGME Milestones framework to evaluate fellows on a semiannual basis, and it is at the Program Director's discretion on how the training activities are set up using program-defined training blocks. The training block defines the areas covered and timeline (rotation schedule), which are subjected to review and approval at the initial ACGME-accreditation process and subsequent annual review for any update or alteration.

There is variation in LGG training from program to program, due at least in part to the laboratory setting (full-menu reference laboratory, academic medical center-affiliated laboratory, or specialty laboratory focusing on a certain area of genetic testing) and expertise areas of the training faculty and laboratories. Clinical PGx is a rapidly growing field in the clinical testing arena, and currently there are no PGx-specific competencies listed in the ACGME LGG Milestones or the LGG Supplemental Guide. It is at the Program Director's discretion to decide the depth of training related to clinical PGx, if any. For example, in Medical Knowledge 1 (Foundations of Medical Genetics and Genomics) and 2 (Testing), the fellows are usually assessed on general aspects of both germline and somatic diseases, but there is no mention of any specific disease or testing areas. However, in the LGG Supplemental Guide, which provides additional guidance and examples for the LGG Milestones, it has "pharmacogenetics" mentioned once as an example for Interpersonal and Communication Skills 3 (Communication within Health Care Systems), Level 4 competence, that is, "organizes a discussion about the inappropriate release of pharmacogenetics testing results in the electronic health record." Finally, a few laboratory directors or training faculty members at different LGG Programs may have had prior training related to pharmacology or PGx. This limits trainees' exposure to clinical PGx testing.

Molecular Genetic Pathology (MGP) Fellowship Programs are also another major training program, typically for pathologists after completion of a residency program in Anatomic and/or Clinical Pathology. There are 42 programs to date (https://apps.acgme.org/ads/Public/Programs/Search, last accessed on April 13, 2024) with an ACGME-required training length of 1 year, although it can be extended to 2 years. All ACGME-accredited MGP programs use the ACGME Milestones framework designed for the MGP fellowship programs to evaluate and document the fellow's training progress like the ACGME-accredited LGG programs.

There is also variation in MGP training in PGx between programs, partially due to laboratory setting and variation in the expertise of training faculty. There is no PGx-specific competency listed in the ACGME-specific MGP Milestones or the Supplemental Guide. Although it is mentioned in the Milestones and the Supplemental Guide under Medical Knowledge 1: Molecular Testing with Various Platforms (Diagnosis, Management, Prognostication) to discuss basic principles and applications of various methodologies and testing platforms in areas including PGx.

Given the wide range of variation in trainee exposure to clinical PGx testing in both types of training programs, this article was written to address these gaps and aid program directors and training faculty with key considerations for clinical PGx testing and useful educational resources.

POINTS TO CONSIDER FOR TRAINING FUTURE PHARMACOGENOMICS LABORATORY DIRECTORS

As clinical PGx testing becomes more widespread, there is an increased need for professionally trained laboratory directors in PGx testing. We propose that training programs design modules or training blocks including didactics on drug metabolism and basic pharmacology of commonly ordered gene–drug pairs (ie, clopidogrel/*CYP2C19*), training in PGx test design, and hands-on experience in interpretation with star (*) allele nomenclature and *CYP2D6* copy number testing, as well as translation from genotype to metabolizer phenotype. As clinical PGx testing is considered a "subspeciality" in molecular genetic laboratories and not all molecular genetic laboratories offer clinical PGx testing, it might be helpful to offer this additional PGx-related training as electives considering the tight training timeline for these fellowship programs. Briefly, we propose the following key skills for PGx including pharmacogenomic interpretation/reporting and basic understanding of the pharmacology of commonly ordered drug–gene PGx tests, as well as understanding of strengths and limitations of targeted and sequencing PGx testing, and awareness of key pharmacogenomic resources. Below, we describe some key strengths and limitations common in PGx testing and available resources.

Understanding the Foundation of Clinical Pharmacology

Clinical Pharmacology is traditionally covered as part of the medical school curriculum for MGP fellows. Although it is not practical to have LGG trainees go through an entire didactic course in Clinical Pharmacology, it is important to understand the following key concepts.

1. PK and PD pathways of drug action
2. Two phases of drug metabolism: Phase I and Phase II, and their contributions to drug efficacy and toxicity
3. Therapeutic index for a drug
4. Drug–drug interactions and the impact on the patient's drug response phenotype
5. Key clinical PGx genes and drug (or drug class) associations, especially those with professional clinical guidelines such as the CPIC
6. General understanding of drug toxicity

Understanding the Strengths and Limitations of Targeted Testing Versus Sequencing Approaches

Clinical PGx testing can either use a targeted or sequencing-based approach. Both approaches of testing have strengths and limitations. Most clinical laboratories currently use a targeted-based approach for PGx testing; however, there is a growing interest in PGx genotyping using sequencing-based platforms as they become more widely used in both constitutional and oncology testing. For laboratory directors, it is important to understand both types of testing as the director may oversee a laboratory currently using targeted testing but the laboratory may later switch to sequencing-based PGx testing or need to interpret reports from other laboratories that may use targeted or sequencing-based PGx testing.

Targeted PGx testing is commonly used by most clinical diagnostic laboratories to test for common clinically relevant variants in pharmacogenes supported by strong clinical evidence with or without clinical guidelines. This approach is technically feasible and more cost-effective compared to sequencing. However, targeted testing has several limitations including the following.

1. Functional rare variants may not be detected with targeted testing since typically only more common, well-characterized variants are interrogated.
2. Some laboratories may not include common variants in underrepresented populations. This can lead to a clinically inaccurate result impacting the genotype and predicted phenotype, ultimately affecting therapeutic management and patient care.
3. Inability to fully characterize complex *CYP2D6* CNVs with quantitative testing. Quantitative testing is used to determine how many copies are present in an interrogated gene region. Common methods include quantitative or digital polymerase chain reaction (PCR). Copy number testing in *CYP2D6* can detect deletions or duplications. However, it may not be sufficient to determine which allele is duplicated, or to detect more complex hybrid alleles depending on how many and which locations are interrogated in the gene [19,20].
4. Inability to phase with targeted testing, such as the *TPMT *1/*3A* diplotype versus *TPMT*3B/*3C* diplotype. There are 3 common haplotypes including *TPMT*3B* (NM_000367.5:c.460G>A, p.Ala154Thr, rs1800460), **3C* (NM_000367.5:c.719A>G, p.Tyr240Cys, rs1142345), and **3A* that includes both variants in cis. If both variants defining the **3B* and **3C* alleles are present, then based on allele frequency data the final diplotype of *TPMT *1/*3A* is assigned, corresponding with an intermediate metabolizer phenotype. The **3B* allele is rare; thus, presence of **3B* and **3C* in trans with a final diplotype of *TPMT*3B/*3C* corresponding to a poor metabolizer phenotype is also rare. Currently, targeted testing cannot phase alleles without subsequent trio or phasing studies [21]. This limitation is common to most other molecular genetic testing for recessive disorders using common molecular techniques.
5. Variability in the PGx alleles incorporated in targeted tests across laboratories. To address this issue, the Association of Molecular Pathology (AMP) PGx Working Group, in collaboration with several other professional societies, has published several recommendations for a minimum set of variants to include for testing in *CYP2C9*, *CYP2C19*, warfarin-response genes, *CYP2D6*, *TPMT*, *NUDT15*, *CYP3A4*, and *CYP3A5* genes [20–25].

Some of the limitations of targeted testing can be addressed with sequencing-based approaches. The main strength of a sequencing-based approach is all variants including common and rare clinically relevant

PGx variants can be detected if there is adequate coverage. Furthermore, sequencing data can be reanalyzed in the future if there is a suspected novel variant in a PGx gene associated with an adverse drug reaction. However, there are several limitations with sequencing-based approaches for clinical PGx laboratory-developed tests.

1. The detection of rare, unclassified variants in PGx genes. Currently, there is no guidance on how to classify or interpret these variants in the setting of clinical PGx testing. The 2015 American College of Medical Genetics and Genomics (ACMG)/AMP guidelines for interpretation of germline variants were not designed for PGx variant classification [26].
2. Reconciling reporting of rare variants with the current star (*) allele nomenclature. Novel haplotypes and those consisting of a collection of variants described by an existing haplotype plus a rare variant (eg, *CYP3A4*37* containing the variants comprising the *CYP3A4*22* and *CYP3A4*3* alleles) can be submitted to PharmVar for consideration of a new star allele [27]. However, there is no process for clinical laboratories to report or interpret rare star alleles beyond what has been annotated by PharmVar experts. There is a need for guidance on how to report these rare variants with existing star allele nomenclature with one system being proposed in one study [15].
3. Short-read sequencing also has a phasing limitation like targeted testing unless the reads contain the variants within the read length. Long-read sequencing has been identified to address this limitation and can be useful for challenging PGx genes such as *CYP2D6* due to the highly homologous neighboring *CYP2D7* and *CYP2D8* pseudogenes that can form complex structural variants with *CYP2D6* [28].
4. CNV testing remains challenging, for *CYP2D6* due to the nearby highly homologous *CYP2D7* and *CYP2D8* pseudogenes. There are bioinformatic star-allele callers available to identify *CYP2D6* copy number from genome sequencing such as Cyrius [29], Stargazer [30], StellarPGx [31], Aldy [32], and PyPGx [33] with good performance in calling deletions, but variability in the performance to accurately call duplications and hybrid alleles from genome sequencing makes them unreliable [19]. Assessment with these star allele callers' ability to assess copy number from exome sequencing is inconsistent which makes copy number analysis not viable at this time [19]. Performance of these star allele callers such as Stargazer, StellarPGx, Aldy, and PyPGx with other PGx genes was found to be highly concordant with consensus calls from well-characterized reference materials [31–34]. With further evaluation, these star allele callers could be validated for PGx genotyping from exome or genome sequencing if there is appropriate read depth and coverage.

Awareness of Key Pharmacogenomic Resources

There are several key publicly available resources important for PGx clinical laboratory directors as mentioned in the following section.

The PharmGKB is an international resource for PGx information that collects, curates, and annotates PGx information including drugs, drug pathways, genes, alleles, gene–drug associations, and genotype–phenotype relationships as well as annotates guidelines by the CPIC, the Canadian Pharmacogenomics Network for Drug Safety, the Dutch Pharmacogenetics Working Group (DPWG), and other professional groups (https://www.pharmgkb.org/) [35]. One of its useful features is its Genotype Selection Interface that allows the user to compare PGx guideline recommendations among CPIC, DPWG, and the US Food and Drug Administration (FDA) label and Table of Pharmacogenetic Associations based on genotypes. In addition, it has PGx gene-specific information tables that provide allele-level information for PGx genes including allele functionality and frequency as well as diplotype–phenotype information.

The PharmVar Consortium catalogs PGx alleles and provides a standardized PGx star allele nomenclature system for the PGx community (https://www.pharmvar.org/) [17,36,37]. It is useful for understanding haplotypes. In addition, PharmVar has published review articles for several genes and most recently a tutorial on *CYP2D6* structural variation testing and recommendations on reporting [3,18,19,38–42].

CPIC serves to provide evidence-based PGx clinical practice guidelines for implementation into routine clinical care. They do not recommend whether PGx testing should be ordered or which variants should be tested but rather focus on how to use available PGx test results in clinical practice (https://cpicpgx.org/) [43]. As of 2020, they have published 23 guidelines that cover 19 genes and 46 drugs [44]. Pertinent to laboratory directors, the CPIC guidelines provide information on clinically actionable variants and associated diplotypes that may lead to a different prescribing decision (ie, dose adjustment or medication change) from standard treatment. In addition to clinical practice guidelines, CPIC has worked on standardization projects including standardization of *CYP2D6* genotype-to-phenotype translation as well as standardization of terms for clinical PGx test results [8,9].

The AMP Clinical Practice Committee Pharmacogenomics Working Group serves to provide recommendations for variants or alleles to include in PGx tests to facilitate standardization of PGx testing across laboratories and ensure the most clinically relevant alleles or variants are included (https://www.amp.org/clinical-practice/practice-guidelines/). To date, the working group has published recommendations for *CYP2C9*, *CYP2C19*, genes related to warfarin response, *CYP2D6*, *TPMT*, *NUDT15*, *CYP3A4*, and *CYP3A5* genes [20–25]. These documents are useful for PGx content at the allele level for relevant pharmacogenes, especially for targeted genotyping-based testing approaches. In addition, other resources include the AMP Certificate Program: Pharmacogenomics: Genes, Drugs, and Genotyping: AMP Pharmacogenomics Guidelines and the "Molecular in My Pocket" reference card for genotyping recommendations for PGx testing.

The Genetic Testing Registry for Reference Materials (GeT-RM) program serves to provide a resource of reference materials with known genotypes for clinical diagnostic testing [45]. The program collaborates with the AMP PGx working group to characterize publicly available genomic DNA reference materials to support clinical PGx testing. To date, GeT-RM has reported their characterization of reference materials for PGx genes including *CYP2C9*, *CYP2C19*, *CYP2C* cluster, *VKORC1*, *GGCX*, *CYP2D6*, *TPMT*, *NUDT15*, *CYP3A4*, and *CYP3A5* [46–52].

The ACMG recently published a technical standard for clinical PGx testing and reporting [7]. This document serves as a resource for clinical laboratory geneticists on the best practices for PGx nomenclature, testing, result interpretation, and reporting as well as summarizing publicly available resources for clinical PGx testing.

The FDA has also published resources in PGx including the "Table of Pharmacogenetic Associations" and the "Table of Pharmacogenomic Biomarkers in Drug Labeling." The Table of Pharmacogenetic Associations is limited to PGx associations that are related to variants in genes encoding drug-metabolizing enzymes, transporters, and variants in other genes known to be related to a predisposition for drug adverse events (https://www.fda.gov/medical-devices/precision-medicine/table-pharmacogenetic-associations). The Table of Pharmacogenomic Biomarkers in Drug Labeling summarizes the PGx information found in the FDA drug labeling (https://www.fda.gov/drugs/science-and-research-drugs/table-pharmacogenomic-biomarkers-drug-labeling). These FDA resources are useful for content selection and interpretation of PGx test results.

Other useful resources or databases include the Pharmacogenomics Global Research Network, where the latest clinical PGx research discoveries and clinical practice can be found through their regularly educational events including annual scientific meetings and webinars (http://www.pgrn.org). For drug–drug interactions, the Flockhart Table is an important teaching and reference tool on understanding cytochrome P450 enzymes-mediated drug–drug interactions (https://drug-interactions.medicine.iu.edu/Home.aspx). For foundational knowledge of clinical pharmacology, many textbooks are available.

SUMMARY

Clinical PGx testing is a niche area in clinical molecular genetics as it lies at the intersection between genetic testing and clinical pharmacology. It is a critical component of personalized medicine with wide applicability in different hospital disciplines such as oncology, cardiology, and psychiatry to identify patients at risk for adverse drug events or inefficacy. The goal of this article is to highlight key areas and resources for clinical fellowship program directors to consider or clinical laboratory directors who may not be familiar with clinical PGx-specific nuances and desire additional exposure. As more clinical molecular laboratories offer PGx tests, it is critical for clinical laboratory directors to be equipped with a basic understanding and foundational knowledge of both pharmacology and genetics, be familiar with the strengths and limitations of different testing approaches used for clinical PGx testing (ie, targeted vs sequencing), and to take advantage of the rich resources including testing recommendations, clinical guidelines, and other information available for clinical PGx testing as described in this article.

DISCLOSURE

R.C. Ly is a member of the PharmVar *CYP2D6* Gene Expert Panel and a member of the AMP Pharmacogenomics Working Group. M.K. Tayeh serves as the director of the Pharmacogenomics Laboratory, Indiana University Genetic Testing Laboratories, United States, a clinical laboratory that offers clinical pharmacogenomic testing on a fee-for-service basis. Y. Ji is a member of the AMP Pharmacogenomics Working Group.

REFERENCES

[1] Wang L, McLeod HL, Weinshilboum RM. Genomics and drug response. N Engl J Med 2011;364(12):1144–53.

[2] Guengerich FP. Cytochrome P450s and other enzymes in drug metabolism and toxicity. AAPS J 2006;8(1): E101–11.
[3] Ramsey LB, Gong L, Lee SB, et al. PharmVar GeneFocus: SLCO1B1. Clin Pharmacol Ther 2023;113(4):782–93.
[4] Group SC, Link E, Parish S, et al. SLCO1B1 variants and statin-induced myopathy–a genomewide study. N Engl J Med 2008;359(8):789–99.
[5] Dean L. Abacavir Therapy and HLA-B*57:01 Genotype. In: Pratt VM, Scott SA, Pirmohamed M, editors. Medical Genetics Summaries. Bethesda (MD): National Center for Biotechnology Information (US); 2015.
[6] Gonsalves SG, Dirksen RT, Sangkuhl K, et al. Clinical pharmacogenetics implementation consortium (CPIC) guideline for the use of potent volatile anesthetic agents and succinylcholine in the context of RYR1 or CACNA1S genotypes. Clin Pharmacol Ther 2019; 105(6):1338–44.
[7] Tayeh MK, Gaedigk A, Goetz MP, et al. Clinical pharmacogenomic testing and reporting: a technical standard of the American College of Medical Genetics and Genomics (ACMG). Genet Med 2022;24(4):759–68.
[8] Caudle KE, Dunnenberger HM, Freimuth RR, et al. Standardizing terms for clinical pharmacogenetic test results: consensus terms from the Clinical Pharmacogenetics Implementation Consortium (CPIC). Genet Med 2017; 19(2):215–23.
[9] Caudle KE, Sangkuhl K, Whirl-Carrillo M, et al. Standardizing CYP2D6 genotype to phenotype translation: consensus recommendations from the clinical pharmacogenetics implementation consortium and dutch pharmacogenetics working group. Clin Transl Sci 2020; 13(1):116–24.
[10] Amstutz U, Henricks LM, Offer SM, et al. Clinical pharmacogenetics implementation consortium (CPIC) guideline for dihydropyrimidine dehydrogenase genotype and fluoropyrimidine dosing: 2017 update. Clin Pharmacol Ther 2018;103(2):210–6.
[11] Huddart R, Fohner AE, Whirl-Carrillo M, et al. Standardized biogeographic grouping system for annotating populations in pharmacogenetic research. Clin Pharmacol Ther 2019;105(5):1256–62.
[12] Hoshitsuki K, Crews KR, Yang W, et al. Challenges in clinical implementation of CYP2D6 genotyping: choice of variants to test affects phenotype determination. Genet Med 2020;22(1):232–3.
[13] Kennedy A, Ma G, Manshaei R, et al. A call for increased inclusivity and global representation in pharmacogenetic testing. NPJ Genom Med 2024;9(1):13.
[14] Devarajan S, Moon I, Ho MF, et al. Pharmacogenomic next-generation DNA sequencing: lessons from the identification and functional characterization of variants of unknown significance in CYP2C9 and CYP2C19. Drug Metab Dispos 2019;47(4):425–35.
[15] Lopes JL, Harris K, Karow MB, et al. Targeted genotyping in clinical pharmacogenomics: what is missing? J Mol Diagn 2022;24(3):253–61.
[16] Luo S, Jiang R, Grzymski JJ, et al. Comprehensive allele genotyping in critical pharmacogenes reduces residual clinical risk in diverse populations. Clin Pharmacol Ther 2021;110(3):759–67.
[17] Gaedigk A, Sangkuhl K, Whirl-Carrillo M, et al. The evolution of PharmVar. Clin Pharmacol Ther 2019;105(1): 29–32.
[18] Nofziger C, Turner AJ, Sangkuhl K, et al. PharmVar GeneFocus: CYP2D6. Clin Pharmacol Ther 2020;107(1): 154–70.
[19] Turner AJ, Nofziger C, Ramey BE, et al. PharmVar tutorial on CYP2D6 structural variation testing and recommendations on reporting. Clin Pharmacol Ther 2023; 114(6):1220–37.
[20] Pratt VM, Cavallari LH, Del Tredici AL, et al. Recommendations for clinical CYP2D6 genotyping allele selection: a joint consensus recommendation of the association for molecular pathology, college of american pathologists, dutch pharmacogenetics working group of the royal dutch pharmacists association, and the european society for pharmacogenomics and personalized therapy. J Mol Diagn 2021;23(9):1047–64.
[21] Pratt VM, Cavallari LH, Fulmer ML, et al. TPMT and NUDT15 genotyping recommendations: a joint consensus recommendation of the association for molecular pathology, clinical pharmacogenetics implementation consortium, college of american pathologists, dutch pharmacogenetics working group of the royal dutch pharmacists association, european society for pharmacogenomics and personalized therapy, and pharmacogenomics knowledgebase. J Mol Diagn 2022; 24(10):1051–63.
[22] Pratt VM, Cavallari LH, Del Tredici AL, et al. Recommendations for Clinical CYP2C9 genotyping allele selection: a joint recommendation of the association for molecular pathology and college of american pathologists. J Mol Diagn 2019;21(5):746–55.
[23] Pratt VM, Del Tredici AL, Hachad H, et al. Recommendations for clinical CYP2C19 genotyping allele selection: a report of the association for molecular pathology. J Mol Diagn 2018;20(3):269–76.
[24] Pratt VM, Cavallari LH, Del Tredici AL, et al. Recommendations for clinical warfarin genotyping allele selection: a report of the association for molecular pathology and the college of american pathologists. J Mol Diagn 2020; 22(7):847–59.
[25] Pratt VM, Cavallari LH, Fulmer ML, et al. CYP3A4 and CYP3A5 genotyping recommendations: a joint consensus recommendation of the association for molecular pathology, clinical pharmacogenetics implementation consortium, college of american pathologists, dutch pharmacogenetics working group of the royal dutch pharmacists association, european society for pharmacogenomics and personalized therapy, and pharmacogenomics knowledgebase. J Mol Diagn 2023;25(9):619–29.
[26] Richards S, Aziz N, Bale S, et al. Standards and guidelines for the interpretation of sequence variants: a joint

consensus recommendation of the american college of medical genetics and genomics and the association for molecular pathology. Genet Med 2015;17(5):405–24.
[27] Powell NR, Shugg T, Ly RC, et al. Life-threatening docetaxel toxicity in a patient with reduced-function CYP3A variants: a case report. Front Oncol 2021;11:809527.
[28] Neu M, Yang Y, Scott SA. Long-read sequencing for germline pharmacogenomic testing. Advances in Molecular Pathology 2023;6(1):99–109.
[29] Chen X, Shen F, Gonzaludo N, et al. Cyrius: accurate CYP2D6 genotyping using whole-genome sequencing data. Pharmacogenomics J 2021;21(2):251–61.
[30] Lee SB, Wheeler MM, Patterson K, et al. Stargazer: a software tool for calling star alleles from next-generation sequencing data using CYP2D6 as a model. Genet Med 2019;21(2):361–72.
[31] Twesigomwe D, Drögemöller BI, Wright GEB, et al. StellarPGx: a nextflow pipeline for calling star alleles in cytochrome P450 Genes. Clin Pharmacol Ther 2021;110(3):741–9.
[32] Hari A, Zhou Q, Gonzaludo N, et al. An efficient genotyper and star-allele caller for pharmacogenomics. Genome Res 2023;33(1):61–70.
[33] Lee SB, Shin JY, Kwon NJ, et al. ClinPharmSeq: a targeted sequencing panel for clinical pharmacogenetics implementation. PLoS One 2022;17(7):e0272129.
[34] Lee SB, Wheeler MM, Thummel KE, et al. Calling star alleles with stargazer in 28 pharmacogenes with whole genome sequences. Clin Pharmacol Ther 2019;106(6):1328–37.
[35] Gong L, Whirl-Carrillo M, Klein TE. PharmGKB, an integrated resource of pharmacogenomic knowledge. Curr Protoc 2021;1(8):e226.
[36] Gaedigk A, Casey ST, Whirl-Carrillo M, et al. Pharmacogene variation consortium: a global resource and repository for pharmacogene variation. Clin Pharmacol Ther 2021;110(3):542–5.
[37] Gaedigk A, Ingelman-Sundberg M, Miller NA, et al. The pharmacogene variation (PHARMVAR) consortium: incorporation of the human cytochrome P450 (CYP) allele nomenclature database. Clin Pharmacol Ther 2018;103(3):399–401.
[38] Yang JJ, Whirl-Carrillo M, Scott SA, et al. Pharmacogene variation consortium gene introduction: NUDT15. Clin Pharmacol Ther 2019;105(5):1091–4.
[39] Botton MR, Whirl-Carrillo M, Del Tredici AL, et al. PharmVar GeneFocus: CYP2C19. Clin Pharmacol Ther 2021;109(2):352–66.
[40] Desta Z, El-Boraie A, Gong L, et al. PharmVar GeneFocus: CYP2B6. Clin Pharmacol Ther 2021;110(1):82–97.
[41] Sangkuhl K, Claudio-Campos K, Cavallari LH, et al. PharmVar GeneFocus: CYP2C9. Clin Pharmacol Ther 2021;110(3):662–76.
[42] Rodriguez-Antona C, Savieo JL, Lauschke VM, et al. PharmVar GeneFocus: CYP3A5. Clin Pharmacol Ther 2022;112(6):1159–71.
[43] Relling MV, Klein TE. CPIC: clinical pharmacogenetics implementation consortium of the pharmacogenomics research network. Clin Pharmacol Ther 2011;89(3):464–7.
[44] Relling MV, Klein TE, Gammal RS, et al. The clinical pharmacogenetics implementation consortium: 10 years later. Clin Pharmacol Ther 2020;107(1):171–5.
[45] Scott SA. The genetic testing reference materials coordination program: over 10 years of support for pharmacogenomic testing. J Mol Diagn 2023;25(9):630–3.
[46] Pratt VM, Zehnbauer B, Wilson JA, et al. Characterization of 107 genomic DNA reference materials for CYP2D6, CYP2C19, CYP2C9, VKORC1, and UGT1A1: a GeT-RM and association for molecular pathology collaborative project. J Mol Diagn 2010;12(6):835–46.
[47] Pratt VM, Everts RE, Aggarwal P, et al. Characterization of 137 Genomic DNA reference materials for 28 pharmacogenetic genes: a GeT-RM collaborative project. J Mol Diagn 2016;18(1):109–23.
[48] Gaedigk A, Turner A, Everts RE, et al. Characterization of reference materials for genetic testing of CYP2D6 alleles: a GeT-RM collaborative project. J Mol Diagn 2019;21(6):1034–52.
[49] Pratt VM, Turner A, Broeckel U, et al. Characterization of reference materials with an association for molecular pathology pharmacogenetics working group tier 2 status: CYP2C9, CYP2C19, VKORC1, CYP2C cluster variant, and GGCX: a GeT-RM collaborative project. J Mol Diagn 2021;23(8):952–8.
[50] Gaedigk A, Boone EC, Scherer SE, et al. CYP2C8, CYP2C9, and CYP2C19 characterization using next-generation sequencing and haplotype analysis: a GeT-RM collaborative project. J Mol Diagn 2022;24(4):337–50.
[51] Pratt VM, Wang WY, Boone EC, et al. Characterization of reference materials for TPMT and NUDT15: A GeT-RM collaborative project. J Mol Diagn 2022;24(10):1079–88.
[52] Gaedigk A, Boone EC, Turner AJ, et al. Characterization of reference materials for CYP3A4 and CYP3A5: A (GeT-RM) collaborative project. J Mol Diagn 2023;25(9):655–64.

Advances in Molecular Pathology 7 (2024) 43–52
ADVANCES IN MOLECULAR PATHOLOGY

Considerations in Clinical Laboratory Development of Pharmacogenomic Testing

Stephen J. Wicks, PhD, Kristy R. Crooks, PhD*
Department of Pathology, University of Colorado Anschutz Medical Campus, 12705 East Montview Boulevard, Suite 400, Aurora, CO 80045, USA

KEYWORDS
• Pharmacogenomics • Pharmacogenetics • Test validation • Genetic testing • Laboratory regulation
• Laboratory developed test (LDT)

KEY POINTS
- Pharmacogenomic testing is commonly incorporated as a component of personalized medicine programs with the aim of improving patient outcomes and reducing health care costs.
- Pharmacogenomic testing has additional complexities compared to most molecular diagnostic genetic testing. Consideration needs to be given to population-dependent allele frequencies, star allele nomenclature, diplotype phasing, multi-genic interpretation of drug interactions, and the potential for genetic variation in pharmacogenes to have additional clinical implications.
- Resources for selecting and validating pharmacogenetic variants are available and should be incorporated in test design and validation studies.
- Pharmacogenomic testing is best implemented in systems with robust clinician and patient education for responsible use of test information. Clinical decision support, patient-friendly information, and a consideration of equitable utility and access to testing across diverse populations are recommended.

INTRODUCTION

Personalized and precision medicine, in which medical care decisions are customized based on an individual's personal characteristics in areas of medical history, environment, lifestyle, and genetics, has emerged as a core element of many current initiatives aiming to reduce health care costs and improve patient outcomes and satisfaction [1–4]. One common component of these initiatives is pharmacogenomics, the study of genetic determinants of drug response, and more specifically the implementation of clinical pharmacogenomic testing to guide prescription management [5–7]. According to the United States Congressional Budget Office, nationwide spending on drug prescriptions increased from $30 billion in 1980 to $335 billion in 2018 [8]. However, commonly prescribed drugs have been found to be ineffective or cause side effects in more than 50% of patients, and prescription drug-related morbidity and mortality is estimated to have contributed to 16% of 2016 US health care expenditures [9,10]. The promise of pharmacogenomics lies in the idea that genetically-informed prescribing will reduce side effects and improve treatment efficacy (and that those improvements may in turn lead to increased patient medication adherence), thereby

*Corresponding author. 12705 East Montview Boulevard, Suite 400, Aurora, CO 80045. *E-mail address:* kristy.crooks@cuanschutz.edu

https://doi.org/10.1016/j.yamp.2024.06.004
www.advancesinmolecularpathology.com
2589-4080/24/

reducing prescription drug-related morbidity, mortality, and health care costs.

Evidence supporting gene-drug interactions and improved treatment outcomes with genotype-guided therapy has long been established [11]. With the ongoing expansion of known gene-drug pairs and clinically relevant genetic variants, pharmacogenomic testing is increasingly recognized as a valuable tool for optimizing prescribing practices. The demand for pharmacogenomic testing panels is rising, prompting laboratories to develop and update existing laboratory-developed tests (LDTs) to meet clinical needs [12]. Here, we present a clinical laboratory perspective of special considerations in pharmacogenomic test development, validation, and implementation.

SPECIAL CONSIDERATIONS IN PHARMACOGENOMIC TESTING

For clinical genetic test validation in the United States, clinical laboratories must at a minimum establish test performance characteristics as required for high-complexity testing under the Clinical Laboratory Improvement Amendments of 1988 (CLIA), which is administered at the state level. These metrics include accuracy, precision, reportable range, and reference intervals/range [13]. For clinical laboratories receiving CLIA certification through an external accreditation agency, there may be additional validation requirements, such as the need to establish test clinical sensitivity and specificity for laboratories accredited through the College for American Pathologists (CAP). These clinical laboratory certification and accreditation agencies as well as molecular pathology and clinical laboratory genetics professional societies (eg, Association for Molecular Pathology [AMP], American College of Medical Genetics [ACMG]) have made available excellent online resources for new test development. These, together with numerous publications for practical guidance and best practices for test validation in the field of molecular pathology, provide an excellent foundation in general principles of molecular pathology LDT validation [14–17], but additional considerations unique to pharmacogenomics often present challenges. The successful implementation of pharmacogenomics goes beyond the performance of the test and generation of results and demands consideration of various factors, including population-specific allele frequencies, allele nomenclature, multigenic drug interaction interpretation, and Mendelian diseases associated with pharmacogenes.

Population-Dependent Allele Frequencies

Population-dependent allele frequencies constitute a critical aspect of pharmacogenomic testing. Allele frequencies can vary significantly among different population groups and ancestries, influencing drug metabolism and response rates [18]. For instance, the *CYP2D6* gene, responsible for the hepatic metabolism of approximately 25% of commonly prescribed drugs, including antidepressants, antipsychotics, antiarrhythmics, opioids, and β-blockers, exhibits notable allele frequency disparities across populations [19]. Understanding these variations is essential for accurate genotype interpretation and clinical decision-making, and there is a need to expand common genotyping approaches when examining understudied or admixed populations. Laboratories should take patient demographics into account to ensure that the test is appropriate for their patient populations. Comprehensive databases compiling population-specific allele frequencies, such as the Pharmacogenomics Knowledgebase (PharmGKB, https://www.pharmgkb.org/), serve as indispensable resources for the interpretation of pharmacogenomic testing.

Star Allele Nomenclature

Unique to the field of pharmacogenomics is the star allele nomenclature system, which provides a standardized framework for characterizing genetic variations associated with pharmacogenes [20,21]. This system of allelic variant classification is designed to facilitate consistent communication and interpretation of pharmacogenomic test results. Star alleles are haplotype patterns at the gene level and are usually associated with protein activity levels. Haplotypes can comprise various types of genetic variants including single nucleotide polymorphisms/variants (SNPs/SNVs), insertions or deletions, and copy number variants (CNVs). For instance, the *CYP2D6**3* defining variant is a single nucleotide deletion (NM_000106.6:c.775del) resulting in a frameshift and premature protein truncation; *CYP2D6**3* is classified as "no function" allele. However, the *3 variant may be found in a haplotype with either the A or G nucleotide at the upstream nucleotide, c.496 A>G.

Typically, *1 denotes the standard reference allele or haplotype, representing the reference (formerly, "wild type") or fully functional variant. However, the designation of the *1 allele is often derived from the subpopulation where the gene was first investigated and might not necessarily be the reference allele nor reflect the most prevalent allele across all populations. Conversely, other star alleles, (eg, *2 or *14) signify haplotypes harboring 1 or more variants [22]. It is important to note that not all haplotypes with a designation other than *1 will have altered protein function, and that all suballeles under each star number are believed to be functionally equal. Thus, even if a test is capable of distinguishing suballeles (eg, *TPMT**3A, *3B, *3C), these are often reported under the same star allele designation [23]. Knowing the combination of variants within a given haplotype, together with the number of gene copies in an individual, is essential for determining likely effects on drug metabolism and drug response, as well as likelihood of adverse drug reactions. The use of pharmacogenomic resources such as the Pharmacogene Variation Consortium (PharmVar, https://www.pharmvar.org), the Clinical Pharmacogenetics Implementation Consortium (CPIC, https://cpicpgx.org/), PharmGKB, and the Dutch Pharmacogenetics Working Group of the Royal Dutch Pharmacists Association is fundamental for accurate utilization of star allele nomenclature and interpretation of genotype profiles to make informed medication decisions [20,24,25].

Multigene-Drug Interactions

Most of the best established, actionable gene-drug interactions link a single pharmacogene to a particular drug, such as *DPYD* and capecitabine, or *UGT1A1* and atazanavir [26,27]. For other drugs, actionable genotypes may exist across multiple genes, and clinical interpretation of the test result and recommended dosing algorithms may be complicated by the need to combine genotypes across genes. The best example of such a multigene-drug interaction effect is warfarin, for which CPIC and AMP guidelines support variant testing in at least *CYP2C9* and *VKORC1*, with the option of adding variants in *CYP4F2* and an intergenic SNV, rs12777823 [28,29]. Importantly, certain variants in the expanded testing recommendations and dosing algorithm are included to bolster the clinical utility of the test in a multi-ethnic patient population, particularly in persons of African ancestry.

Multigenic interpretation of gene-drug interactions underscores the interplay between multiple genes influencing drug metabolism, transport, and pharmacodynamics. Pharmacogenomic interactions involving multiple genes can have a significant impact on drug efficacy and safety, necessitating a comprehensive understanding of their combined effects.

Non-pharmacogenomic Clinical Implications Associated with Pharmacogenes

In rare cases, pharmacogenomic testing can result in a finding consistent with an increased risk of a clinical condition independent of the gene-drug interaction of interest. Examples include *UGT1A1*-associated hyperbilirubinemia syndromes and *G6PD* deficiency.

*UGT1A1**6 and *28 pharmacogenetic testing is recommended on the United States Federal Drug Administration-approved drug label for irinotecan, a chemotherapeutic topoisomerase I inhibitor, as patients with poor or intermediate metabolizer phenotype for *UGT1A1* are at an increased risk for irinotecan-related toxicity, which can range from mild to life-threatening. The most common decreased function allele, *28, is within a polymorphic dinucleotide TA repeat in the *UGT1A1* promoter and has 1 additional TA repeat compared to the reference allele. Homozygosity for the *28 variant causes an approximately 70% reduction in enzyme activity and is associated with Gilbert syndrome, a typically benign, reduced penetrance condition of mild intermittent jaundice. A more severe condition associated with complete absence of UGT1A1 activity, Crigler-Najjar syndrome, is caused by homozygosity or compound heterozygosity for loss-of-function variants in *UGT1A1*. Depending on the methodology, laboratories performing *UGT1A1* testing may identify an incidental finding consistent with an increased risk of Crigler-Najjar syndrome, and policies regarding whether or how to address such a finding in the report should be established. Alternatively, laboratories may find that providers mistakenly or inappropriately order *UGT1A1* pharmacogenetic testing for the purpose of investigating the genetic cause of a patient's hyperbilirubinemia when the test is not validated for that indication.

Similar considerations apply to *G6PD* testing. Glucose 6-phosphate dehydrogenase (G6PD) deficiency is an X-linked recessive disorder caused by reduced enzymatic activity of the *G6PD* protein product. Individuals with G6PD deficiency are at risk of acute hemolytic anemia not only in the context of drug-induced oxidative stress (eg, rasburicase, pegloticase, etc.), but with also exposure to certain chemicals or foods (eg, fava beans). It is also associated with an increased risk of neonatal jaundice. Laboratories should set policies for reporting *G6PD* testing that include non-pharmacogenomic implications for severe cases of G6PD deficiency and that include a recommendation for the consideration of genetic counseling when appropriate.

VALIDATION CONSIDERATIONS

Commonly, laboratories develop new or expanded pharmacogenomic tests to meet specific clinical needs of their client base, and these needs differ based on patient population, clinical indications for testing, prescribing practices, health care payor distribution, and reimbursement landscape, among other factors.

Laboratory directors must balance competing interests, such as reducing costs versus building capacity for flexibility and growth or leveraging economies of scale by running larger batches of samples less frequently versus meeting rapid turnaround times. The design of an assay, including the methodology used, genes and variants included, bioinformatics analyses, and reporting choices, must be considered in the context of the clinical needs of the health care providers and patients that the laboratory serves (Fig. 1).

Gene and Allele Selection

The landscape of known pharmacogenomic gene-drug interactions is dynamic, with new associations continually emerging. It is the responsibility of the CLIA director to ensure that each gene and allele included in the laboratory's pharmacogenomic tests has sufficient data underlying the gene-drug interactions of interest to justify its inclusion in clinical testing and reporting. Three related freely available online resources mentioned earlier, PharmGKB, PharmVar, and CPIC, are useful references for gene and allele selection, although they differ in the types of information they curate.

PharmGKB catalogs information related to the relationships between genetic variants, drugs, and clinical outcomes. It provides data on how genetic variation affects drug response, including information on drug metabolism, efficacy, and adverse reactions. In the setting of clinical laboratory test development, PharmGKB is an excellent resource for exploring and weighing the evidence supporting associations between specific genetic variants and drug response.

PharmVar is a consortium that catalogs and interprets genetic variation in pharmacogenes with a focus on haplotype structure. It is responsible for establishing and annotating the relationship between individual variants in a gene, its haplotypes, and star allele designations, where applicable. For each gene, PharmVar publishes versioned reference files, such as allele functionality tables, phenotype tables, diplotype-phenotype tables, and frequency tables that are useful in determining which variants need to be tested to detect haplotypes of interest. PharmVar tables are particularly useful in confirming that the alleles selected for testing within a gene are sufficiently comprehensive to be unambiguously interpreted and reported in the appropriate standardized nomenclature and classification system.

CPIC is a consortium dedicated to reducing barriers to clinical implementation of pharmacogenetic testing. It publishes clinical practice guidelines for particular gene-drug pairs that include variant information useful for clinical assay design. These guidelines, which are indexed in PubMed, are regularly updated and linked to associated PharmGKB reference files. CPIC guidelines are also helpful references for documenting clinical utility of the test content.

In addition to the above resources, AMP, in collaboration with CPIC, CAP, PharmGKB, the Dutch Pharmacogenetics Working Group of the Royal Dutch Pharmacists Association, and the European Society for Pharmacogenomics and Personalized Therapy, has published a series of 6 guidelines detailing genotyping recommendations and variant selection within 8 genes to date (*CYP2C19*, *CYP2C9*, *CYP2D6*, *CYP3A4*, *CYP3A5*, *NUDT15*, *TPMT*, and *VKORC1*) [28,30–34]. Each guideline establishes recommendations for pharmacogenetic testing allele selection. Alleles are categorized into tiers, with Tier 1 alleles representing the minimum set recommended for inclusion in clinical pharmacogenomics genotyping tests. Tier 2 alleles typically represent a more comprehensive genotyping panel for which there is sufficient scientific evidence for clinical implementation, but which do not meet all criteria for Tier 1 (eg, availability of reference material for validation studies).

Platform Considerations

Laboratories often experience practical constraints in the selection of test methodology for new tests, with a heavy reliance on existing instrumentation and infrastructure. Fortunately, most pharmacogenomic alleles are simple sequence variants amenable to detection by a variety of common sequencing and genotyping methodologies, including Sanger sequencing, short-read and long-read sequencing, allelic discrimination genotyping, SNP microarray genotyping, and others [35]. Where the chosen platform has poor performance for the accurate detection of 1 or more variants under development, a complementary assay must be considered. Variants that commonly pose challenges for particular technologies include discrimination of the *UGT1A1* dinucleotide repeat size underlying the *28, *36, and *37 alleles and *CYP2D6* copy-number assignment, particularly in the setting of gene conversion events [36,37].

Validation Sample Selection and Sourcing

Once the panel content and methodology have been chosen, validation typically begins with the testing of reference samples of known genotype. Identifying and sourcing these samples can be challenging, but here again, the AMP guidelines are useful; each has 1 or more tables listing available appropriate reference samples for the variants, haplotypes, or diplotypes of interest [28,30–34]. For genes or variants not included in AMP guidelines, the Center for Disease Control and

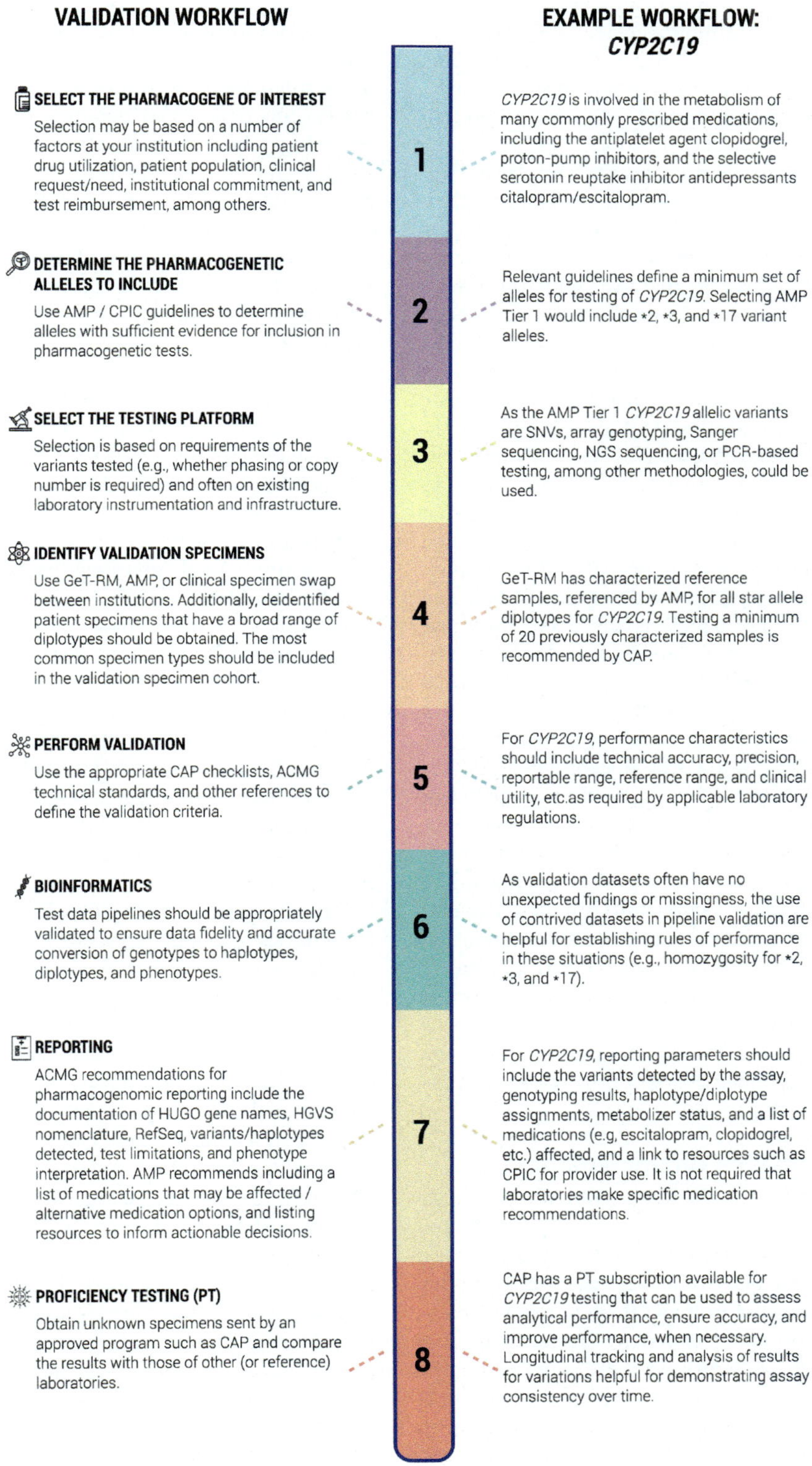

FIG. 1 Common steps in the development and validation of a pharmacogenomic test (*left*) and a practical example of how each step might be applied for *CYP2C19* testing (*right*).

Prevention's Genetic Testing Reference Materials (GeT-RM) Pharmacogenomics resource (https://www.cdc.gov/labquality/get-rm/inherited-genetic-diseases-pharmacogenetics/pharmacogenetics.html) has additional curations [38–42].

For any variants for which reference samples are unavailable, options include requesting deidentified samples from other clinical laboratories or identifying commercially available cell lines with the needed genotypes. It is important to note that the standard for reference samples is that the genotype must have been established with clinical certainty. This is most commonly achieved by using samples that have been previously clinically tested or that have appropriate annotation in the literature (eg, AMP and GeT-RM). Alternatively, one can leverage broader research cell line repositories and associated research sequencing data to identify potential reference samples; it is important that the expected genotypes are confirmed by a validated assay before being used as validation or control samples.

One of the challenges for the development of broad pharmacogenomic test panels is the need, for those methodologies for which a platform-based or methods-based validation is inappropriate, to perform individual variant-specific analytical validation. For example, a panel of 100 diallelic SNPs would, at its least, require 200 validation samples to cover all genotypes (AA/AB/BB for each SNP). In this theoretic, maximally inefficient sample set, each sample has a homozygous reference genotype for 99 SNPs and is either heterozygous or homozygous for the variant allele for the single remaining SNP. This single-variant approach to building a validation cohort is time consuming and increases validation costs. Bioinformatics approaches can be used to identify the minimum set of samples within a larger cohort of samples that will cover all 3 genotypes at each locus [43]. The reduced set of validation samples can later be implemented as a panel of rotating positive controls for the assay.

Clinical Performance Characteristics

As for other molecular genetic tests, validation testing is used to establish the technical and clinical performance characteristics of a pharmacogenomic test. Analytical (or technical) validation determines the degree to which the test method reliably discriminates the genotypes of interest. Analytical accuracy, sensitivity, and specificity, and measures of uncertainty around these point estimates (eg, 95% confidence intervals) are typically determined by the testing of previously characterized samples of known genotype. Clinical validation establishes that the evidence underlying the association between the variant(s) and medical outcomes of interest (eg, drug response, adverse events) is robust enough to justify clinical implementation of the test. Typically, laboratories cite existing data in the literature and in reference databases (eg, CPIC, PharmGKB, etc.) to establish clinical validity and do not perform association studies to generate data for this purpose. A comprehensive discussion of the generation and analysis of association studies to support clinical validity and utility of novel drug-gene interactions is beyond the scope of this review. Other publications provide a thorough and detailed exploration of these topics [44–46].

Bioinformatics and Data Analysis

Clinical interpretation of pharmacogenes is complicated by the required conversion of genotypes at multiple loci into haplotypes, which may then be assigned a star allele designation and/or activity score. The 2 haplotypes for each gene are usually converted to a diplotype before a final interpretation with respect to the protein product function (eg, metabolizer or transporter status) is determined.

Bioinformatics pipelines that convert the genotype calls to haplotypes, diplotypes, activity scores, and phenotypes are commercially available or can be laboratory developed. Regardless of the sophistication of the software used, the pipeline itself should be validated as part of test development. A mock validation dataset covering all possible (and unexpected) genotypes is useful, as is establishing decision parameters in the setting of missingness for 1 or more data points.

Phasing analysis is typically not performed, except by laboratories leveraging long-range sequencing methods, and the assignation of genotypes to haplotypes is typically done by inference of phasing using data in the literature regarding the likelihood of multiple heterozygous variants appearing on the same haplotype (*in cis*) or on opposite haplotypes (*in trans*). The interpretation in the report may therefore represent the most likely phenotype rather than a definite phenotype.

Consider, for example, a test for the 3 AMP Tier 1 alleles in *CYP2C19* (**2*, **3*, and **17*), for which a patient sample is determined to be heterozygous for the *2 variant and the *3 variant, both "no function" alleles. Population data demonstrate that these 2 variants are almost always observed *in trans*, meaning that the patient would have 2 copies of a "no function" allele and an expected "poor metabolizer" phenotype [34,47]. However, one can imagine a very rare haplotype with these 2 variants *in cis*, in which case the patient would have 1 normal function allele and 1 no function allele, with an expected phenotype of "intermediate metabolizer."

For this very rare patient, the diplotype and interpretation would be inaccurate if phasing were not performed. Test development should take into consideration the current data on variant phasing across haplotypes and determine for each possible allele combination whether the result is interpretable and reportable without phasing analysis.

Resources for Proficiency Testing

A part of test validation that should not be overlooked is the development of a plan for ongoing assay proficiency testing (PT) after test launch. Currently, CAP offers 3 PT subscriptions in the area of pharmacogenomics, covering a limited number of variants in 17 genes: *COMT, CYP2B6, CYP2C19, CYP2C9, CYP2D6, CYP3A4, CYP3A5, CYP4F2, DPYD, G6PD, IFNL3, NUDT15, OPRM1, SLCO1B1, TPMT, UGT1A1*, and *VKORC1*. Human Leukocyte Antigen (HLA) alleles are also available in PT designed for this locus. For additional genes and variants or as an alternative to CAP subscriptions, laboratories should establish a PT plan for ongoing assessment of assay performance.

CONSIDERATIONS REGARDING THE RESPONSIBLE IMPLEMENTATION OF PHARMACOGENOMIC TESTING

Pharmacogenomic testing is best implemented in systems with robust clinician and patient support for the responsible use of test information. Clinical decision support (CDS), patient-friendly information, and laboratory support of end-users are recommended.

The utility of pharmacogenomic findings extends across diverse health care settings, encompassing both large academic medical centers and smaller physician-led community clinics where the findings can inform treatment decisions for both inpatients and outpatients [48–50]. Moreover, pharmacogenomic testing can be conducted through 2 modalities: Reactive, at the time the drug is prescribed; or preemptive, which establishes pharmacogenomic data for future use when needed [51–54].

Advancements in genotyping technologies, coupled with expanding knowledge of gene-drug interactions, have led to the increasing accessibility and cost-effectiveness of pharmacogenomic testing. Despite these advances, obstacles persist in integrating pharmacogenomics into routine clinical practice. The widespread adoption of pharmacogenomic testing has been hindered by a relative lack of standardized testing protocols, interpretation guidelines, CDS tools, and provider and patient education.

Regardless of the health care setting or testing modality employed, successful clinical implementation necessitates careful consideration of several key areas.

- At the point of delivery within health care systems, modification of existing clinical pathways to accommodate pharmacogenomic results is required to ensure their prompt availability to health care providers. This can mean creating new pathway checkpoints where other health care professionals, such as pharmacists, help in individual case management.
- To effectively implement and make use of pharmacogenomic findings, integration of CDS tools into electronic health record (EHR) systems is needed. The use of CDS facilitates the translation of pharmacogenomic findings into actionable clinical recommendations and can reduce the burden on health care providers of providing pharmacogenomics-informed care. Depending on the EHR capabilities, CDS may take a number of forms. For more severe potential outcomes, interruptive alerts are often used at the time of prescribing and are designed to inform the health care provider of the gene-drug interaction and can suggest patient-specific alternative medications or dosing strategies. For less worrisome potential adverse events, passive approaches may require the health care provider to access a link or dedicated site within the EHR to find information relating to the pharmacogenomic finding and cross-reference to the drug in question [55]. Fuller integration of CDS tools into EHR systems and the use of interruptive alerts can help optimize medication selection and dosing for improved patient outcomes. However, creating such tools can be costly and time-consuming and often needs creative use of EHR system capabilities [56]. Nevertheless, these integrative approaches hold promise for enhancing the accessibility and utility of pharmacogenomic testing in real-world clinical settings.
- There is currently a significant knowledge gap among health care providers regarding pharmacogenomics. A lack of standardization in the field, complex information about gene-drug interactions, and limited pharmacogenomics medical education mean that poor uptake in the use of pharmacogenomic findings and understanding of their clinical actionability is hindering implementation [57]. Improved training programs and continuous education are essential to equip health care providers with the necessary skills to interpret pharmacogenomic findings and effectively apply them in the management and treatment of patients.

- Standardization of approaches to pharmacogenomic testing and applicability are required, as there can be varying opinions on the level of evidence needed to support clinical implementation which may influence how providers manage patient medication selection and management [58]. Without defined frameworks for result interpretation and clinical actionability, health care providers may struggle to effectively use genetic information in treatment decisions [59].
- The application of pharmacogenomic testing to guide medication selection and dosing in diverse medical specialties such as psychiatry and cardiology underscores the requirement to develop frameworks that address particular clinical needs and that can be implemented into specialist treatment pathways [60].
- Alongside the requirements of greater health care provider pharmacogenomic education, there is a concurrent need to educate patients on the pharmacogenomic findings and how they may help manage medication selection and dosage [61,62]. This is important so that patients understand, on receiving pharmacogenomic test results, that they should not suddenly stop taking medication or change dosing without the oversight of a health care professional.
- Additionally, consideration must be given to addressing systemic barriers such as limited insurance coverage and variable reimbursement policies for pharmacogenomic testing which may limit the ability of health care providers to personalize medication selection and management for their patients [63–65]. As in other areas of medical study, the majority of pharmacogenomic research has been conducted in people of European ancestry, so a deliberate and particular focus on equitable access, improved multi-racial utility, and patient privacy protections in the utilization of pharmacogenomic information is required [11].

SUMMARY

The implementation of pharmacogenomic testing as a component of personalized and precision medicine initiatives is an emerging approach to health care improvement. Pharmacogenomic testing offers the potential to mitigate adverse drug reactions and improve treatment efficacy and presents an opportunity to reduce prescription drug-related morbidity and mortality and their associated costs.

In addition to the regulations and guidelines that apply to the development of molecular genetic tests in general, the validation and implementation of pharmacogenomic testing requires unique considerations, including population-specific allele frequencies, a distinct nomenclature system, multigene-drug interactions, and non-pharmacogenomic clinical implications associated with pharmacogenes. Furthermore, the responsible integration of pharmacogenomic information into routine clinical practice requires addressing knowledge gaps among health care providers, improving patient education, standardizing testing protocols, addressing reimbursement, and overcoming systemic barriers to equitable utility of pharmacogenomic information across populations. Moving forward, interdisciplinary collaboration, continuing education, payor engagement, and laboratory and health record system innovations will be needed to begin realizing the potential of pharmacogenomics to improve patient outcomes and reduce health care costs.

DISCLOSURE

The authors have nothing to disclose.

REFERENCES

[1] Jakka S, Rossbach M. An economic perspective on personalized medicine. HUGO J 2013;7:1–6.

[2] Luzum JA, Petry N, Taylor AK, et al. Moving pharmacogenetics into practice: it's all about the evidence. Clin Pharmacol Therapeut 2021;110(3):649–61.

[3] Mathur S, Sutton J. Personalized medicine could transform healthcare. Biomedical reports 2017;7(1):3–5.

[4] Shabaruddin FH, Fleeman ND, Payne K. Economic evaluations of personalized medicine: existing challenges and current developments. Pharmacogenomics Personalized Med 2015;8:115–26.

[5] Naik H, O'Connor MY, Sanderson SC, et al. Pharmacogenomic knowledge and awareness among diverse patients treated with angiotensin converting enzyme inhibitors. Pharmacogenomics 2023;24(18):921–30.

[6] Wiley LK, Shortt JA, Roberts ER, et al. Building a vertically integrated genomic learning health system: The biobank at the Colorado Center for Personalized Medicine. Am J Hum Genet 2024;111(1):11–23.

[7] Uber R, Wright E. Pharmacogenomics implementation and multidisciplinary genomics collaboration: Real-world experience from Geisinger. Am J Health Syst Pharm 2022;79(13):1038–41.

[8] Congressional Budget Office. Prescription Drugs: Spending, Use, and Prices. 2022. Available at: https://www.cbo.gov/system/files/2022-01/57050-Rx-Spending.pdf.

[9] Watanabe JH, McInnis T, Hirsch JD. Cost of Prescription Drug-Related Morbidity and Mortality. Ann Pharmacother 2018;52(9):829–37.

[10] Schork NJ. Personalized medicine: time for one-person trials. Nature 2015;520(7549):609–11.

[11] Morris SA, Alsaidi AT, Verbyla A, et al. Cost Effectiveness of Pharmacogenetic Testing for Drugs with Clinical Pharmacogenetics Implementation Consortium (<scp>CPIC</scp>) Guidelines: A Systematic Review. Clin Pharmacol Therapeut 2022;112(6):1318–28.

[12] Moyer AM, McMillin GA, Long TA, et al. Genotype and Phenotype Concordance for Pharmacogenetic Tests Through Proficiency Survey Testing: An Update. Arch Pathol Lab Med 2020;144(9):1057–66.

[13] Clinical Laboratory Improvement Amendments of 1988, 42 U.S.C. § 493.1253 (1988).

[14] Jennings L, Van Deerlin VM, Gulley ML. Recommended principles and practices for validating clinical molecular pathology tests. Arch Pathol Lab Med 2009;133(5):743–55.

[15] Mattocks CJ, Morris MA, Matthijs G, et al. A standardized framework for the validation and verification of clinical molecular genetic tests. Eur J Hum Genet 2010;18(12): 1276–88.

[16] Bean L, Funke B, Carlston CM, et al. Diagnostic gene sequencing panels: from design to report—a technical standard of the American College of Medical Genetics and Genomics (ACMG). Genet Med 2020;22(3):453–61.

[17] South ST, McClure M, Astbury C, et al. Risk categorization for oversight of laboratory-developed tests for inherited conditions: an updated position statement of the American College of Medical Genetics and Genomics (ACMG). Genet Med 2020;22(6):983–5.

[18] Qiao W, Martis S, Mendiratta G, et al. Integrated CYP2D6 interrogation for multiethnic copy number and tandem allele detection. Pharmacogenomics 2019;20(1):9–20.

[19] Owen RP, Sangkuhl K, Klein TE, et al. Cytochrome P450 2D6. Pharmacogenetics Genom 2009;19(7):559–62.

[20] Caudle KE, Dunnenberger HM, Freimuth RR, et al. Standardizing terms for clinical pharmacogenetic test results: consensus terms from the Clinical Pharmacogenetics Implementation Consortium (CPIC). Genet Med 2017; 19(2):215–23.

[21] Hoffman JM, Dunnenberger HM, Kevin Hicks J, et al. Developing knowledge resources to support precision medicine: principles from the Clinical Pharmacogenetics Implementation Consortium (CPIC). J Am Med Inf Assoc 2016;23(4):796–801.

[22] Robarge JD, Li L, Desta Z, et al. The Star-Allele Nomenclature: Retooling for Translational Genomics. Clin Pharmacol Therapeut 2007;82(3):244–8.

[23] Kalman L, Agúndez J, Appell ML, et al. Pharmacogenetic allele nomenclature: International workgroup recommendations for test result reporting. Clin Pharmacol Therapeut 2016;99(2):172–85.

[24] Relling MV, Klein TE. CPIC: Clinical Pharmacogenetics Implementation Consortium of the Pharmacogenomics Research Network. Clin Pharmacol Ther 2011;89(3):464–7.

[25] Swen JJ, Nijenhuis M, de Boer A, et al. Pharmacogenetics: from bench to byte–an update of guidelines. Clin Pharmacol Ther 2011;89(5):662–73.

[26] Amstutz U, Henricks LM, Offer SM, et al. Clinical Pharmacogenetics Implementation Consortium (CPIC) Guideline for Dihydropyrimidine Dehydrogenase Genotype and Fluoropyrimidine Dosing: 2017 Update. Clin Pharmacol Ther 2018;103(2):210–6.

[27] Gammal RS, Court MH, Haidar CE, et al. Clinical Pharmacogenetics Implementation Consortium (CPIC) Guideline for UGT1A1 and Atazanavir Prescribing. Clin Pharmacol Ther 2016;99(4):363–9.

[28] Pratt VM, Cavallari LH, Del Tredici AL, et al. Recommendations for clinical warfarin genotyping allele selection: a report of the Association for Molecular Pathology and the College of American Pathologists. J Mol Diagn 2020;22(7):847–59.

[29] Johnson JA, Caudle KE, Gong L, et al. Clinical Pharmacogenetics Implementation Consortium (CPIC) Guideline for Pharmacogenetics-Guided Warfarin Dosing: 2017 Update. Clin Pharmacol Ther 2017;102(3):397–404.

[30] Pratt VM, Cavallari LH, Del Tredici AL, et al. Recommendations for Clinical CYP2D6 Genotyping Allele Selection. J Mol Diagn 2021;23(9):1047–64.

[31] Pratt VM, Cavallari LH, Del Tredici AL, et al. Recommendations for Clinical CYP2C9 Genotyping Allele Selection. J Mol Diagn 2019;21(5):746–55.

[32] Pratt VM, Cavallari LH, Fulmer ML, et al. TPMT and NUDT15 genotyping recommendations: a joint consensus recommendation of the association for molecular pathology, clinical pharmacogenetics implementation consortium, college of American pathologists, Dutch pharmacogenetics working group of the royal Dutch pharmacists association, European society for pharmacogenomics and personalized therapy, and pharmacogenomics knowledgebase. J Mol Diagn 2022;24(10):1051–63.

[33] Pratt VM, Cavallari LH, Fulmer ML, et al. CYP3A4 and CYP3A5 genotyping recommendations: a joint consensus recommendation of the association for molecular Pathology, clinical pharmacogenetics implementation Consortium, College of American pathologists, Dutch pharmacogenetics working Group of the royal Dutch pharmacists association, European society for pharmacogenomics and personalized therapy, and pharmacogenomics Knowledgebase. J Mol Diagn 2023;25(9):619–29.

[34] Pratt VM, Del Tredici AL, Hachad H, et al. Recommendations for clinical CYP2C19 genotyping allele selection: a report of the Association for Molecular Pathology. J Mol Diagn 2018;20(3):269–76.

[35] van der Lee M, Kriek M, Guchelaar H-J, et al. Technologies for pharmacogenomics: a review. Genes 2020; 11(12):1456.

[36] Gaedigk A. Complexities of CYP2D6 gene analysis and interpretation. Int Rev Psychiatr 2013;25(5):534–53.

[37] Turner AJ, Aggarwal P, Boone EC, et al. Identification of CYP2D6 haplotypes that interfere with commonly used assays for copy number variation characterization. J Mol Diagn 2021;23(5):577–88.

[38] Gaedigk A, Boone EC, Scherer SE, et al. CYP2C8, CYP2C9, and CYP2C19 characterization using next-generation

sequencing and haplotype analysis: a GeT-RM collaborative project. J Mol Diagn 2022;24(4):337–50.

[39] Gaedigk A, Boone EC, Turner AJ, et al. Characterization of Reference Materials for CYP3A4 and CYP3A5. J Mol Diagn 2023;25(9):655–64.

[40] Gaedigk A, Turner A, Everts RE, et al. Characterization of Reference Materials for Genetic Testing of CYP2D6 Alleles. J Mol Diagn 2019;21(6):1034–52.

[41] Pratt VM, Everts RE, Aggarwal P, et al. Characterization of 137 Genomic DNA Reference Materials for 28 Pharmacogenetic Genes. J Mol Diagn 2016;18(1):109–23.

[42] Pratt VM, Wang WY, Boone EC, et al. Characterization of Reference Materials for TPMT and NUDT15. J Mol Diagn 2022;24(10):1079–88.

[43] Scott ER, Bansal V, Meacham C, et al. VarCover: Allele Min-Set Cover Software. J Mol Diagn 2020;22(2):123–31.

[44] Tonk ECM, Gurwitz D, Maitland-van der Zee AH, et al. Assessment of pharmacogenetic tests: presenting measures of clinical validity and potential population impact in association studies. Pharmacogenomics J 2017;17(4):386–92.

[45] Jansen ME, Rigter T, Rodenburg W, et al. Review of the reported measures of clinical validity and clinical utility as arguments for the implementation of pharmacogenetic testing: a case study of statin-induced muscle toxicity. Front Pharmacol 2017;8:555.

[46] Hertz DL, Arwood MJ, Stocco G, et al. Planning and conducting a pharmacogenetics association study. Clin Pharmacol Therapeut 2021;110(3):688–701.

[47] Ionova Y, Ashenhurst J, Zhan J, et al. CYP2C19 Allele Frequencies in Over 2.2 Million Direct-to-Consumer Genetics Research Participants and the Potential Implication for Prescriptions in a Large Health System. Clin Transl Sci 2020;13(6):1298–306.

[48] Weitzel KW, Elsey AR, Langaee TY, et al. Clinical pharmacogenetics implementation: approaches, successes, and challenges. Am J Med Genet C Semin Med Genet 2014;166c(1):56–67.

[49] Klein ME, Parvez MM, Shin JG. Clinical Implementation of Pharmacogenomics for Personalized Precision Medicine: Barriers and Solutions. J Pharm Sci 2017;106(9):2368–79.

[50] Dunnenberger HM, Crews KR, Hoffman JM, et al. Preemptive clinical pharmacogenetics implementation: current programs in five US medical centers. Annu Rev Pharmacol Toxicol 2015;55:89–106.

[51] Van Driest SL, Shi Y, Bowton EA, et al. Clinically actionable genotypes among 10,000 patients with preemptive pharmacogenomic testing. Clin Pharmacol Therapeut 2014;95(4):423–31.

[52] Haidar CE, Crews KR, Hoffman JM, et al. Advancing pharmacogenomics from single-gene to preemptive testing. Annu Rev Genom Hum Genet 2022;23:449–73.

[53] Peruzzi E, Roncato R, De Mattia E, et al. Implementation of pre-emptive testing of a pharmacogenomic panel in clinical practice: Where do we stand? Br J Clin Pharmacol 2023.

[54] Obeng AO, Samwald M, Scott SA. Reactive, point-of-care, preemptive, and direct-to-consumer pharmacogenomics testing. Pharmacogenomics. London, UK: Elsevier; 2019. p. 369–84.

[55] Aquilante CL, Kao DP, Trinkley KE, et al. Clinical implementation of pharmacogenomics via a health system-wide research biobank: the University of Colorado experience. Pharmacogenomics 2020;21(6):375–86.

[56] Roden DM, McLeod HL, Relling MV, et al. Pharmacogenomics. Lancet 2019;394(10197):521–32.

[57] Ta R, Cayabyab MA, Coloso R. Precision medicine: a call for increased pharmacogenomic education. Per Med 2019;16(3):233–45.

[58] Luzum JA, Petry N, Taylor AK, et al. Moving Pharmacogenetics Into Practice: It's All About the Evidence. Clin Pharmacol Ther 2021;110(3):649–61.

[59] Barker CIS, Groeneweg G, Maitland-van der Zee AH, et al. Pharmacogenomic testing in paediatrics: Clinical implementation strategies. Br J Clin Pharmacol 2022;88(10):4297–310.

[60] Sanghvi S, Ferner RE, Scourfield A, et al. How to assess pharmacogenomic tests for implementation in the NHS in England. Br J Clin Pharmacol 2023;89(9):2649–57.

[61] Haga SB. Educating patients and providers through comprehensive pharmacogenetic test reports. Future Medicine 2017;18(11):1047–50.

[62] Mills R, Ensinger M, Callanan N, et al. Development and initial assessment of a patient education video about pharmacogenetics. J Personalized Med 2017;7(2):4.

[63] Keeling NJ, Rosenthal MM, West-Strum D, et al. Preemptive pharmacogenetic testing: exploring the knowledge and perspectives of US payers. Genet Med 2019;21(5):1224–32.

[64] Lemke LK, Alam B, Williams R, et al. Reimbursement of pharmacogenetic tests at a tertiary academic medical center in the United States. Front Pharmacol 2023;14:1179364.

[65] Rogers SL. The current state of pharmacoeconomics and reimbursement for pharmacogenomics. Advances in Molecular Pathology 2023;6(1):87–97.

Hematopathology

Advances in Molecular Pathology 7 (2024) 53–61
ADVANCES IN MOLECULAR PATHOLOGY

Advances in Structural Variant Detection in Hematolymphoid Malignancies

Optical Genome Mapping

Soma Roy Chakraborty, MD*, Wahab A. Khan, PhD, Prabhjot Kaur, MD, Jeremiah Karrs, DO
Dartmouth Hitchcock Medical Center, 1 Medical Center Drive, Lebanon, NH 03766, USA

KEYWORDS

• Optical genome mapping • Structural variants • Leukemia • Lymphoma

KEY POINTS

- Optical genome mapping (OGM) is a new genome-wide technology that simplifies lab workflow by revealing both structural genomic changes and copy number variants in a single assay.
- This review comprehensively describes the OGM technique, outlining its unique strengths and weaknesses compared to standard-of-care techniques for hematologic malignancies.
- This review also explains how the OGM technique has the potential to transform front-line testing for various hematologic malignancies, including acute myeloid leukemia, myelodysplastic syndromes, acute lymphoblastic leukemia, multiple myeloma, and chronic lymphocytic leukemia.

INTRODUCTION

Structural variants (SVs) play a key role in biological processes and are known to impact gene expression, potentially resulting in altered phenotypes and diseases. Therefore, identifying SVs and copy number variants (CNVs) from human genomes is crucial in disease diagnosis, especially in the era of precision medicine. Diagnosis of hematological malignancies utilizes a combination of cytogenetic and molecular testing for appropriate classification. The conventional diagnostic tests to identify SVs and CNVs include karyotyping, fluorescence in situ hybridization (FISH), and chromosomal microarrays (CMA) each having their own benefits and limitations. To compensate for each assay's limitations, they are often combined, but this complicates workflows and still has inherent limitations. OGM is a technology that offers a simplified workflow by detecting SVs and CNVs across the genome in 1 test and which has the potential to replace the earlier-mentioned multiple testing modalities. Recent scientific studies show that optical genome mapping (OGM) appears concordant with standard cytogenetic techniques while simultaneously detecting additional valuable biomarkers. An additional benefit to utilizing 1 platform for cytogenetic testing is cost-effectiveness and better turnaround time. With the ability of producing whole genome results with gene-level resolution, OGM offers efficient classification, prognostic, and therapeutic stratification in hematological malignancies.

*Corresponding author, *E-mail address:* smcshoma@gmail.com

https://doi.org/10.1016/j.yamp.2024.06.002 www.advancesinmolecularpathology.com
2589-4080/24/

APPLICATION OF OPTICAL GENOME MAPPING IN HEMATOLOGICAL MALIGNANCIES

The genomic complexity in hematolymphoid malignancies ranges from chromosomal aberrations to driver point mutations, contributing to the fine-tuning of diagnostic criteria. Actionable biomarkers with therapeutic and prognostic significance play a pivotal role in classifying hematolymphoid malignancies.

Undoubtedly, OGM holds significant potential in refining diagnostics of intricate diseases. We review the literature with a focus on OGM specifically for hematologic malignancies.

Acute Myeloid Leukemia

Acute myeloid leukemia (AML) is an aggressive hematologic cancer that affects a considerable number of people worldwide including up to 4 cases per 100,000 in the United States [1]. Major challenges in treating AML include the complexity of genomic alterations, which have a substantial impact on prognosis and clinical treatment. Therefore, comprehensive genetic testing is essential for accurate diagnosis and risk stratification of AML patients. Fortunately, new genetic testing methods, such as OGM, have been developed to provide more precise and comprehensive information about this disease. A growing body of research has shown that OGM can help identify genetic abnormalities that may not be detected by a standard diagnostic genomic workup. This additional information can be crucial in developing effective treatment plans for AML patients.

Gerding and colleagues [2] used the OGM platform as a diagnostic tool in a group of 27 AML and myelodysplastic syndromes (MDS) cases with excessive blasts. A high concordance of 93% was observed with other cytogenetic methods, along with the detection of cytogenetically cryptic rearrangements including *NUP98::NSD1*, *MECOM::MSI2*, and *DDX3X::MLLT10*. *NUP98::NSD1* rearrangement is seen in about 1% of all AML cases and is found to be associated with poor prognosis in pediatric patients [3]. *MLLT10* rearrangement is rare in AML and associated with a worse prognosis independent of the fusion partner [4,5]. OGM analysis also detected rare SVs and CNVs in selected myeloid genes (*KMT2A-PTD*, *ETV6*, *JAK2*, and *RUNX1*) with potential clinical relevance [6–9].

A multicenter study by Levy and colleagues performed OGM in a cohort of 100 AML cases previously characterized by karyotype alone or karyotype and FISH or CMA [10]. OGM identified clinically relevant genomic abnormalities with 98.4% concordance to routine cytogenetic analysis when clones were present in ≥5% of cells. OGM was also able to identify chromoplexy (characterized by multiple translocations and deletions) which was not detected by conventional cytogenetic analysis. In 6.3% of the cases (3 out of 48 cases) with normal karyotypes reported, OGM uncovered hidden translocations resulting in clinically significant gene fusions. These cases included 2 with a t(5;11)(q35.3;p15.4) translocation leading to a *NUP98::NSD1* fusion and 1 with a t(3;12) (q26.2;p13.2) translocation resulting in an *ETV6::MECOM* fusion. After being initially reported as 46,XY, a subsequent MECOM break-apart FISH probe study identified a MECOM rearrangement without a defined fusion partner by FISH in the t(3;12) (q26.2;p13.2) case. There were 5 cases where the use of OGM resulted in a change in the European Leukemia Net (ELN)-2022 risk classification and could have potentially changed treatment. In one of the cases, cytogenetic studies initially showed a simple karyotype, which led to an intermediate risk classification. However, OGM identified additional chromosomal aberrations, including a 7q deletion, which met the criteria for a complex karyotype. This upgraded the patient's risk from intermediate to adverse. In another case, the ELN risk was upgraded from intermediate to adverse due to the detection of a cryptic *ETV6::MECOM* fusion which was not visible during karyotyping. OGM testing also identified the presence of inv(16) in a case that was not detected by karyotyping, lowering the risk category from intermediate to favorable. In a case, OGM uncovered a cryptic unbalanced der(5)t(4;5) (q26;q21.3) and del(8) (q21.3q22.1) in addition to the classic t(8;21) (q22;q22) translocation leading to *RUNX1::RUNX1T1*. In 8% of the cases, OGM identified additional genomic events that made those cases eligible for clinical trial enrollment. These included the newly detected fusions, as well as additional alterations resulting in a complex karyotype. In a specific case, a *TP53* deletion was suspected in a simple karyotype due to an abnormal banding pattern at 17p. However, OGM changed the designation from simple to complex (which indicates adverse risk) by identifying a deleted 12p that involved *ETV6* and resolving the abnormal 17p as a balanced t(1;17) translocation without any loss of *TP53*. Although this did not change the risk category, it provided crucial information to the clinician that the patient's adverse risk was independent of *TP53*. As a result, the patient could potentially be enrolled in multiple trials that target complex karyotypes in patients with AML.

Tembrink and colleagues [11] used OGM to identify a previously unrecognized fusion of *NUP98* and *ASH1L* in an adult patient with secondary AML, which was a result of a complex structural rearrangement between chromosomes 1 and 11. The case discussed in that study involves secondary AML that developed from a *JAK2*-mutated myelodysplastic syndrome/myeloproliferative neoplasm (MDS/MPN). According to the current World Health Organization (WHO) guidelines, *NUP98* rearrangements are considered a defining genetic abnormality for AML regardless of the fusion partner even if the blast counts are below 20%. However, *NUP98* structural variations are often cryptic in conventional cytogenetic analysis. Although standard FISH diagnostic tests can detect the *NUP98* break-apart, the novel fusion partner would not be routinely detected with standard cytogenetic diagnostic procedures and FISH-panels. This case highlights the benefit OGM provides to deciphering unusual structural variants.

Suttorp and colleagues [12] conducted a study comparing classical cytogenetics to OGM in 24 pediatric patients diagnosed with AML, bi-lineage leukemia, and mixed-phenotype acute leukemia. Due to OGM's higher resolution and whole-genome approach, new alterations were identified and validated to be used as patient-specific markers for minimal residual disease. These alterations include a deletion on chromosome 19 involving the *MEF2B* gene and 2 translocations, t(2;12) and t(8;12), affecting the *ETV6* gene.

Myelodysplastic Syndromes

MDS are a group of myeloid neoplasms that are characterized by cytopenias and a high degree of genetic alterations, ranging from single nucleotide variation (SNVs) to intermediate and large-sized SVs. Recent research in MDS has emphasized the significance of evaluating both somatic mutations and SVs in genomic regions of interest for precise prognosis. A study conducted by Bernard and colleagues [13] delved into the detailed characterization of the *TP53* allelic state in 3,324 MDS patients, examining its implications for disease biology, clinical presentation, and outcomes. The study revealed that two-thirds of *TP53*-mutated patients had multiple hits, such as more than 1 gene SNV, SNV and deletion, or SNV and copy-neutral loss-of-hyperzygosity (CN-LOH), indicating biallelic impact. The study showed that genome instability, treatment resistance, disease progression, and poor outcomes are associated with the multi-hit *TP53* state in MDS, relative to the presence of any 1 *TP53* event.

Yang and colleagues [14] conducted the initial and most comprehensive research to date on the pan-genomic profiling of MDS patients using OGM at diagnosis. The study employed high-resolution structural variant profiling (SVP) via OGM and targeted deep next-generation sequencing (NGS) to assess clinical prognostication and mutation profiling. The group assessed the clinical value of SV detection by OGM in 101 newly diagnosed patients with MDS from a single medical center. The patients underwent standard-of-care cytogenetic and targeted NGS studies. The study found that OGM detected 383 recurrent and novel SVs that were clinically significant. Of these, 224 SVs (51%) were cryptic by chromosomal banding analysis (CBA), which included rearrangements involving *MECOM*, *NUP98::PRRX2*, *KMT2A* partial tandem duplications, among others. These cryptic SVs were observed in 34% of the patients, meaning about a third of them demonstrated such a finding. The study identified 4030 unique somatic variant calls, out of which 383 (9.5%), including 222 CNVs and 161 SVs, were classified as "clinically significant" based on overlap with a gene or region of interest. The study found that OGM identified at least 1 clinically significant SV in 70 out of 101 MDS patients (70%), higher than the 62% identified by CBA. In addition to gene-level alterations, significant structural alterations at the exon-level such as partial tandem duplications involving *KMT2A (KMT2A-PTD)* were detected. Overall, the study demonstrated a 16% decrease in the percentage of MDS patients with normal karyotype (NK) compared to CBA. Specific structural variants in NK cases identified by OGM included *MECOM*, *NUP98:PRRX2*, *KMT2A-PTD*, and deletions encompassing *TET2*, *KMT2A*, and *ETV6*. The integration of data from both NGS and OGM proved to be highly effective in detecting driver alterations in most patients (97 out of 101). The combined SNV and SV profiling was successful in identifying biallelic *TP53* alterations in 3 patients, including a patient with wild-type *TP53* by NGS. Moreover, notable associations such as double *RAS/FLT3* mutations in 2 out of 3 patients with *KMT2A-PTD* were also identified. The study also discovered clinically informative biomarkers, including *TP53* for allele state, *MECOMr*, *NUP98r*, and *KMT2A* alterations, all using solely OGM technology. Overall, OGM-derived results led to modification of the cytogenetic risk for 21% of patients, leading to an overall change in Revised International Prognostic Scoring System (R-IPSS) risk category for 17 (~17%) patients.

Acute Lymphoblastic Leukemia/Lymphoma

Genetic abnormalities are the primary basis for categorizing B-cell lymphoblastic leukemia/lymphoma (B-ALL). The sub-classification of B-ALL/-LBL by the WHO is based on primary genomic abnormalities and defines distinct subgroups. It is worth noting that although only B-ALL has subgroups defined by genetic variants, there are known recurrent genetic events in T-cell lymphoblastic leukemia/lymphoma (T-ALL). These genetic abnormalities can be identified through various techniques such as traditional karyotype or FISH analysis, NGS, or transcriptomics. These ancillary techniques help in identifying, often hidden, abnor malities. Therefore, a comprehensive classification and risk assessment of ALL requires using a combination of genetic techniques in addition to traditional morphologic assessment and immunophenotyping.

Rack and colleagues [15] applied OGM to the diagnostic work-up of 41 ALL cases. Compared to the standard testing pathway, OGM identified all recurrent copy number alterations (CNAs) and SVs and the resulting fusion genes. Based on the results, 32 patients were assigned to a significant cytogenetic risk group, compared to 23 when using the standard approach, which identified 24 out of 34 recurrent chromosomal abnormalities, while OGM identified 33 out of 34. OGM misinterpreted 1 case of low hypodiploidy but was able to identify 10 recurrent SVs in addition to the other SVs detected by standard testing methods. In 1 case of B-ALL, OGM detected a *PAX5* rearrangement which was not identified by karyotype analysis attributable to low-resolution banding. Another case of B-ALL showed an isochromosome for the long arms of chromosome 9 [i(9q)] in poor-quality metaphases which was not identified by OGM, which revealed a t(1;19) *TCF3::PBX1* which was missed by CBA. OGM also solely detected a *EP300::ZNF384* fusion gene, and other translocations involving *PAX5* and *FOXO1*, which may influence the B-ALL outcome. FISH detected gene rearrangements in 7 out of 12 T-ALL cases, but identifying the partner chromosome was difficult even after extensive testing. OGM confirmed these rearrangements and identified the partner gene in all cases.

Vieler and colleagues [16] used OGM to study 9 patients with B-ALL and 2 patients with T-ALL at the time of diagnosis or when the disease was progressing. The results showed that all the genetic alterations previously identified by karyotyping and FISH were confirmed or redefined by OGM. After filtering the data, OGM analysis identified 101 rare SVs and 27 CNVs in the patients studied. The number of clinically significant SVs varied between 1 and 11 per patient, while for CNVs, the range was from 0 to 8 per patient. In 2 patients, aneuploidies of more than 3 chromosomes were detected. In that study, classical karyotyping detected 5 translocations; 1 of them was a t(12;22) (p13;q13) translocation characterized by FISH as a *ZNF384* rearrangement and shown using OGM to have the fusion partner *EP300*. It has been estimated that around 1% of pediatric patients have the rare fusion partner *EP300* [17]. A separate study found that a distinct immune phenotype exists for fusion genes related to *ZNF384*, with low or negative expression for *CD10* and abnormal expression of *CD13* and/or *CD33*, further supporting a unique subtype of B-ALL [18]. *EP300::ZNF384* fusions respond better to steroid monotherapy and conventional chemotherapy, and they do not cause significant elevation of WBC. On the other hand, *ZNF384*-fusions with a different partner gene, *TCF3*, result in an elevated white blood cell (WBC) level and a poor response to prednisolone and conventional chemotherapy [19]. Hence, OGM is also a useful tool for enabling personalized therapy. In this study, OGM was able to detect a ring chromosome 9, which was missed by karyotyping and FISH, through manual inspection of the data. Additionally, in 1 patient, OGM data suggested the presence of an idic(8q), which represents another potential aberration that was not detected in the initial chromosome analysis. In a different patient, who was 35 years old, OGM revealed the presence of a *CUX1::NUTM1* fusion that was not identified during karyotyping. Previously, *NUTM1* rearrangements were only reported in childhood ALL, with a prevalence ranging from 3% to 5% in infants to less than 1% in children and seem to have a favorable prognosis [20].

Lestringant and colleagues [21] compared the effectiveness of OGM to standard techniques (CBA, FISH, single nucleotide polymorphism (SNP)-microarray, multiple ligation-dependent probe amplification [MLPA]) in 10 selected cases of B or T-ALL. The study found that 90% of the anomalies identified using standard techniques were also identified using OGM, which detected 16 anomalies not detected by standard techniques, 7 of which were significant. Standard techniques often overlook some of these anomalies, which are frequently observed in ALL. OGM found a translocation resulting in *MYC* overexpression in 1 case of T-ALL and identified a complex rearrangement involving 3 genes, including *LMO2*, which was overexpressed due to the T-cell receptor alpha (α) (TRA) insertion in a case with *TLX1-TRA*. This study's findings suggest that OGM can be used as a single tool to detect ALL-related cytogenetic anomalies and leads to a better understanding of these complex diseases with the potential for more targeted treatments.

Chronic Lymphocytic Leukemia

Chronic Lymphocytic Leukemia (CLL) is an indolent B cell lymphoproliferative disorder that displays significant clinical and biologic heterogeneity. It can be mild or rapidly progressing, and its severity varies from patient to patient. Fortunately, the development of targeted treatments has significantly improved clinical outcomes for CLL patients. The most common genetic alterations found in patients with CLL/small lymphocytic lymphoma (SLL) are del(11q), del(13q), del(17p), and trisomy 12 [22]. When *TP53* disruption occurs with del(17p), there is frequently accompanying mutations of the other *TP53* allele although a significant portion of cases display *TP53* mutations without del(17p) [23]. Therefore, before initiating any targeted therapy, it is crucial to investigate both *TP53* deletions and other mutations, given such findings can serve as a biomarker that predicts resistance to chemoimmunotherapy. Hence, del(17p) and/or *TP53* mutations have the most significant impact on prognosis and the prediction of therapeutic outcomes, even when targeted agents are used. Clinical studies have also demonstrated the significance of examining the entire genome for SVs in CLL. This is especially important for identifying complex karyotypes or SVs, which are associated with a poor prognosis, and can be involved in the development and progression of CLL. It has been observed in previous studies that CLL is commonly associated with phenomena like chromothripsis and chromoplexy [24]. As such, OGM has been explored as an alternative to classical cytogenetic testing for several types of hematological malignancies, including CLL/SLL, due to its ability to provide high-resolution and comprehensive genome-wide analysis.

The study conducted by Valkama and colleagues [25] provides valuable insights into the accuracy of OGM. The study evaluated 2 techniques, standard-of-care FISH and OGM, and found that the latter was able to reproduce FISH findings in all 18 CLL samples. However, the OGM analysis also revealed novel structural variations and large aberrations outside the FISH-targeted loci in 78% (14/18) of the samples, which were missed by the standard-of-care testing. OGM also identified complex events, including chromothripsis, chromoplexy, and CN-LOH, which are significant in disease diagnosis and progression. Importantly, OGM was able to identify cytogenetic alterations in 4 of the 5 FISH-negative samples, demonstrating the diagnostic value of this technique. These findings highlight the advantages of OGM over the traditional FISH technique for baseline workup of CLL.

Ramos-Campoy et al. [26] conducted a study to compare microarrays and OGM for detecting chromothripsis patterns in CLL patients with complex karyotypes. The study found that OGM technology detected the majority (74/84; 88.1%) of CNAs identified by microarray. In addition, OGM identified more abnormalities than conventional methods including rearrangements involving chromothriptic regions. Puiggros and colleagues [27] studied 42 CLL patients with complex karyotypes using OGM technology which identified 90% of known alterations and provided additional structural information about these aberrations in 55% of the patients. These 2 studies show how OGM can add nuanced differentiation to complex structural aberrations in CLL.

OPTICAL GENOME MAPPING TECHNIQUE AND ANALYSIS

As part of the workflow, ultra-high molecular weight (UHMW) DNA is extracted, labeled, and loaded onto a chip. The current generation (G3 chips) can process up to 3 samples at a time (across 2 chips for a total of 6 in 1 batch). The next generation of OGM instrumentation is poised to do this at scale. Namely, UHMW DNA is enzymatically labeled at specific hexamers motifs (CTTAGG) iterated along the length of the chromosome. This motif repeats every 5000 to 6000 base pairs. The labeled DNA molecules are then loaded onto a chip that further elongates them. The molecules are subsequently passed through a nanochannel array where they are imaged as individual DNA molecules. Each image has a unique pattern of bands, which are then converted into a digital representation that can be bioinformatically processed and assembled into a genome to detect all types of structural rearrangements [28].

There are 2 ways to analyze the digital molecules for structural variations: rare variant assembly and de novo assembly. The main difference between these 2 methods is their ability to detect low-frequency variants and structurally resolve complex events. The rare variant assembly compares the collection of hybrid molecules to the reference genome to identify structural variants, making this method highly sensitive down to about 5% variant allele fraction at 400 $\times$ coverage depth. On the other hand, de novo assembly self-aligns the digitized molecules in a genome assembly, resulting in chromosome structure assembly. While the de novo assembly is less sensitive to rare events, it can detect smaller structural variations and reveal complex structure compared to the rare variant pipeline.

Data visualization is an essential aspect in OGM technology that can be achieved through various methods. Three of the most common methods are the Circos plot, genome browser view, and whole-genome plot. The Circos plot provides a high-level view of the

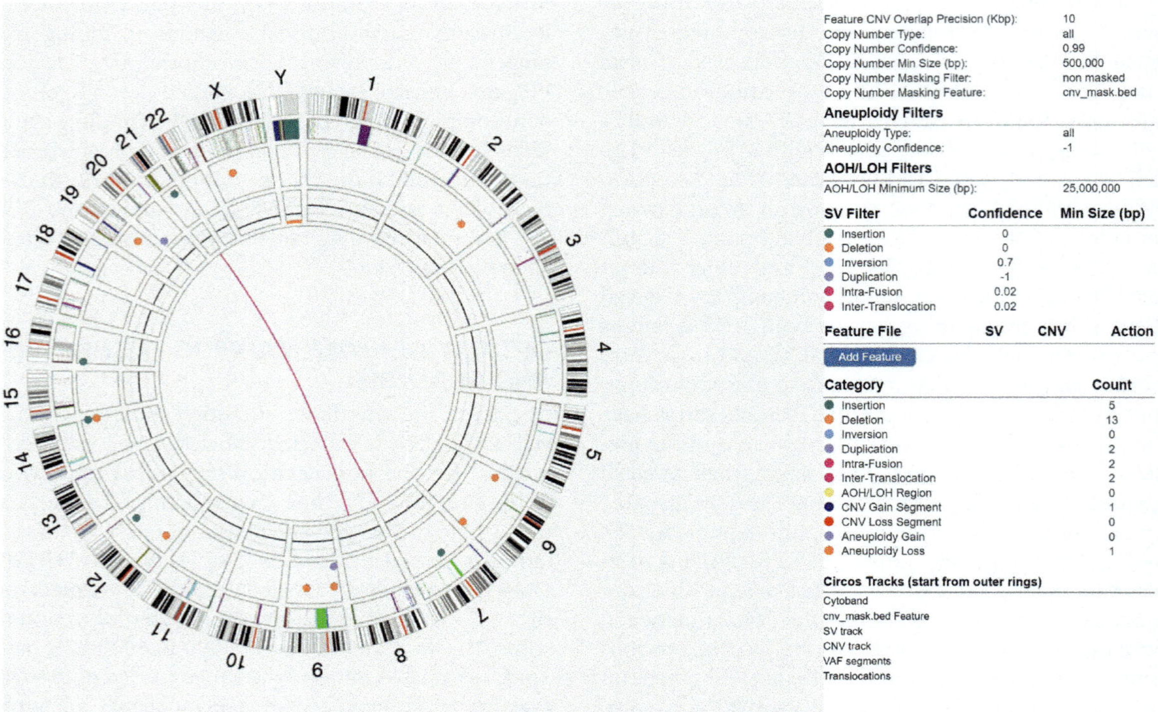

FIG. 1 The optical genome mapping circos plot depicts the classical t(8;21) translocation leading to RUNX1::RUNX1T1 in an acute myeloid leukemia patient.

detected variants, along with the chromosome number, cytobands, structural variant track, CNV track, variant allele fraction profile, and translocation information (Fig. 1). The genome browser view is an interactive visualization tool which enables analysis and visualization of the test molecules against the reference, as well as the ability to zoom into the genes, assess confidence quality scores, and examine number of self-molecules overlapping a given call. Finally, the whole-genome view provides a comprehensive display of aneuploidy, partial gains and losses, LOH, and variant allele fraction (VAF) in 3 separate plots [29]. Recently, the ability to interface these data into separate visualization software (VIA), where structural variant analysis decision trees can be constructed based on disease type, has further streamlined the analysis.

Advantages of Optical Genome Mapping Technique

OGM provides a highly effective way to assess genomic alterations on a genomic scale, which helps complement cytogenetic testing. Chromosome banding analysis typically analyzes 20 metaphases and can be affected by culture bias or artifacts. It also has a banding resolution of about 3 to 10 Mb, depending on the haploid band length, sample type, and chromosome location. However, metaphase chromosome analysis allows single cell resolution with true context that allows reconstructing clonal and sub-clonal events with high sensitivity versus bulk DNA applications. FISH only examines a targeted genomic region, albeit can provide faster turnaround times for diagnostic and prognostic markers of interest. Chromosomal microarrays allow genome-wide copy number detection but cannot detect balanced chromosomal rearrangements such as translocations or inversions.

By using UHMW DNA, OGM approach creates long molecules that result in detection of structural variants ranging from 500 bp to chromosome length alterations while revealing gene-level information. Further, OGM does not rely on polymerase chain reaction (PCR) amplification or tissue culture, bypassing culture or PCR-based artifacts. The ability to detect both balanced and unbalanced events along with aneuploidy and smaller copy number changes in a single assay is a strong advantage of OGM. OGM is particularly useful in identifying rearrangements, including novel ones, involving genes with multiple potential partners in hematological malignancies. When analyzing these rearrangements, traditional methods such as FISH with break-apart probes may require multiple hybridizations, when searching for the partner gene, which can be costly and prohibitive.

OGM compared to standard 30 × whole genome sequencing (WGS) provides higher coverage, enabling the detection of clonal populations in acquired disease as well as low variant allele frequencies more robustly. Furthermore, OGM technology with its user-friendly interface enables intuitive visualization of cytogenomics data making it a reliable tool for detecting structural variations in the genome.

Limitations of Optical Genome Mapping Technique

While the OGM technique has many advantages, it also has some limitations. It cannot detect changes in the haploid sets of chromosomes in a cell, also known as "ploidy changes." To accurately identify ploidy changes impacting the entire chromosome set (eg, tetrasomy), context-based CBA analysis can be pursued. Ploidy changes play a significant role in hematological malignancies, particularly in the diagnosis and prognostic stratification of pediatric ALL or multiple myeloma. Current work is being pursued to enrich plasma cells prior to OGM applications to bridge the gap in hyperdiploidy detection in myelomas, but this also relies on the amount of plasma cell content of the sample.

OGM technology cannot evaluate specimens that have undergone fixation (eg, FFPE) or DNA extracted by conventional methods. Furthermore, OGM does not provide data at the sequence level. This means that additional sequence-based methods are necessary to identify small (<50 bp) variants and insertion/deletion events. Moreover, OGM's ability to identify a large body of SVs may lead to the detection of genomic variations with unknown significance, which poses challenges to current interpretive capabilities. OGM is unable to detect certain chromosome rearrangements, such as balanced whole arm translocations near centromeric regions, and end-to-end telomere fusions. Therefore, these chromosomal changes may not be represented in the Circos plot.

Alternative Technologies to Optical Genome Mapping

Other modern technologies have been explored for the advanced detection of structural variants (Table 1). One example of this is RNA Sequencing (RNA-seq), which involves analyzing transcriptomes to reveal gene expression patterns as well as RNA-based processes. Advantages include evaluation of expression levels in addition to fusion calling [30]. Disadvantages include a suboptimal ability to evaluate copy number alterations [31]. High-through chromosome conformation capture (Hi-C) studies the 3D structure of chromatin, uncovering genome organization and spatial proximity of regulatory elements [32]. Unlike OGM, this assay can be performed on paraffin-embedded tissues. A

TABLE 1
Advantages and Disadvantages of Structural Variant Detection Methods

	Optical Genome Mapping	RNA-seq	High-Through Chromosome Conformation Capture	Whole Genome Sequencing
Advantages	Genome-wide structural and copy number variant analysis	Ability to obtain expression data and structural events (fusions); works on formalin-fixed paraffin-embedded (FFPE).	Ability to reconstruct 3D structural domains (TADs); works on FFPE	Comprehensive technique which obtains single base pair and structural variants resolution
Disadvantages	Incompatible with formalin-fixed tissue and does not have single base resolution	Problems with CNA; RNA abundance	Only capable of providing chromatin interactions—does not provide true structure. Limited analysis and experience in the clinical space	Coverage issues; limitations in separating clonal events

Abbreviations: CNA, copy number alterations; TAD, topologically associating domain.

disadvantage Hi-C is that analysis relies on visual inspection limiting its use to predefined regions [33]. Bioinformatic pipelines and packages continue to evolve for Hi-C data analysis [34]. Whole Genome Sequencing (WGS) examines entire genomes, providing comprehensive data analysis including single base pair resolution, as well as structural variants. Disadvantages include depth of coverage issues limiting sensitivity for structural alterations, some of which can be overcome with deeper sequencing [35]. In summary, optical genome mapping focuses on DNA structure, RNA-seq captures gene expression, and Hi-C reveals chromatin organization and topology, while WGS offers detailed sequence-level information. From a research standpoint, combining these techniques can allow holistic insights into genome structure, function, and regulation.

SUMMARY

Diagnosing hematological malignancies can be challenging, and it often requires a cascade of cytogenetic and molecular tests to analyze multiple clinically significant genomic variants, including genome-wide structural variation. OGM provides the ability to more efficiently and comprehensively diagnose, prognosticate, and treat hematolymphoid neoplasms. OGM is a cost-effective, non-sequencing-based technique that offers a high-resolution and comprehensive approach to detect structural variations in a single test. This system can also overcome several limitations of standard techniques, making it an attractive solution for clinical laboratories toward a more constructive and beneficial outcome for patients.

DISCLOSURE

No financial or commercial conflicts of interests to declare.

REFERENCES

[1] Shallis RM, Wang R, Davidoff A, et al. Epidemiology of acute myeloid leukemia: Recent progress and enduring challenges. Blood Rev 2019;36:70–87.
[2] Gerding WM, Tembrink M, Nilius-Eliliwi V, et al. Optical genome mapping reveals additional prognostic information compared to conventional cytogenetics in AML/MDS patients. Int J Cancer 2022;150(12):1998–2011.
[3] Mohanty S, Jyotsana N, Sharma A, et al. Targeted Inhibition of the NUP98-NSD1 Fusion Oncogene in Acute Myeloid Leukemia. Cancers (Basel) 2020;12(10):2766.
[4] Ries RE, Leonti AR, Triche TJ Jr, et al. Structural Variants Involving MLLT10/AF10 Are Associated with Adverse Outcome in AML Regardless of the Partner Gene - a COG/Tpaml Study. Blood 2019;134(Supplement_1): 461.
[5] Forgione MO, McClure BJ, Yeung DT, et al. MLLT10 rearranged acute leukemia: incidence, prognosis, and possible therapeutic strategies. Genes Chromosomes Cancer 2020; 59(12):709–21.
[6] Döhner K, Tobis K, Ulrich R, et al. Prognostic significance of partial tandem duplications of the MLL gene in adult patients 16 to 60 years old with acute myeloid leukemia and normal cytogenetics: a study of the Acute Myeloid Leukemia Study Group Ulm. J Clin Oncol 2002; 20(15):3254–61.
[7] Steudel C, Wermke M, Schaich M, et al. Comparative analysis of MLL partial tandem duplication and FLT3 internal tandem duplication mutations in 956 adult patients with acute myeloid leukemia. Genes Chromosomes Cancer 2003;37(3):237–51.
[8] Dicker F, Haferlach C, Sundermann J, et al. Mutation analysis for RUNX1, MLL-PTD, FLT3-ITD, NPM1 and NRAS in 269 patients with MDS or secondary AML. Leukemia 2010;24(8):1528–32.
[9] Antherieu G, Bidet A, Huet S, et al. Allogenic Stem Cell Transplantation Abrogates Negative Impact on Outcome of AML Patients with KMT2A Partial Tandem Duplication. Cancers (Basel) 2021;13(9):2272.
[10] Levy B, Baughn LB, Akkari Y, et al. Optical genome mapping in acute myeloid leukemia: a multicenter evaluation. Blood Adv 2023;7(7):1297–307.
[11] Tembrink M, Gerding WM, Wieczorek S, et al. Novel NUP98::ASH1L Gene Fusion in Acute Myeloid Leukemia Detected by Optical Genome Mapping. Cancers 2023; 15(11):2942.
[12] Suttorp J, Lühmann JL, Behrens YL, et al. Optical Genome Mapping as a Diagnostic Tool in Pediatric Acute Myeloid Leukemia. Cancers (Basel) 2022;14(9):2058.
[13] Bernard E, Nannya Y, Hasserjian RP, et al. Implications of TP53 allelic state for genome stability, clinical presentation and outcomes in myelodysplastic syndromes. Nat Med 2020;26(10):1549–56.
[14] Yang H, Garcia-Manero G, Sasaki K, et al. High-resolution structural variant profiling of myelodysplastic syndromes by optical genome mapping uncovers cryptic aberrations of prognostic and therapeutic significance. Leukemia 2022;36(9):2306–16.
[15] Rack K, De Bie J, Ameye G, et al. Optimizing the diagnostic workflow for acute lymphoblastic leukemia by optical genome mapping. Am J Hematol 2022;97(5):548–61.
[16] Vieler LM, Nilius-Eliliwi V, Schroers R, et al. Optical Genome Mapping Reveals and Characterizes Recurrent Aberrations and New Fusion Genes in Adult ALL. Genes (Basel) 2023;14(3):686.
[17] Gocho Y, Kiyokawa N, Ichikawa H, et al. A novel recurrent EP300-ZNF384 gene fusion in B-cell precursor acute lymphoblastic leukemia. Leukemia 2015;29(12):2445–8.

[18] Hirabayashi S, Ohki K, Nakabayashi K, et al. ZNF384-related fusion genes define a subgroup of childhood B-cell precursor acute lymphoblastic leukemia with a characteristic immunotype. Haematologica 2017; 102(1):118–29.

[19] Zhu L, Bai W, Cheng Q, et al. ZNF384-Related Fusion Genes in Acute Lymphoblastic Leukemia. Cancer Control 2023;30:10732748231182787.

[20] Boer JM, Valsecchi MG, Hormann FM, et al. Favorable outcome of NUTM1-rearranged infant and pediatric B cell precursor acute lymphoblastic leukemia in a collaborative international study. Leukemia 2021;35(10): 2978–82.

[21] Lestringant V, Duployez N, Penther D, et al. Optical genome mapping, a promising alternative to gold standard cytogenetic approaches in a series of acute lymphoblastic leukemias. Genes Chromosomes Cancer 2021; 60(10):657–67.

[22] Döhner H, Stilgenbauer S, Benner A, et al. Genomic aberrations and survival in chronic lymphocytic leukemia. N Engl J Med 2000;343(26):1910–6.

[23] Campo E, Cymbalista F, Ghia P, et al. TP53 aberrations in chronic lymphocytic leukemia: an overview of the clinical implications of improved diagnostics. Haematologica 2018;103(12):1956–68.

[24] Zavacka K, Plevova K. Chromothripsis in Chronic Lymphocytic Leukemia: A Driving Force of Genome Instability. Front Oncol 2021;11:771664.

[25] Valkama A, Vorimo S, Kumpula TA, et al. Optical Genome Mapping as an Alternative to FISH-Based Cytogenetic Assessment in Chronic Lymphocytic Leukemia. Cancers (Basel) 2023;15(4):1294.

[26] Ramos-Campoy S, Puiggros A, Kamaso J, et al. TP53 Abnormalities Are Underlying the Poor Outcome Associated with Chromothripsis in Chronic Lymphocytic Leukemia Patients with Complex Karyotype. Cancers (Basel) 2022;14(15):3715.

[27] Puiggros A, Ramos-Campoy S, Kamaso J, et al. Optical Genome Mapping: A Promising New Tool to Assess Genomic Complexity in Chronic Lymphocytic Leukemia (CLL). Cancers (Basel) 2022;14(14):3376.

[28] Smith AC, Neveling K, Kanagal-Shamanna R. Optical genome mapping for structural variation analysis in hematologic malignancies. Am J Hematol 2022;97(7): 975–82.

[29] Genomics B. Visualizing-Different-Classes-of-Structural-Variants-in-Bionano-Access-Software. 2022. Bionano Genomics Inc website.

[30] Tran TH, Langlois S, Meloche C, et al. Whole-transcriptome analysis in acute lymphoblastic leukemia: a report from the DFCI ALL Consortium Protocol 16-001. Blood Advances 2022;6(4):1329–41.

[31] Brown LM, Lonsdale A, Zhu A, et al. The application of RNA sequencing for the diagnosis and genomic classification of pediatric acute lymphoblastic leukemia. Blood Advances 2020;4(5):930–42.

[32] Denker A, de Laat W. The second decade of 3C technologies: detailed insights into nuclear organization. Genes & Development 2016;30(12):1357–82.

[33] Lestringant V, Guermouche-Flament H, Jimenez-Pocquet M, et al. Cytogenetics in the management of hematological malignancies: an overview of alternative technologies for cytogenetic characterization. Current Research in Translational Medicine 2024;103440.

[34] Serizay J, Matthey-Doret C, Bignaud A, et al. Orchestrating chromosome conformation capture analysis with Bioconductor. Nat Commun 2024;15(1):1072.

[35] Duncavage EJ, Schroeder MC, O'Laughlin M, et al. Genome Sequencing as an Alternative to Cytogenetic Analysis in Myeloid Cancers. N Engl J Med 2021; 384(10):924–35.

Advances in Molecular Pathology 7 (2024) 63–75
ADVANCES IN MOLECULAR PATHOLOGY

Recent Advances in the Molecular Pathogenesis and Diagnosis of Chronic Myelomonocytic Leukemia

Michele Anderson, DO[a], Rajeswari Jayakumar, MD[a,*]
[a]Department of Pathology, Virginia Commonwealth University, 1101 East Marshall Street, Richmond, VA 23298-0662, USA

KEYWORDS
• Chronic myelomonocytic leukemia • CMML • Monocytosis • Post-CMML acute leukemia
• Prognostication of CMML

KEY POINTS

- Purpose of Review: Chronic myelomonocytic leukemia (CMML) is a clonal hematopoietic malignancy defined by both proliferative and dysplastic features, monocytosis and a predilection for leukemic transformation. CMML is a poorly understood neoplasm with an overall dismal prognosis, and minimal treatment options.
- This review aims to summarize the diagnostic features in the updated World Health Organization 5th Edition (WHO5), molecular findings in CMML, and current prognostic models, as well as provide recommendations for future studies.
- The 2022 WHO5 and the International Consensus Classification have both demonstrated emphasis on molecular studies and this will likely only increase in future as targeted therapy continues to develop.

INTRODUCTION

Chronic myelomonocytic leukemia (CMML) is a clonal hematopoietic stem cell neoplasm characterized by monocytosis, dysplasia, evidence of clonality, and acquired somatic mutations [1]. It is currently classified as a myelodysplastic/myeloproliferative neoplasm (MDS/MPN) and is the most common hematologic malignancy in this category. The overall incidence of CMML is 12.8 cases per 100,000 persons per year with a male predominance and average age of 65 to 75 year old and a median survival of 20 to 40 months [1]. CMML has an inherent risk of transformation to acute myeloid leukemia (AML), with transformation occurring in ∼15-30% of patients [1]. It is heterogenous in disease presentation and can demonstrate morphologic and clinical overlap with other MDS and MPN [2,3]. At this time, a defining molecular event has not been identified, thus CMML diagnosis and subsequent risk stratification relies on a thorough assessment of clinical findings, morphologic features, cytogenetic aberrations, and molecular alterations. Recurrent somatic mutations have been found in up to 90% of cases of CMML and most commonly include *TET2*, *SRSF2*, *ASXL1*, and *RAS* [1–3]. To date, treatment options are limited. This literature review will discuss updates to the World Health Organization (WHO) classification, describe any variation from the International Consensus Classification (ICC) guidelines and review the cytogenetic and molecular landscape of CMML.

*Corresponding author. VCU Health, CSC 6th floor, Room 665k, 403 North 13th street, Richmond, VA 23298. *E-mail address:* rajeswari.jayakumar@vcuhealth.org

https://doi.org/10.1016/j.yamp.2024.07.001 www.advancesinmolecularpathology.com
2589-4080/24/

DIAGNOSIS AND CLASSIFICATION

In 2022, the WHO released the beta version of the 5th edition of the WHO Classification of Haematolymphoid Tumors (WHO5). Included in this update, is a revision of the diagnostic criteria of CMML. The current requirements are presented in Box 1. The first prerequisite is the presence of persistent absolute (greater than or equal to 0.5 x 10^9/L) and relative (≥10%) peripheral blood monocytosis [1]. This decrease in the cutoff for absolute monocytosis from greater than or equal to 1 x 10^9/L to greater than or equal to 0.5 x 10^9/L is meant to include cases that were formally referred to as "oligomonocytic CMML" [1,4,5]. The second requirement is a blast count of less than 20% in both the peripheral blood and bone marrow. The third and fourth requirements are the absence of diagnostic criteria of chronic myeloid leukemia or MPN and myeloid/lymphoid neoplasms with tyrosine kinase fusions or molecular abnormalities of *PDGFRA, PDGFRB* and *PCM1::JAK2* [1].

The supporting criteria are also displayed in Box 1 and include: (1) Dysplasia involving greater than 1 myeloid lineage, (2) Acquired clonal cytogenetic or molecular abnormality, and (3) Abnormal partitioning of peripheral blood monocyte subsets. Regarding the second supporting criterion, both the ICC and the WHO5 include the presence of mutations and cytogenetic abnormalities as evidence of clonality [1,6]. The third supporting criteria is new in the WHO5 and is included as most patients with CMML show an expansion of classical monocytes (MO1-, CD14+/CD16-) [1,7]. The number of supporting criteria required for diagnosis is determined based on the level of absolute monocytosis, requiring at least one supporting criterion if the absolute monocytosis is greater than or equal to1 x 10^9/L, and requiring supporting criteria #1 and #2 if absolute monocytosis is less than 1 x 10^9/L to enhance diagnostic accuracy [1].

In 2001 and 2008, the WHO classification scheme recognized CMML as a MDS/MPN with subclassification

BOX 1
The World Health Organization (WHO) 2022 Diagnostic Criteria for Chronic Myelomonocytic Leukemia (CMML)

Diagnostic Criteria WHO5

Pre-requisite Criteria

- Persistent absolute (greater than or equal to 0.5 x 10^9/L) and relative (≥10%) peripheral blood monocytosis.
- Blasts less than 20% in PB and BM.
- Not meeting diagnostic criterion of CML or other MPN[a].
- Not meeting diagnostic criterion of myeloid/lymphoid neoplasms with eosinophilia and defining gene rearrangements[b].

Supporting criteria

- Dysplasia involving greater than or equal to 1 myeloid lineage.
- Acquired clonal cytogenetic or molecular abnormality[c].
- Abnormal partitioning of peripheral blood monocyte subsets.

Requirements for diagnosis

- Pre-requisite criteria must be present in all cases.
- If monocytosis is greater than or equal to 1 x 10^9/L; greater than or equal to 1 supporting criterion must be met.
- If monocytosis is less than 1 x 10^9/L; supporting criteria 1 and 2 must be met.

Subtyping criteria

- MDS CMML (MD-CMML): WBC count less than 13 x 10^9/L.
- Myeloproliferative CMML (MP-CMML): WBC count greater than or equal to 13 x 10^9/L.

Subgrouping criteria (based on percentage of blasts and promonocytes)

- CMML-1: less than 5% PB and less than 10% BM.
- CMML-2: 6% to 19% PB and 10% to 19% BM.

Abbreviations: BM, bone marrow; CML, chronic myeloid leukemia; MPN, myeloproliferative neoplasms; PB, peripheral blood.[a] A documented history of MPN excludes a diagnosis of CMML, and the presence of MPN features or high burden of MPN associated mutations (JAK2, CALR or MPL) favor an MPN.[b] Defining gene rearrangements include PDGFRA, PDGFRB, FGFR1, or JAK2[c] See Box 4.

Khoury, J.D., Solary, E., Abla, O. et al. The 5th edition of the World Health Organization Classification of Haematolymphoid Tumours: Myeloid and Histiocytic/Dendritic Neoplasms. Leukemia 36, 1703–1719 (2022). https://doi.org/10.1038/s41375-022-01613-1

of CMML-1 and CMML-2 based on percentages of blasts in peripheral blood and bone marrow. In the 2016 update, the WHO included further classification into myeloproliferative CMML (MP-CMML) and MDS CMML (MD-CMML), as well as a 3-tier classification defined by percentage of blasts (CMML-0, CML-1, and CMML-2). In the updated WHO5 and 2022 ICC, the 3-tier blast count subgrouping was reversed to the 2-tier system, as the prognostic impact was not found to be significant between CMML-0 and CMML-1 [1,4,6]. The WHO5 subgrouping defines CMML-1 as less than 5% in peripheral blood and less than 10% in the bone marrow, and CMML-2 as 6% to 19% in the peripheral blood and 10% to 19% in the bone marrow. Included in the 5th edition is the official recognition of 2 defined subtypes of MDS CMML (defined by white blood cell [WBC] count of less than 13 x 10^9/L) and a myeloproliferative CMML (defined by WBC count $\geq$13 x 10^9/L) [1]. The specific cutoff, however, is debated as it is often viewed as arbitrary [8,9] and was initially suggested in 1994 by the French-American-British cooperative group [10]. To date, no specific molecular or cytogenetic findings have been identified as defining alterations to distinguish the subtypes MD-CMML versus MP-CMML, however there are studies [2,9,11] which have investigated and determined that there are true biologic differences between these 2 entities [9]. There have been several studies demonstrating their different prognostic, molecular and clinical presentations [2,9,11,12]. The 2022 WHO diagnostic criteria for CMML are summarized in Box 1 [1].

In contrast to the WHO5 criteria, the ICC requires the presence of a persistent monocytosis, defined as greater than or equal to 0.5 $\times$ 10^9/L and greater than or equal to 10%, the presence of cytopenia, and evidence of clonality with either abnormal cytogenetics or an associated mutation with a variant allele frequency (VAF) of greater than or equal to 10%. The ICC diagnostic criteria are summarized in Box 2 [6]. Additionally, in cases that do not fulfill CMML criteria, but present with a persistent monocytosis, absence of cytopenia, or no significant dysplasia or a VAF of less than 10% are instead classified as clonal monocytosis of undetermined significance (CMUS) [6]. The criteria by the ICC for CMUS are presented in Box 3.

It is important to differentiate CMML from other causes of monocytosis including infectious causes, autoimmune, or connective tissue disorders [1,3]. Additionally, identification of monocytosis can be associated with MPN such as chronic myeloid leukemia or myeloid/lymphoid neoplasms with defined genetic rearrangements such as *PDGFRA* mutations [1,3]. These specific cases have been re-defined due to their response to targeted treatments. In the updated WHO guidelines, the absolute monocyte count has been reduced from greater than or equal to 1 x 10^9/L to greater than or equal to 0.5 x 10^9/L. This has potential impacts on the diagnostic and, by association, the molecular and prognostic distinctions of previously defined "myeloproliferative neoplasms with monocytosis." This is particularly important for patients with monocytosis associated with polycythemia vera who are more commonly been found to have unfavorable cytogenetic abnormalities, *TET2* and *SRSF2* mutations, and patients with primary myelofibrosis associated with monocytosis and a higher frequency of *ASXL1* mutations [3,13].

CYTOGENETIC ABNORMALITIES

Clonal cytogenetic alterations are detected in a subset of cases of CMML, accounting for 20% to 30% of cases [14–18]. These alterations most commonly include trisomy 8, -Y, −7/del(7q), −21 and complex karyotype [3]. Of these, trisomy 8 and monosomy 7 are most frequent, with complex karyotypes being rarely identified. Though these are non-specific to CMML, they may aid in the establishment of a clonal neoplastic process. It is notable that these karyotypic abnormalities are more commonly identified in secondary or therapy related CMML versus *de novo* CMML [3]. These findings were utilized by the Spanish CMML specific cytogenetic risk stratification system to aid in prognostication [3]. The Spanish CMML specific risk stratification system is summarized in Table 1. In 2018 recommendations from the European LeukemiaNet and European Hematology Association were published and included 5 risk stratification systems which include CMML-specific prognostic scoring system (CPSS-Mol) [2], Mayo Molecular Model [19], Groupe Francophone des Myelodysplasies (GFM) [20], MD Anderson Prognostic Score (MDAPS) [14] and CMML Prognostic Scoring System (CPSS) [16]. Of these, only 3 include both cytogenetic abnormalities and recurrent somatic mutations and are the preferred risk stratification models, these are CPSS-Mol, Mayo Molecular Model and GFM [21]. Both CPSS-Mol and the Mayo Molecular Model incorporate *ASXL1* only with specific mutational variation including frameshift or nonsense mutations, while GFM includes any *ASXL1* mutations [21]. This has been criticized as further data involving prognosis of specific mutations have been discovered. Of note, only the CPSS-Mol incorporates mutations other than *ASXL1* mutations, and includes *NRAS*, *RUNX1*, and *SETBP1* in addition to *ASXL1* [2].

BOX 2
ICC Diagnostic Criteria for CMML

- Monocytosis defined as monocytes greater than or equal to 0.5×10^9/L and greater than or equal to 10% of the WBC.
- Cytopenia (thresholds same as MDS)[a].
- Blasts (including promonocytes) less than 20% of the cells in blood and bone marrow.
- Presence of clonality: abnormal cytogenetics and/or presence of at least 1 myeloid neoplasm associated mutation of at least 10% allele frequency.
- In cases without evidence of clonality,
  - Monocytes greater than or equal to 1.0×10^9/L and greater than 10% of the WBC and increased blasts (including promonocytes) greater than or equal to 5% in the bone marrow and/or greater than or equal to 2% in the peripheral blood.

    Or
  - Morphologic dysplasia, or an abnormal immunophenotype consistent with CMML would be required for its diagnosis.
- Bone marrow examination with morphologic findings consistent with CMML (hypercellularity due to a myeloid proliferation often with increased monocytes), and lacking diagnostic features of AML, MPN or other conditions associated with monocytosis[a].
- No BCR::ABL1 or genetic abnormalities of myeloid/lymphoid neoplasms with eosinophilia and tyrosine kinase gene fusions.

[a] In such cases, a diagnosis of CMUS could be considered. If cytopenia is present, a diagnosis of clonal cytopenia with monocytosis of undetermined significance (CCMUS) could be entertained. In these diagnostic settings, however, an alternative cause for the observed monocytosis would have to be excluded based on appropriate clinicopathologic correlations.

Adapted from Arber, D. A., et al., (2022). International Consensus Classification of Myeloid Neoplasms and Acute Leukemias: integrating morphologic, clinical, and genomic data. Blood, 140(11), 1200–1228.

Molecular Landscape

In recent years, there has been a dramatic increase in the molecular evaluation of CMML, due to routine next generation sequencing. CMML has a complex genetic landscape which is important to evaluate for prognosis, risk assessment and treatment strategies. Routine sequencing of suspected CMML cases is recommended. No single mutation defines CMML, but it has been shown that in roughly 90% of cases, at least 1 molecular abnormality/mutation can be identified [3,18,22]. Historically, CMML has been described as a disease of aging and some mutations have been found in elderly patients who previously did not fulfill the diagnostic criteria for CMML. However, these patients had similar immunophenotype and overall survival, irrespective of CMML diagnosis [7,23]. In ~20% of cases of CMML, patients present with an autoimmune or systemic inflammatory syndrome prior to diagnosis [1,24]. It is suspected that, as this is also seen in Clonal hematopoiesis of indeterminate potential (CHIP) and other MDS syndromes, systemic inflammation may be involved

BOX 3
ICC Diagnostic Criteria for Clonal Monocytosis of Undetermined Significance

- Persistent monocytosis defined as monocytes greater than or equal to 0.5×10^9/L and greater than or equal to 10% of the WBC.
- Absence or presence of cytopenia (thresholds same as for MDS).
- Presence of at least 1 myeloid neoplasm associated mutation of appropriate allele frequency (ie, $\geq$2%).
- No significant dysplasia, increased blasts (including promonocytes) or morphologic findings of CMML on bone marrow examination.
- No criteria for a myeloid or other hematopoietic neoplasm are fulfilled.
- No reactive condition that would explain a monocytosis is detected.

Adapted from Arber, D. A., et al., (2022). International Consensus Classification of Myeloid Neoplasms and Acute Leukemias: integrating morphologic, clinical, and genomic data. Blood, 140(11), 1200–1228.

TABLE 1
Summary of Spanish CMML Specific Cytogenetic Risk Stratification System [3]

Risk Category	Cytogenetic Findings
Low	Normal karyotype or -Y
Intermediate	All other abnormalities not defined as high or low risk
High	+8, abnormalities of chromosome 7 and complex karyotype

Adapted from Patnaik, M. M., & Tefferi, A. (2022). Chronic myelomonocytic leukemia: 2022 update on diagnosis, risk stratification, and management. American journal of hematology, 97(3), 352–372. https://doi.org/10.1002/ajh.26455

in the pathogenesis of these [24]. Mutations may be seen at low VAF in the setting of CHIP, and several different cutoffs have been suggested to differentiate CHIP versus MDS or MDS/MPN [25]. It has been demonstrated that greater than or equal to 2 mutations at a VAF of greater than or equal to 10% or greater than or equal to 1 mutation at a VAF of greater than or equal to 20% have a positive predictive value of 100%, negative predictive value of 38%, sensitivity of 60% and specificity of 100%. Presence of greater than or equal to 1 mutation or abnormal cytogenetics/FISH improve the sensitivity and negative predictive value (96%) without reducing the positive predictive value (96%) [23].

The ICC has identified CMUS and clonal cytopenia with monocytosis of undetermined significance (CCMUS) to be CMML precursor conditions. This entity was introduced in the 2022 ICC Hematopathology update to classify a neoplastic process, not yet meeting the criteria for CMML. The diagnostic criteria include the following.

- Persistent monocytosis (>0.5 x10^9/L and >10% of white blood cells).
- Absence or presence of cytopenias.
- Presence of 1 myeloid neoplasm-associated mutation of appropriate allele frequency as determined by the International Consensus Group Conference, Vienna, 2018.
- No significant dysplasia, increased blasts or morphologic findings of CMML on bone marrow.
- Absence of reactive conditions leading to a monocytosis.
- Not meeting criteria for other myeloid or hematopoietic neoplasm [6,23].

Mutations acquired by patients with diagnoses of CMML have been found in the following categories: epigenetic modifiers, cell signaling, mRNA splicing, DNA repair and transcription factors [2,3,26]. The most common mutations in CMML are *TET2* (60%), *SRSF2* (50%), *ASXL1* (40%), and genes of the *RAS* pathway (*KRAS, NRAS, PTPN11, NF1*) (30%) [3]. It has been shown that over 90% of individuals with CMML will have somatic gene mutations, while about 30% exhibit clonal cytogenetic abnormalities [3].

Several studies have identified the most common ancestral mutations to be found in *TET2* and *ASXL1* [27,28]. In a study by Palomo and colleagues, it was found that ancestral *TET2* mutations were found most frequently, followed by *SRSF2* and *ASXL1*. *TET2* ancestral mutations were found frequently associated with a combination of bi-allelic *TET2* and *TET2-SRSF2* mutations [27]. Current studies suggest a stepwise accumulation of mutations with *TET2* or *ASXL1* first, followed by spliceosome component mutations (eg, *SRSF2*), followed by transcription factor mutations (*RUNX1*) and then signal pathway mutations (eg, *RAS, CBL*) [28]. However, in a recent study by Carr, and colleagues, it was shown that specifically in MP-CMML, *RAS* pathway mutations appear early in the disease course, rather than a secondary mutation [9]. Mutations in *RUNX1, NRAS, SETBP1,* and *ASXL1* are all independently associated with impact on overall survival [2,3,23]. A schematic representation of the pathway of CMML is presented in Fig. 1.

A recommended minimal next-generation sequencing panel has been modified from the WHO5 and is presented in Box 4.

Post-Chronic Myelomonocytic Leukemia Acute Leukemia

There is an inherent risk of leukemic transformation in ~13-30% of CMML cases [3]. In a recent study by Montalban-Bravo et. el., they examined the genomic profiles and clonal evolution of CMML in 189 patients [29]. They identified 3 distinct pathways of AML with blast phenotypes including monocytic (Mo-AML), myeloid (My-AML) and erythroid (Ery-AML). Mo-AML is defined by the presence of *SRSF2, TET2,* and *RAS* pathway co-dominance and were more likely to evolve from *SRSF2-TET2* co-mutation. In My-AML, *CEBPA* mutations were more frequent, and Ery-AML is defined by complex karyotypes and *TP53* mutations [29]. The most common chromosomal abnormality for post-CMML AML was trisomy 8. Mo-AML demonstrated specific cytogenetic abnormalities including trisomy 1 and der [1]q [10,29]. These findings are significant and highlight potential therapeutic targets.

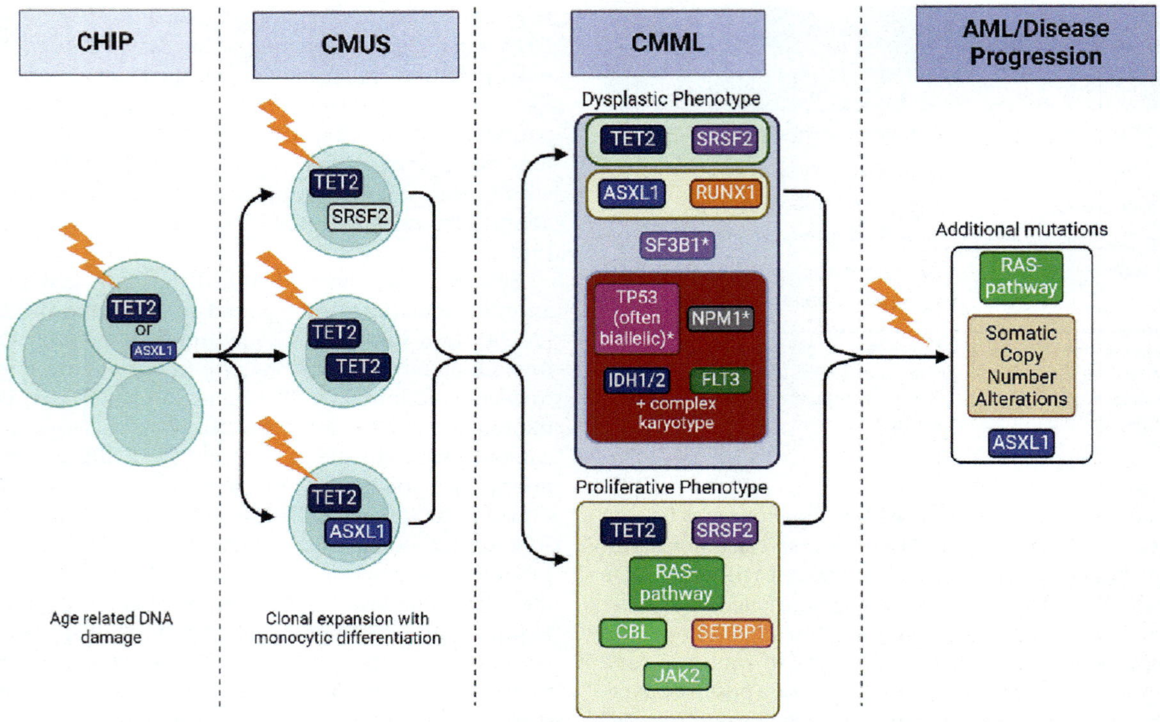

FIG. 1 Schematic representation of current CMML pathways. Large boxes represent risk group and include low risk (*light green*), intermediate risk (*yellow*), and high risk (*red*). Smaller boxes represent class of mutation. Cell signaling-green, Epigenetic modifiers—blue, mRNA splicing-purple, DNA repair—pink, Transcription factors—orange and Other—gray. * Mutations defined in AML and MDS neoplasms. (Created with BioRender.com)

MYELOPROLIFERATIVE-CHRONIC MYELOMONOCYTIC LEUKEMIA VERSUS MYELODYSPLASTIC-CHRONIC MYELOMONOCYTIC LEUKEMIA

MP-CMML is an aggressive subtype of CMML presenting with higher leukocyte counts and an overall worse prognosis compared to the MDS subtype [1–3,8,12]. Patients with MP-CMML typically present with organomegaly, cachexia, and constitutional symptoms including night sweats and weight loss [1–3], with higher bone marrow cellularity, and lower median survival versus the MDS subtype (31 months vs 16 months) [12]. MP-CMML is commonly, and uniquely characterized by mutations in the *RAS/MAPK* pathway, specifically the *RAS-KMT2A-PLK1* axis as a potential founding mutation [3,9], and ~70% of cases demonstrate mutations in this pathway [4]. MP-CMML also demonstrated a higher frequency of *ASXL1* and *JAK2* mutations as well as cytogenetic findings of trisomy 8 as compared to MDS CMML (MD-CMML) [4]. Importantly, *ASLX1* mutations have been associated with an overall poor survival and more frequent progression to acute leukemia [3,19]. In a study by Bhumika, and colleagues ancestral mutations involving *SETBP1*, *JAK2*, *SRSF2* and *NRAS* were only identified in cases of MP-CMML. Other studies have identified similar findings, implicating *TET2*, *SRSF2* or *RAS* mutations [3,30].

MD-CMML is a subtype of CMML, defined by a white blood cell count of less than 13 x 10^9/L, along with the previously described findings. MD-CMML more commonly exhibits mutations in *SF3B1* and *U2AF1* [30]. MD-CMML also demonstrated a slightly higher frequency of *TET2* mutations (54% vs 43% in MP-CMML) [3]. In a study of 150 CMML patients, next generation sequencing evaluation identified ancestral mutations involving *SF3B1*, *DNMT3A*, *STAG2*, and *CBL* in cases of MD-CMML and not MP-CMML [30]. In analysis of individual mutations, *SF3B1* mutations were also associated with improved outcomes and better overall survival [31,32]. It is notable, however, that in the updated WHO and ICC guidelines, in the presence of an *SF3B1* mutation, these cases may be more appropriately categorized as MDS with low blasts [1] or MDS with *SF3B1* mutation.

BOX 4
Recurrent Mutations and Frequencies Found in CMML

Molecular Abnormalities in CMML

Epigenetic Modifiers
- *TET2* (29%–61%)
- *ASXL1*[a] (32%–44%) [b]
- *DNMT3A* (2%–12%)[b]
- *EZH2*[a] (5%–13%)
- *IDH1* (1%–2%)
- *IDH2* (6%–7%)
- *BCOR*[a] (6%–7%)

Cell Signaling
- *CBL*[a](8%–22%)
- *NRAS*[a] (4%–22%)
- *KRAS*[a] (7%–16%)
- *JAK2* (1%–10%)
- *FLT3* (1%–3%)

mRNA splicing
- *SRSF2*[a] (29%–52%)
- *SF3B1*[a] (6%–10%)
- *U2AF1*[a] (4%–10%)
- *ZRSR2*[a] (4%–8%)

DNA repair
- *PHF6* (5%)
- *TP53* (<1%)

Transcription Factors
- *RUNX1*[a] (8%–23%)[b]
- *SETBP1*[a] (4%–18%)[b]

Other
- *NPM1*[a] (1%–3%)[b,c]

[a] 1 or more required for diagnosis if monocytosis is less than 1 x 10^9/L.[b] Have been associated with poor prognosis (Hussein).[c] Unclear implications of finding this mutation, due to re-classification of AML categories with defined genetic abnormalities.

Khoury, J.D., Solary, E., Abla, O. et al. The 5th edition of the World Health Organization Classification of Haematolymphoid Tumours: Myeloid and Histiocytic/Dendritic Neoplasms. Leukemia 36, 1703–1719 (2022). https://doi.org/10.1038/s41375-022-01613-1

A recent study presented at the 65th American Society of Hematology Annual Meeting in 2023 demonstrated a proof of concept for a molecular classification of CMML [33]. This study evaluated 2471 patients with CMML and identified 5 distinct subgroups with varying phenotypic, molecular features, overall survival and leukemia-free survival.

MUTATIONS IN EPIGENETIC REGULATOR GENES AFFECTING DNA METHYLATION AND HYDROXY METHYLATION (*TET2, DNMT3A, IDH1 AND IDH2*)

10-11 translocation 2 (*TET2*) is a tumor suppressor gene located on chromosome 4q24 [18,34,35] and is mutated in CMML with an incidence of ~60% [3]. *TET2* catalyzes the conversion of 5-methyl-cytosine to 5-hydroxy-methyl-cytosine (5-hmc), which is most commonly found at transcription start sites and within gene bodies [20,36]. *TET2* deletions on CD34+/CD38+ cells have demonstrated to promote monocyte expansion and is thought to be involved in the process of lineage commitment [18,35]. Several studies have identified *TET2* mutations to be the most frequent and are often associated with *SRSF2* mutations or bi-allelic *TET2* with secondary acquisition of mutations involving signaling pathways, epigenetic regulation, transcription factors and pre mRNA splicing [27,37,38]. This suggests that *TET2* mutations occur in the initial stages of CMML with secondary accumulation of other mutations, such as *SRSF2* and *ASXL1*, prompting disease progression [8,27,34]. Patients with *TET2* mutations tended to be older, presenting with MD-CMML [22]. Data regarding the impact on overall survival or leukemia-free survival have been highly debated [22,28]. However, Patnaik, and colleagues demonstrated that multiple *TET2* mutations or truncating *TET2* mutations imparted a survival advantage [20,39]. In fact, the absence of *TET2* mutations, as documented in a recent study, negatively impacted overall survival [39]. This is contrary to the findings of *TET2* mutations in MDS or AML, in which these mutations are associated with a negative prognostic impact [38]. The presence of *TET2* mutations has been found to improve the negative prognostic impact of an additional *ASXL1* mutation [20], at least partially. Cases with the mutation phenotype of wild type/non-mutated *ASXL1* and mutated *TET2* were found to have an improved response to hypomethylating agents [20,39].

DNA methylation is mediated by a group of DNA methyltransferase enzymes (DNMT), including *DNMT3A* which is found on chromosome 2p23 and functions to carry out *de novo* DNA methylation [40]. The mutational hot spot in this gene is Arginine882 and accounts for 40% to 60% of *DNMT3A* mutations, with some reports suggesting loss of methyltransferase activity in *in-vitro* assays [3]. This hotspot is not specific to CMML, however. *DNMT3A* mutations are seen in ~5% of CMML cases and have been found to independently and adversely affect overall (OS) and leukemia-free (LFS) survival [41].

Isocitrate dehydrogenase 1 (*IDH1*), found on chromosome 2q34 and isocitrate dehydrogenase 2 (*IDH2*) found on chromosome 15q26.1 are participants of the citric acid cycle and convert isocitrate to 5-alpha-ketoglutarate [3,36]. IDH1/2 are cofactors of TET2 that can produce alpha keto glutarase [3,36]. Fig. 2 depicts this pathway. *IDH1/2* mutations are uncommon in CMML, with *IDH2* mutations accounting for most. These are mutually exclusive with *TET2* mutations, as mutations in *IDH1/2* result in the development of 2-hydroxyglutarate which, in turn, impairs other enzymes including *TET2*, which contributes to leukemogenesis. In these cases, *IDH1/2* inhibitors may be beneficial, including ivosidenib and enasidenib [42].

MUTATIONS IN EPIGENETIC REGULATOR GENES AFFECTING HISTONE MODIFICATION (ASXL1, EZH2)

ASXL1 (additional sex combs-like 1) encodes a chromatin binding protein found on chromosome 20q11 and regulates the function of polycomb group complex repressive complex proteins (PRC1 and PRC2). PRC2 functions to recruit chromatin and results in the trimethylation of the H3K27 mark (H3K27me3) [36,43]. Mutations of *ASXL1* result in up-regulation of homeobox A genes involved in the hematopoietic stem cell self-renewal [34]. *ASXL1* mutations have been found in ~40% of cases of CMML [1,3]. Mutations in *ASXL1* have been found to be an independent poor prognostic marker in CMML, specifically nonsense or frameshift mutations leading to the truncation of *ASXL1* [3]. In ~50% of cases of CMML with an *ASXL1* mutation, the most frequent mutation is of c.1934dupG; p.G646WfsX12 [19,44,45]. In myeloid neoplasms, including AML and other MDS, MPN or MDS/MPN syndromes, *ASXL1* has been found to have an extremely poor prognosis [46]. In the germline *GATA-2* MDS/AML predisposition syndrome, the occurrence of *ASXL1* mutations is common and in a study of 5 patients, 4 progressed to MP-CMML [34].

EZH2 (enhancer of zeste homolog2) found on chromosome 7q23 [47] is an enzymatic catalytic subunit of PRC2 [36]. Mutation of *EZH2* is an infrequent finding in CMML, but almost always co-occurs with *ASXL1* mutations and present with MP-CMML [36]. Mutations of *EZH2* alone have not been shown to affect overall survival, however co-mutated patients demonstrate a higher risk and shorter survival compared to *ASXL1* mutated cases without *EZH2* mutations and it is suspected that the co-mutational status results in synergistic activity leading to unrestricted transcription [48].

MUTATIONS AFFECTING CELLULAR SIGNALING AND TYROSINE KINASE PATHWAYS (*NRAS, KRAS, NPM1, FLT3, CBL, AND JAK2*)

Mutations affecting signaling pathways and tyrosine kinase pathways are more commonly associated with MP-CMML and mostly affect granulocyte-macrophage-colony stimulating factor (GM-CSF). The prototypical mutation of these, in CMML, and the most mutated of these are of the *RAS* pathway [1–3].

RAS proteins drive growth, proliferation, and migration of cells. Point mutations in codons 12, 13, and 61 of the *NRAS* or *KRAS* oncogenes are identified in 20%

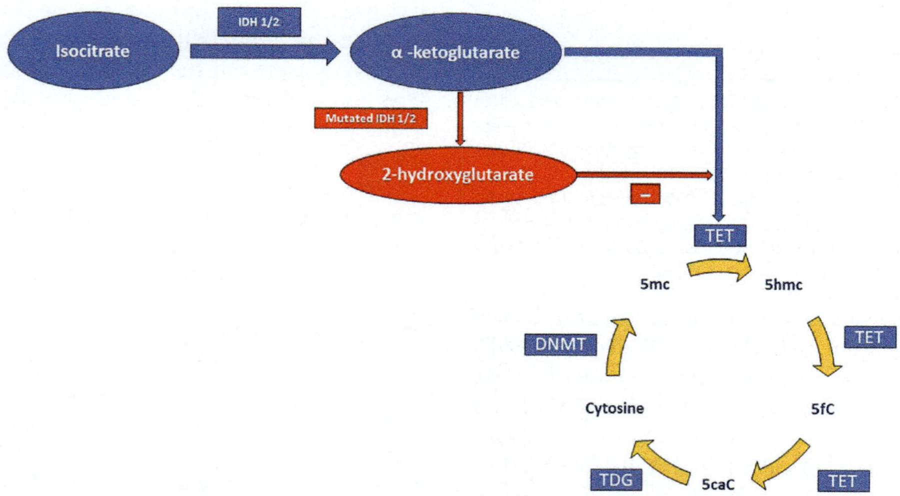

FIG. 2 Depiction of epigenetic mutations affecting the conversion of 5mc to 5-hmc.

to 40% of CMML [8]. Mutations in *RAS* lead to activation of Ras proteins and uncontrolled cell proliferation. *RAS* mutations in CMML are associated with MP-CMML, poor prognosis, and shorter survival [14]. *RAS* mutations were found to increase the expression of mitotic check point kinase *PLK1* through lysine methyltransferase *KMT2A* (MLL1), in association with enrichment of H3K4me1 at its promoter. It has also been shown that pharmacologic inhibition of *PLK1* decreases monocytosis and hepatosplenomegaly. Mutations in the *RAS* pathway were also found more commonly in the leukemic transformed cases versus chronic phase CMML. Though *NRAS* mutations are found in both MD-CMML and MP-CMML, the VAF was notably different, 38% versus 15%, respectively [49]. This finding suggests that *NRAS* knockdown may be related to clonal versus sub clonal nature of *NRAS* mutations. Additionally, it has been shown that plasmacytoid dendritic cells are present in ~20% of cases of CMML and are strongly associated with the *RAS* pathway mutations and may be an early predictor of leukemic transformation [49]. In the case of secondary *NRAS* mutations, these were most commonly identified in MD-CMML cases, mainly when co-occurring with *STAG2* mutations [30]. MP-CMML cases with *NRAS* mutations were the most aggressive subtype, demonstrating a shorter OS and LFS [2,3].

NPM1 (nucleophosmin gene) is located on chromosome 5q and engages in many basic cellular processes including ribosome biogenesis, cell proliferation and regulation of p53/TP53. *NPM1* mutations have been seen in a rare subset of CMML cases (1%–3%) and are associated with poor prognosis [50]. Of note, *NPM1* is listed in the suggested mutation profiling (see Box 4) for CMML, however, given the new diagnostic category of AML with defining genetic abnormalities (blasts need not be $\geq$ 20%), the presence of an *NPM1* mutation or other acute leukemia defining gene rearrangement designates the categorization of these cases as such as *de novo* AML per WHO5 [1]. The ICC, in contrast to WHO5, still requires a blast count of greater than 10% in the setting of an *NPM1* mutation to be considered AML [6]. Though the ICC does not consider this to be a *de novo* AML, the presence of an *NPM1* mutation has an aggressive clinical course, with overall survival found to be 12.5 months versus 20.5 months in *NPM1*—wild type cases [4,49]. In the setting of a secondary accumulation of *NPM1* at the time of transformation, this represents an adverse prognosis, and the adverse prognosis of secondary AML is not negated by the presence of an *NPM1* mutation [6,31].

FLT3 (Fms-like tyrosine kinase 3) gene is found on chromosome 13q12.2 and codes for a type III receptor tyrosine kinase involved in differentiation, proliferation, and survival of hematopoietic progenitor cells. *FLT3* mutations are rare in CMML [1] and have not been found to have an impact on OS or LFS, however implications of the impact on leukemia free and overall survival are challenging to elucidate because of the small subset of CMML patients with this mutation [51].

CBL (Casitas B-cell lymphoma gene) is found on chromosome 11q23.3 and encodes for E3 ubiquitin ligase, which is involved in the degradation of activated tyrosine kinases including *FLT3*, *PDGFR* and *JAK2*. The *CBL* family E3 ubiquitin ligases act to decrease *JAK2* stability and signaling via the adaptor protein LNK/SH2B3 [3]. Mutations of *CBL*, then, can cause the prolongation of *JAK2* half-life, protein levels and signaling. These mutations are found in 8% to 22% of cases of CMML, and mutations of the RING finger domain are frequently associated with uniparental disomy. *CBL* mutations are commonly associated with monosomy 7 and *TET2* mutations. Of note, it has been shown in several studies that mutations in *CBL* have resulted in elevated signaling of *FLT3* because of impaired *CBL* downregulation, suggesting a potential use of *FLT3* inhibition therapy [49,52]. *CBL* mutations have been found as ancestral mutational events in MD-CMML, however, secondary acquisition of these mutations was found in MP-CMML cases [3,53].

JAK2 (Janus kinase 2) mutations, specifically *JAK2V617 F* mutations, are mutations most commonly of proliferative phenotypes. In CMML, they commonly co-occur with *TET2* mutations and a normal karyotype [36,54]. Mutations of *JAK2V617 F* mutations in CMML were not found to have an increase in thrombotic events, as commonly seen in clonal hematopoiesis of indeterminate potential (CHIP) or MPN, and these mutations did not have any impact on leukemia-free or overall survival [54].

Cases with mutations in these categories may benefit from targeted therapies such as ruxolitnib (*JAK1/2* inhibitor), momelotinib (*JAK2* inhibitor), pacritinib (*JAK/FLT3* inhibitor), or inhibitors such as midostaurin, gilteritinib, and sorafenib (*FLT3* inhibitors) [36,42]. Data from phase I/II clinical trials of ruxolitnib are promising and demonstrate improved overall survival (69 vs 21 months) [55]. *FLT3* inhibitors [49], such as quizartinib may be beneficial in both *FLT3* mutated and *CBL* mutated cases and is currently in phase I/II [21]. Due to the presence of plasmacytoid dendritic cells identified in *RAS* mutated cases, there is a potential role of anti-CD123 therapies such as tagraxofusp or flotuzumab [49]. Additionally, in *RAS* mutated cases, PLK1 inhibitors may be beneficial [49,56]. GM-CSF antibodies including lenzilumab have been shown to inhibit the growth factor independent myeloid colony formation in vitro, which is a characteristic of CMML cases with *RAS* mutations [21]. Lenzilumab is currently in phase 2/3 trials; however, early data are promising [21]. Many of these targeted treatments have not been studied among CMML patients thus far.

MUTATIONS AFFECTING PRE-mRNA SPLICEOSOME PATHWAYS (*SRSF2, U2AF1, SF3B1, ZRSR2*)

Spliceosome component mutations (*SRSF2, U2AF1, SF3B1,* and *ZRSR2*) all affect pre-mRNA splicing, and involving the 3′ splice site recognition of pre-mRNA [3]. *SRSF2* (serine/arginine-rich splicing factor 2) is a splicing factor, found on chromosome 17q25.2. Mutations of *SRSF2* are found in other myeloid neoplasms including AML, MDS and are seen in much higher frequency in CMML (~50% of CMML cases vs 15%–20% in MDS and AML) [3]. *SRSF2* mutations (and other spliceosome mutations including *SF3B1* and *U2AF1*) are frequently associated with monocytosis [57]. Of note, *SRSF2-TET2* co mutations are most seen in CMML, whereas when *SRSF2* is co-mutated with *SETBP1*, the presentation is more commonly associated with MDS/MPN with neutrophilia (previously called atypical CML in prior WHO classifications ref. 1) [27]. The combination of *SRSF2* mutation and *TET2* mutations leads to a proliferative outcome and is most found in MP-CMML [9]. While *SRSF2* mutations when found in cases of MDS have been associated with significantly reduced OS, the impact on survival and prognostic impact of mutations of *SRSF2* in CMML is contradictory [3,58]. To date, they have not been found to have an independent prognostic impact [58].

SF3B1 (splicing factor 3B, subunit 1) is found on chromosome 2q33.1 and is very commonly found in MDS and has a high frequency of ringed sideroblasts. Mutations in *SF3B1* have no impact on overall survival or leukemia free survival but are the only genetic predictor of high hemoglobin levels [2]. It is important to consider MDS with low blasts and *SF3B1* mutations in these cases [1].

U2AF1 (U2 small nuclear RNA auxiliary factor) found on chromosome 21q22 is seen in a smaller percentage of CMML cases, (4%–10%) and has not been shown to have an independent prognostic effect [36].

ZRSR2 (zinc finger CCCH-type, RNA binding motif and serine/arginine rich 2) is found on chromosome Xp22.2. Mutations of *ZRSR2* are infrequent and have, thus far, not been shown to have prognostic effect in CMML [36,59].

MUTATIONS AFFECTING TRANSCRIPTION FACTORS (*RUNX1, SETBP1*)

RUNX1 (RUNX family transcription factor 1) is found on chromosome 21q22.12 and is a transcription factor which forms a complex with cofactor *CBFB* and is involved in the generation of hematopoietic stem cells and their differentiation. These mutations occur in 8% to 23% of CMML patients and are associated with an unfavorable prognosis and shorter LFS [36,42]. The effect of mutations in *RUNX1* however, have not been consistently found to impact OS and are included in the CPSS-Mol as a poor prognostic indicator, and carries a higher score compared to mutations in *ASXL1, NRAS,* and *SETBP1* [2,36,60]. As seen in *SRSF2* mutations, the partner mutation with *RUNX1* may impact the presentation. *RUNX1* co-mutations with *SRSF2* are more commonly identified in CMML cases, whereas *RUNX1* co-mutations with *EZH2* are more commonly seen in MDS/MPN with neutrophilia [27].

SETBP1 (SET binding protein 1) found on chromosome 18q21.1 is a protein localized predominantly in the nucleus and expressed in hematopoietic stem cells and committed progenitors [28,61]. Mutations in *SETBP1* are most commonly found in MP-CMML and are also associated with lower overall survival and more frequent progression to AML [2,62]. Patnaik, and colleagues, found *NRAS, RUNX1* and *SETBP1* protein mutations to have an overall worse prognosis in CMML [3].

MUTATIONS INVOLVING DNA REPAIR (TP53 AND PHF6)

The tumor suppressor *TP53* mutations have an incidence of less than 1% in CMML [1] and are associated with complex cytogenetics and response to decitabine [36]. *TP53* mutations, in small studies, have demonstrated poor prognosis [41,63]. However, many of these studies are either too small (41) or fail to differentiate between treatment related cases [63] and *de-novo* CML cases in statistical analysis of outcomes.

PHF6 is a chromatin adaptor, found in 5% of CMML [1] and to date has not been associated with significance in prognosis [36].

SUMMARY

CMML is a myeloid neoplasm with a relatively homogeneous molecular profile [3] and markedly heterogenous presentation and subsequent outcomes [2,3]. Though significant advances have been made in determination of the underlying genetic pathways of CMML, it is evident that further research is needed. Due to the rarity of CMML

[1], large cohorts for clinical trials are challenging, and the frequent changes to diagnostic criteria [1,6] further complicates the retrospective analysis of the molecular and cytogenetic profiles, prognosis, outcomes, and response to novel targeted therapies. The re-classification of MD-CMML and MP-CMML, along with removal of cases which may be better characterized under new distinct categories such as MDS with *SF3B1* or AML with *NPM1* may aid to further characterize these entities. Given the recent data from large studies as demonstrated by Carr, and colleagues [9] and Lanino, and colleagues [33] it may soon be possible to separate MD-CMML and MP-CMML as 2 distinct entities. The 2022 WHO5 and the ICC classifications have both demonstrated emphasis on molecular studies and this will likely only increase in future as targeted therapy continues to develop.

CLINICS CARE POINTS

- Myeloproliferative-chronic myelomonocytic leukemia (MP-CMML) is aggressive and has worse prognosis than myelodysplastic-chronic myelomonocytic leukemia (MD-CMML).
- Expansion of classic monocytes in monocyte repartition flow cytometry helps distinguish neoplastic monocytosis from reactive monocytosis.

ACKNOWLEDGMENTS

The authors would like to acknowledge Dr Akanksha Gupta for her support and contribution of BioRender publication rights.

DISCLOSURE

Authors do not have any financial or commercial conflicts of interest.

REFERENCES

[1] Khoury JD, Solary E, Abla O, et al. The 5th edition of the World Health Organization Classification of Haematolymphoid Tumours: Myeloid and Histiocytic/Dendritic Neoplasms. Leukemia 2022;36:1703–19.

[2] Elena C, Gallì A, Such E, et al. Integrating clinical features and genetic lesions in the risk assessment of patients with chronic myelomonocytic leukemia. Blood 2016;128(10):1408–17.

[3] Patnaik MM, Tefferi A. Chronic myelomonocytic leukemia: 2022 update on diagnosis, risk stratification, and management. Am J Hematol 2022;97(3):352–72.

[4] Fontana D, Elli EM, Pagni F, et al. Myelodysplastic Syndromes/Myeloproliferative Overlap Neoplasms and Differential Diagnosis in the WHO and ICC 2022 Era: A Focused Review. Cancers 2023;15(12):3175.

[5] Calvo X, Garcia-Gisbert N, Parraga I, et al. Oligomonocytic and overt chronic myelomonocytic leukemia show similar clinical, genomic, and immunophenotypic features. Blood advances 2020;4(20):5285–96.

[6] Arber DA, Orazi A, Hasserjian RP, et al. International Consensus Classification of Myeloid Neoplasms and Acute Leukemias: integrating morphologic, clinical, and genomic data. Blood 2022;140(11):1200–28.

[7] Cargo C, Cullen M, Taylor J, et al. The use of targeted sequencing and flow cytometry to identify patients with a clinically significant monocytosis. Blood 2019;133(12):1325–34.

[8] Ricci C, Fermo E, Corti S, et al. RAS mutations contribute to evolution of chronic myelomonocytic leukemia to the proliferative variant. Clin Cancer Res 2010;16(8):2246–56.

[9] Carr RM, Vorobyev D, Lasho T, et al. RAS mutations drive proliferative chronic myelomonocytic leukemia via a KMT2A-PLK1 axis. Nat Commun 2021;12:2901.

[10] Bennett JM, Catovsky D, Daniel MT, et al. The chronic myeloid leukaemias: guidelines for distinguishing chronic granulocytic, atypical chronic myeloid, and chronic myelomonocytic leukaemia. Proposals by the French-American-British Cooperative Leukaemia Group. British journal of haematology 1994;87(4):746–54.

[11] Patel BJ, Przychodzen B, Thota S, et al. Genomic determinants of chronic myelomonocytic leukemia. Leukemia 2017;31(12):2815–23.

[12] Nösslinger T, Reisner R, Grüner H, et al. Dysplastic versus proliferative CMML–a retrospective analysis of 91 patients from a single institution. Leuk Res 2001;25(9):741–7.

[13] Morsia E, Gangat N. Myeloproliferative neoplasms with monocytosis. Current hematologic malignancy reports 2022;17(1):46–51.

[14] Onida F, Kantarjian HM, Smith TL, et al. Prognostic factors and scoring systems in chronic myelomonocytic leukemia: a retrospective analysis of 213 patients. Blood 2002;99(3):840–9.

[15] Patnaik MM, Lasho TL, Finke CM, et al. Spliceosome mutations involving SRSF2, SF3B1, and U2AF35 in chronic myelomonocytic leukemia: prevalence, clinical correlates, and prognostic relevance. Am J Hematol 2013;88(3):201–6.

[16] Such E, Cervera J, Costa D, et al. Cytogenetic risk stratification in chronic myelomonocytic leukemia. Haematologica 2011;96(3):375–83.

[17] Tang G, Zhang L, Fu B, et al. Cytogenetic risk stratification of 417 patients with chronic myelomonocytic leukemia from a single institution. Am J Hematol 2014;89(8):813–8.

[18] McCullough KB, Patnaik MM. Chronic myelomonocytic leukemia: a genetic and clinical update. Current hematologic malignancy reports 2015;10(3):292–302.
[19] Patnaik MM, Itzykson R, Lasho TL, et al. ASXL1 and SETBP1 mutations and their prognostic contribution in chronic myelomonocytic leukemia: a two-center study of 466 patients. Leukemia 2014;28(11):2206–12.
[20] Coltro G, Mangaonkar AA, Lasho TL, et al. Clinical, molecular, and prognostic correlates of number, type, and functional localization of TET2 mutations in chronic myelomonocytic leukemia (CMML)-a study of 1084 patients. Leukemia 2020;34(5):1407–21.
[21] Chan O, Renneville A, Padron E. Chronic myelomonocytic leukemia diagnosis and management. Leukemia 2021;35(6):1552–62.
[22] Itzykson R, Kosmider O, Renneville A, et al. Clonal architecture of chronic myelomonocytic leukemias. Blood 2013;121(12):2186–98.
[23] Patwardhan PP, Aarabi M, Aggarwal N. Genomics of myelodysplastic/myeloproliferative neoplasm. Semin Diagn Pathol 2023;40(3):195–201.
[24] Weeks LD, Marinac CR, Redd R, et al. Age-related diseases of inflammation in myelodysplastic syndrome and chronic myelomonocytic leukemia. Blood 2022;139(8):1246–50.
[25] Mangaonkar AA, Swoboda DM, Coltro G, et al. Clinicopathologic characteristics, prognostication and treatment outcomes for myelodysplastic/myeloproliferative neoplasm, unclassifiable (MDS/MPN-U): Mayo Clinic-Moffitt Cancer Center study of 135 consecutive patients. Leukemia 2020;34(2):656–61.
[26] El Hussein S, Wang SA, Pemmaraju N, et al. Chronic myelomonocytic leukemia: hematopathology perspective. J Immunother Precis Oncol 2021;4(3):142–9.
[27] Palomo L, Meggendorfer M, Hutter S, et al. Molecular landscape and clonal architecture of adult myelodysplastic/myeloproliferative neoplasms. Blood 2020;136(16):1851–62.
[28] Patnaik MM, Tefferi A. Cytogenetic and molecular abnormalities in chronic myelomonocytic leukemia. Blood Cancer J 2016;6(2):e393.
[29] Montalban-Bravo G, Kanagal-Shamanna R, Li Z, et al. Phenotypic subtypes of leukaemic transformation in chronic myelomonocytic leukaemia. Br J Haematol 2023;203(4):581–92.
[30] Bhumika J Patel, Huang Dayong, Thota Swapna, et al. Chronic myelomonocytic leukemia (CMML) can be categorized by ancestral mutational events. Blood 2014;124(21):1893.
[31] Prakash S, Arber DA, Bueso-Ramos C, et al. Advances in myelodysplastic/myeloproliferative neoplasms. Virchows Arch 2023;482(1):69–83.
[32] Falantes JF, Márquez-Malaver FJ, Carrillo E, et al. SF3B1, RUNX1 and TP53 mutations significantly impact the outcome of patients with lower-risk myelodysplastic syndrome. Clin Lymphoma, Myeloma & Leukemia 2022;22(12):e1059–66.
[33] Lanino L, Hunter AM, Sala C, et al. Molecular classification of chronic myelomonocytic leukemia: results of the analysis of an international cohort of 2,471 patients. Blood 2023;142(Supplement 1):3244.
[34] Carr RM, Patnaik MM. Genetic and epigenetic factors interacting with clonal hematopoiesis resulting in chronic myelomonocytic leukemia. Curr Opin Hematol 2020;27(1):2–10.
[35] Feng Y, Li X, Cassady K, et al. TET2 function in hematopoietic malignancies, immune regulation, and DNA repair. Front Oncol 2019;9:210.
[36] Jian J, Qiao Y, Li Y, et al. Mutations in chronic myelomonocytic leukemia and their prognostic relevance. Clin Transl Oncol 2021;23(9):1731–42.
[37] Hochman MJ, Savani BN, Jain T. Examining disease boundaries: Genetics of myelodysplastic/myeloproliferative neoplasms. EJHaem 2021;2(3):607–15.
[38] Gurney M, Greipp PT, Gliem T, et al. TET2 somatic copy number alterations and allelic imbalances in chronic myelomonocytic leukemia. Leuk Res 2023;134:107391.
[39] Patnaik MM, Lasho TL, Vijayvargiya P, et al. Prognostic interaction between ASXL1 and TET2 mutations in chronic myelomonocytic leukemia. Blood Cancer J 2016;6(1):e385.
[40] Yang L, Rau R, Goodell MA. DNMT3A in haematological malignancies. Nat Rev Cancer 2015;15(3):152–65.
[41] Patnaik MM, Vallapureddy R, Yalniz FF, et al. Therapy related-chronic myelomonocytic leukemia (CMML): Molecular, cytogenetic, and clinical distinctions from de novo CMML. Am J Hematol 2018;93(1):65–73.
[42] Castaño-Díez S, López-Guerra M, Bosch-Castañeda C, et al. Real-World data on chronic myelomonocytic leukemia: clinical and molecular characteristics, treatment, emerging drugs, and patient outcomes. Cancers 2022;14(17):4107.
[43] Kwon J. Diagnosis and treatment of chronic myelomonocytic leukemia. Blood research 2021;56(S1):S5–16.
[44] Itzykson R, Kosmider O, Renneville A, et al. Prognostic score including gene mutations in chronic myelomonocytic leukemia. J Clin Oncol 2013;31(19):2428–36.
[45] Patnaik MM, Padron E, LaBorde RR, et al. Mayo prognostic model for WHO-defined chronic myelomonocytic leukemia: ASXL1 and spliceosome component mutations and outcomes. Leukemia 2013;27(7):1504–10.
[46] Zhang A, Wang S, Ren Q, et al. Prognostic value of ASXL1 mutations in patients with myelodysplastic syndromes and acute myeloid leukemia: A meta-analysis. Asia Pac J Clin Oncol 2023;19(5):e183–94.
[47] Duan R, Du W, Guo W. EZH2: a novel target for cancer treatment. J Hematol Oncol 2020;13(1):104.
[48] Patnaik MM, Vallapureddy R, Lasho TL, et al. EZH2 mutations in chronic myelomonocytic leukemia cluster with ASXL1 mutations and their co-occurrence is prognostically detrimental. Blood Cancer J 2018;8(1):12.

[49] Hammond D, Montalban-Bravo G. Management and outcomes of blast transformed chronic myelomonocytic leukemia. Current hematologic malignancy reports 2021;16(5):405–17.

[50] Vallapureddy R, Lasho TL, Hoversten K, et al. Nucleophosmin 1 (NPM1) mutations in chronic myelomonocytic leukemia and their prognostic relevance. Am J Hematol 2017;92(10):E614–8.

[51] Daver N, Strati P, Jabbour E, et al. FLT3 mutations in myelodysplastic syndrome and chronic myelomonocytic leukemia. Am J Hematol 2013;88(1):56–9.

[52] Reindl C, Quentmeier H, Petropoulos K, et al. CBL exon 8/9 mutants activate the FLT3 pathway and cluster in core binding factor/11q deletion acute myeloid leukemia/myelodysplastic syndrome subtypes. Clin Cancer Res 2009;15(7):2238–47.

[53] Gelsi-Boyer V, Cervera N, Bertucci F, et al. Molecular similarity between myelodysplastic form of chronic myelomonocytic leukemia and refractory anemia with ring sideroblasts. Haematologica 2013;98(4):576–83.

[54] Patnaik MM, Pophali PA, Lasho TL, et al. Clinical correlates, prognostic impact and survival outcomes in chronic myelomonocytic leukemia patients with the JAK2V617F mutation. Haematologica 2019;104(6):e236–9.

[55] Padron E, Dezern A, Andrade-Campos M, et al, Myelodysplastic Syndrome Clinical Research Consortium. A multi-institution Phase I trial of ruxolitinib in patients with chronic myelomonocytic leukemia (CMML). Clin Cancer Res 2016;22(15):3746–54.

[56] Bewersdorf JP, Zeidan AM. Polo-like kinase inhibition as a therapeutic target in acute myeloid leukemia. Oncotarget 2021;12(13):1314–7.

[57] van Zeventer IA, de Graaf AO, Koorenhof-Scheele TN, et al. Monocytosis and its association with clonal hematopoiesis in community-dwelling individuals. Blood advances 2022;6(14):4174–84.

[58] Arbab Jafari P, Ayatollahi H, Sadeghi R, et al. Prognostic significance of SRSF2 mutations in myelodysplastic syndromes and chronic myelomonocytic leukemia: a meta-analysis. Hematology (Amsterdam, Netherlands) 2018;23(10):778–84.

[59] Yoshida K, Sanada M, Shiraishi Y, et al. Frequent pathway mutations of splicing machinery in myelodysplasia. Nature 2011;478(7367):64–9.

[60] Kuo MC, Liang DC, Huang CF, et al. RUNX1 mutations are frequent in chronic myelomonocytic leukemia and mutations at the C-terminal region might predict acute myeloid leukemia transformation. Leukemia 2009;23(8):1426–31.

[61] Cristóbal I, Blanco FJ, Garcia-Orti L, et al. SETBP1 overexpression is a novel leukemogenic mechanism that predicts adverse outcome in elderly patients with acute myeloid leukemia. Blood 2010;115(3):615–25.

[62] Nguyen N, Vishwakarma BA, Oakley K, et al. Myb expression is critical for myeloid leukemia development induced by Setbp1 activation. Oncotarget 2016;7(52):86300–12.

[63] Gurney M, Mangaonkar AA, Lasho T, et al. Somatic TP53 single nucleotide variants, indels and copy number alterations in chronic myelomonocytic leukemia (CMML). Leukemia 2023;37(8):1753–6.

Advances in Molecular Pathology 7 (2024) 77–87
ADVANCES IN MOLECULAR PATHOLOGY

Molecular Profiling of Small Mature B Cell Lymphomas; New Insights on Diagnosis and Treatment

Jonathan Wilcock, MD, Ifeyinwa E. Obiorah, MD, PhD*
Department of Pathology, Division of hematopathology, University of Virginia Health, 1215 Lee Street, Charlottesville, VA 22903, USA

KEYWORDS
• B cell lymphoma • Molecular • Mutations • Translocations • Next-generation sequencing (NGS)

KEY POINTS
- The use of high throughput next-generation sequencing has identified the most common somatic genetic alterations associated with the lymphomagenesis of mature small B cell lymphomas.
- Specific recurrent genetic aberrations detect cellular pathways and provide biomarkers for clinical prognosis and prediction of treatment response.
- Modern prognostic models can incorporate molecular mutations with clinical information to create novel treatment algorithms for the clinical management of patients with small B cell lymphomas.

INTRODUCTION

Mature small B cell lymphomas (SBCL) are clinically and biologically heterogeneous tumors characterized by small to medium-sized atypical lymphoid cells. Recognized by the World Health Organization (WHO) [1] and international consensus classification (ICC) [2], this group includes chronic lymphocytic leukemia/small lymphocytic lymphoma (CLL/SLL), follicular lymphoma (FL), mantle cell lymphoma(MCL), marginal zone lymphomas (MZL) (including splenic, nodal, and extranodal), lymphoplasmacytic lymphoma (LPL), and hairy cell leukemia (HCL). The diagnosis of SBCL requires a comprehensive approach involving histologic morphology, immunohistochemistry, flow cytometry, cytogenetics, and molecular studies [3]. Genetic sequencing advances have revealed genetic alterations marking specific SBCL subtypes, elucidating the molecular basis of these diseases, and allowing establishment of SBCL disease models [4]. These activities could also prove useful clinically in disease diagnosis, subtyping, or assessment of prognosis, providing a deeper understanding of the oncogenic drives of progression and therapy refractoriness. Fluorescence in situ hybridization (FISH) is an important diagnostic tool used in the detection of certain SBCL, including MCLs with t (11;14) (q13;q32) and FLs with t(14;18) (q32;q21) [5,6]. However, t(14;18) may be negative in FL or identified in other SBCLs, limiting the distinction of FL from follicular colonization of nodal MZL [7]. The advent of sequencing analysis has led to the discovery of somatic mutations of chromatin modifiers like *CREBBP* and *EZH2*, which are readily demonstrated in FL and not in MZL [8]. The detection of *BRAF* V600 E is helpful in distinguishing HCL from hairy cell leukemia variant, otherwise known as splenic B-cell lymphoma/leukemia with prominent nucleoli [9]. In LPL, the most frequent driver mutation

*Corresponding author. Department of Pathology, Division of Hematopathology, University of Virginia Health, Charlottesville, VA 22903. *E-mail address:* jnp5qm@uvahealth.org

https://doi.org/10.1016/j.yamp.2024.07.002 www.advancesinmolecularpathology.com
2589-4080/24/

is the driver mutation is *MYD88*, and additional mutations in *CXCR4* have prognostic and therapeutic implications [10,11]. This review summarizes our current understanding of the molecular pathogenesis of mature small B cell lymphoma and details the impact of the genomic abnormalities on diagnosis, prognosis, and treatment.

CHRONIC LYMPHOCYTIC LEUKEMIA/ SMALL LYMPHOCYTIC LYMPHOMA

Chronic lymphocytic leukemia (CLL) is defined by the presence of $\geq 5 \times 10^9$/L clonal B-lymphocytes with CLL phenotype in the peripheral blood, or by the detection of its non-leukemic variant, small lymphocytic lymphoma (SLL). Based on the mutational status of immunoglobulin heavy chain variable region (*IGHV*) genes, which encode part of the B cell receptor (BCR), 2 major molecular subgroups have been identified. The *IGHV*-mutated group is thought to be derived from germinal center cell–memory B cells, while the *IGHV*-unmutated subtype develops from either naive or germinal center-independent memory B cells [12,13]. The *IGHV*-mutated lymphomas typically run an indolent course with a good prognosis [14]. In contrast, the *IGHV*-unmutated lymphomas are often aggressive, with poor treatment response and shorter survival times. BCR signaling is essential for the pathogenesis of CLL/SLL and is the central driver for neoplastic proliferation. BCR signaling may be activated by binding with autoantigens or exogenous antigens or in an antigen-independent manner driven by homotypic BCR-to-BCR interactions [14,15]. A third of patients with CLL show a remarkable BCR restriction, so-called stereotypic BCR that represents a highly homologous *IGHV* rearrangement that occurs independent of *IGHV* mutational status [16]. For instance, stereotyped BCR subset 2 is characterized by an *IGHV3-21* rearrangement that includes both mutated and unmutated *IGHV* genes [17]. Subset 2 is associated with a poor outcome irrespective of the *IGHV* mutational status. In addition, stereotyped subsets #6 and #8 express unmutated *IGHV* genes but subset #6 is less aggressive compared to subset #8, which has the highest risk for Richter's transformation among all CLL subsets [18].

The genomic landscape of CLL/SLL is heterogeneous and involves numerous genetic aberrations. The most common chromosomal abnormalities (Table 1) are deletions of 13q14.3 (miR-16–1 and miR-15a), followed by trisomy 12, then del11q22-q23 (*ATM* and *BIRC3*), deletion in 17p13 (*TP53*), or deletion in 6q21.11q[12,19]. Del13q14 is involved in the regulation of the cell cycle and apoptosis [20], while del11q (*ATM*) and del17p (*TP53*) affect the response to DNA damage [21]. Isolated del 13q is associated with a more favorable clinical outcome, whereas del 17p and del 11 confer a worse overall survival [19]. Genetic mutations are observed in 3% to 15% of CLL/SLL cases. The most frequently mutated genes in CLL/SLL are *NOTCH1*, *ATM*, *SF3B1*, *TP53*, *BIRC3*, *POT1*, and *MYD88* [19,21,22]. The clinical heterogeneity of CLL/SLL requires the detection of biological correlates of high-risk CLL, to identify the patients at risk for CLL progression. Mutated *NOTCH1*, *ATM*, *SF3B1*, and *TP53* are associated with poorer progression-free and overall survival in treatment-naïve CLL patients [23]. Treatment with chemoimmunotherapy contributes to the inactivation of these tumor suppressors, the acquisition of chromosomal aberrations, and clonal evolution. *SF3B1* and *NOTCH1* mutations are associated with a higher risk of disease progression and recurrence after chemotherapy-based CLL therapy [23,24]. *TP53* alterations, including del17p13 and *TP53* mutations, are predictive of a lack of response to fludarabine-containing regimes [25]. The majority of patients with Richter's transformation (RT) have mutations in genes involved in cellular proliferation, chromatin modification, MYC, NF-κB, and NOTCH signaling pathways [26]. Risk factors for the development of RT (Table 2) include *TP53* disruption, *NOTCH1* mutations, *CDKN2A* loss, and *MYC* activation [26]. DNA methylation studies have identified 3 CLL epigenetic subtypes based on their methylation profiles; naive B-cell-like, memory B-cell-like, and intermediate CLL [27]. These distinct subtypes indicate the developmental maturation state of the putative normal B-cell counterpart from which the different CLL epitypes are derived. The naive-like CLL, which is less epigenetically mature, is associated with an unfavorable prognosis, whereas the memory-like CLL has the best outcome [27]. DNA hypomethylation-induced upregulation of *TP63*, *ZAP70*, *PAX9*, and *NFATc1* and downregulation of *DUSP22* and *KLF4* are thought to be responsible for aggressive disease courses [3,18,27].

MANTLE CELL LYMPHOMA

Mantle cell lymphoma (MCL) is an aggressive subtype of non-Hodgkin lymphoma. Conventional MCLs harbor unmutated or minimally/borderline mutated *IGHV* genes. They are enriched in naïve B-cell signatures, overexpression of SOX-11, high genomic complexity, and nodal disease with an aggressive disease course [28]. A minority of cases have highly mutated *IGHV* with memory B cell signatures, SOX11 negativity, and non-nodal

TABLE 1
Summary of Major Cytogenetic and Molecular Features of Small Mature B Cell Lymphomas

B Cell Lymphoma Subtype	Main Cytogenetic Features	Major Molecular Mutations and Affected Pathways
Chronic lymphocytic leukemia/small lymphocytic lymphoma	del13q14.3, +12, del11q22-q23, del17p13, 6q21.11q	Cell cycle and DNA damage (*ATM, TP53, POT1*) NOTCH1 signaling (*NOTCH1*) RNA splicing (*SF3B1*) BCR signaling (*BIRC3, MYD88*)
Mantle cell lymphoma	t(11;14) (q13;q32) CCND2, CCND3 rearrangements	Cell cycle and DNA damage (*ATM, TP53, CDKN2A, CCND1*) Recurrent mutations (*NSD2, MT2A, SP140, KMT2D, CARD11,S1PR1, NOTCH1*)
Conventional Follicular lymphoma (FL)	t(14;18) (q32;q21), del1p36, (3q27) rearrangements	Epigenetic modifiers (*CREBBP, KMT2D, EZH2, ARID1A*) TNFR family (*TNFRSF14*) Apoptosis (*BCL2*)
Diffuse FL	del1p36	STAT signaling (*STAT6*) TNFR family (*TNFRSF14*) Epigenetic modifiers (*CREBBP*)
Pediatric FL	del1p36	MAPK/ERK signaling (*MAP2K1*) TNFR family (*TNFRSF14*) Transcription factor (*IRF8*)
Extranodal marginal zone lymphoma	+3, +12, +18, t(11;18) (q21;q21), t(3;14) (p14;q32), t(1;14) (p22;q32), t(14;18) (q32;q21), t(X;14) (p11;q32)	NFkB signaling (*TNFAIP3*) *NOTCH1* signaling (*NOTCH1, SPEN*) Epigenetic modifiers (*KMT2C, CREBBP, EP300, KMT2D*) DNA methylation (*TET2*) PI3K/AKT pathway (*TBL1XR1*) Tumor suppressor (*PRDM1*)
Nodal marginal zone lymphoma	+3, +18, del6q23	Epigenetic modifiers (*KMT2D*) TNFR family (*TNFRSF14*) Tumor suppressor (*PTPRD*) DNA methylation (*TET2*) Transcription factors (*KLF2*) Recurrent mutations (*LRP1B*) Apoptosis (*FAS*) NFkB signaling (*TNFAIP3, CARD11*) *NOTCH2* signaling (*NOTCH2*) PI3K/AKT pathway (*TBL1XR1*) MEK-ERK signaling (*BRAF*)
Splenic marginal zone lymphoma	del7q31, t(2;7) (p12;q21), +3q	Transcription factors (*KLF2*) *NOTCH* signaling (NOTCH1, *NOTCH2*) DNA damage (*TP53*) Epigenetic modifiers (*KMT2D*) NFkB signaling (*TNFAIP3*)
Pediatric marginal zone lymphoma	del1p36	MAPK/ERK signaling (*MAP2K1*) TNFR family (*TNFRSF14*) Transcription factor (*IRF8*)

(*continued on next page*)

TABLE 1
(*continued*)

B Cell Lymphoma Subtype	Main Cytogenetic Features	Major Molecular Mutations and Affected Pathways
Lymphoplasmacytic lymphoma	del6q	BCR signaling (*MYD88*) Recurrent mutations *CXCR4, TP53*
Hairy cell leukemia (HCL)	del7q	MAPK/ERK signaling (*BRAF-V600E*)
HCL variant/splenic B-cell lymphoma/leukemia with prominent nucleoli	del7q, del17p	MAPK/ERK signaling (*MAP2K1*) DNA damage (*TP53*)
Splenic diffuse red pulp small B-cell lymphoma	-	BCR signaling (*BCOR*) Cell cycle (*CCND3*) *NOTCH* signaling (*NOTCH1, NOTCH2, SPEN*)

Abbreviations: BCR, B cell receptor; MAPK/ERK, mitogen-activated protein kinase/extracellular signal-regulated kinase; TNFR, tumor necrosis factor receptor.

presentations, which correspond to a more indolent subtype [28]. The pathogenesis of MCL is complex and involves various molecular aberrations in genes and pathways involving the cell cycle machinery and senescence, DNA damage response, and cell survival [29]. The primary oncogenic event in MCL is the t(11;14)(q13;q32), between *IGH* and *CCND1*, resulting in cyclin D1 overexpression [30]. In a small subset of cases, the translocation partner for *CCND1* is the immunoglobulin light chain kappa (*IGK*) or lambda (*IGL*) gene. Additionally, another small subset of cases do not harbor *CCND1* translocation (Cyclin D1-Negative MCL) but often exhibit *CCND2* or *CCND3* translocations [31]. *CCND1* rearrangements have been detected in the peripheral blood of healthy individuals, suggesting that secondary genetic alterations are necessary for the oncogenesis of MCL [32].

TABLE 2
Major Genetic Alterations Implicated in Large Cell Transformation in Select Small B Cell Lymphoma

B Cell Lymphoma Category	Major Genetic Alterations
Chronic lymphocytic leukemia/small lymphocytic lymphoma	*TP53* disruption, *NOTCH1* mutations, *CDKN2A* loss, and *MYC* alterations
Conventional Follicular lymphoma	*TP53* and *CDKN2A* mutations as well as *MYC* translocations
Nodal marginal zone lymphoma	*TNFAIP3* and *TP53* mutations
Splenic marginal zone lymphoma	*TNFAIP3* and *TP53* mutations, loss of 9p21.3, and gains of 6p
Lymphoplasmacytic lymphoma	Wildtype *MYD88*, *TP53* mutations

More than 90% of MCLs display frequent chromosomal alterations, especially SOX11-positive MCL, resulting in multiple gains and losses of 13q (*RB1*), 9p (*CDKN2A*), 10p (*BMI1*), 12q (*CDK4*), 11q (*ATM*),12q (*MDM2*),17p (*TP53*), 18q(*BCL2*),6q (*TNFAIP3*) and 11q (*BIRC3*) [33]. Next-generation sequencing (NGS) studies of samples taken at diagnosis or baseline showed *ATM* was the most frequently mutated gene (43.5%) followed by *TP53* (26.8%), *CDKN2A* (23.9%), *CCND1* (20.2%) *NSD2* (15.0%), *KMT2A* (8.9%), *S1PR1* (8.6%), and *CARD11* (8.5%) [34]. In MCL, it is hypothesized that multiple molecular driver events contribute to resistance to therapy and disease recurrence and progression. *TP53* mutations predict an aggressive course and inferior outcomes [35]. Mutations in *KMT2D, SMARCA4, SMARCA2,* and *ARID2* genes, and diminished H3K4 methylation levels are associated with resistance to ibrutinib-venetoclax [36]. DNA methylation studies have identified 2 distinct clusters of MCL patients. Cluster 1, is associated with unmutated IGHV and an aggressive disease course, whereas cluster 2 is associated with mutated *IGHV* and indolent MCL [37]. A recent study [38] divided MCL patients into 4 prognostic clusters based on a comprehensive genomic and transcriptomic analysis. C1 includes mutated *IGHV, CCND1* mutation, amp(11q13), and active BCR signaling. C2 is characterized by del(11q), *ATM* mutations and upregulated

NF-kB, and DNA repair pathways. C3 is enriched in mutations in *SP140, NOTCH1, KMT2D,* and *NSD2,* with and downregulated TNF-α, NF-kB, BCR signaling, and MYC target pathways. C4 exhibits del(17p)/*TP53* mutations, del(13q), and del(9p), and active MYC pathway and hyperproliferation signatures. Patients with the C1 subtype had a more favorable outcome (- year overall survival [OS], 100%) than those with C2 (56.7%), C3 (48.7%), and C4 (14.2%) subtypes. These defined subtypes of MCL form the basis for designing precision therapies for aggressive MCL.

FOLLICULAR LYMPHOMA AND SUBTYPES

Follicular lymphoma (FL) is an indolent, incurable, heterogeneous germinal center B cell neoplasm. The WHO and ICC classifications identify multiple variants, including conventional nodal FL, in situ follicular neoplasia/in-situ follicular B cell neoplasm (ISFN), duodenal-type FL, testicular FL, diffuse subtype/BCL2-R–negative, CD23-positive follicle center lymphoma (dFL), primary cutaneous follicle center lymphoma (PCFCL), and pediatric type. FL is derived from transformed germinal center B (GCB) cells, which is supported by morphologic, immunophenotypic, and gene expression of GCB cells. This association includes activation-induced cytidine deaminase (AID) expression, somatic hypermutation, and class switch recombination [39]. Conventional nodal FL (cFL) is the most common, characterized by the translocation t(14;18)(q32;q21) (*BCL2*-R), which is present in most cases of grade 1 to 2/3A FL (otherwise known as classic FL) [40]. BCL2-R is typically negative in grade 3B FL/follicular large B cell lymphoma. Furthermore, *BCL2*-R is almost uniformly negative in testicular FL, PCFCL, dFL, and pediatric FL [40]. *BCL6* rearrangements, involving chromosome 3q25, can be observed in any type of FL [41]. cFL often harbors recurrent gains in chromosomal regions 1q, 2p15, 7, 8q, 12q, 18p, and 18q, as well as losses in 1p36, 3q, 6q, 9p, 10q, 11q, 13q, and 17p [42]. Mutations in epigenetic regulators and chromatin remodelers, such as *CREBBP, KMT2D, EZH2, ARID1A,* and *MEF2B,* are present in up to 85% of FL cases [8,43]. These mutations likely occur early in FL development, suggesting the importance of epigenetic alterations as important pathogenic mechanisms [43]. Additional "hits" include loss of function mutations and deletions in *TNFRSF14,* involving the 1p36 region, found in virtually all FL cases [44]. *BCL2* mutations are also common due to AID activity [45]. *TP53* and *CDKN2A* mutations, as well as *MYC* translocations, are frequent in large cell-transformed lymphoma compared to preceding FL [46,47]. The mutational profiles of ISFN and duodenal-type FL, though similar to cFL, are less complex, exhibiting lower frequencies of large losses, chromosomal copy-number abnormalities, and *KMT2D* mutations [48]. BCL2-R and negative BCL2-R FL often show overlapping mutational profiles and chromosomal abnormalities. Kalmbach and colleagues [49] demonstrated that mutations in *KMT2D, BCL2, ABL2, IGLL5,* and *ARID1A* are enriched in BCL2-R FL, while *STAT6* mutations more frequently occur in BCL2-R negative FL. *CREBBP* and *STAT6* co-mutations, along with a high frequency of 1p36/*TNFRSF14* abnormalities and *KMT2D* mutations, are observed in dFL [44,50]. In PCFCL, BCL2-R is seen in 10% to 40% of cases, while 1p36/*TNFRSF14* alterations are mutually exclusive with BCL2-R and occur in 20% to 30% of BCL2-R negative patients [40]. Mutations detected in PCFCL are similar to those seen in BCL2-R cFL. Unlike other BCL2-R negative FL, there is minimal overlap between the mutational profiles of pediatric FL and cFL. Mutations in epigenetic modifiers as well as *STAT6* mutations are uncommon in pediatric FL. Abnormalities in *MAP2K1* and 1p36/*TNFRSF14* are the most frequent genetic alterations in pediatric FL [51]. A hot-spot mutation affecting *IRF8* has been identified, co-existing with *TNFRSF14* but not with *MAPK21,* suggesting 2 divergent pathways in the lymphomagenesis of pediatric FL [52].

MARGINAL ZONE LYMPHOMA AND SUBTYPES

Marginal zone lymphomas (MZL) have highly altered variable *IGHV* and *IGLV* genes, suggesting GCB or post-GCB origin. Despite shared histologic and immunophenotypic features, extranodal marginal zone lymphoma of mucosa-associated lymphoid tissue (EMZL), nodal marginal zone lymphoma (NMZL), and splenic marginal zone lymphoma (SMZL) have distinct etiologies. Molecular advances have detected significant differences in the mutational landscapes among the MZL subtypes. Primary cutaneous marginal zone lymphoma or lymphoproliferative disorder (PCMZL) is recognized as a distinct entity from other EMZL [1,2]. Similarly, pediatric nodal marginal zone lymphoma is recognized as a distinctive type of lymphoma. EZML, the most frequent subtype, usually exhibits an indolent behavior. The pathogenesis involves recurrent chromosomal aberrations, some including trisomies of chromosomes 3, 12, and 18 in 20% to 30% of EMZL [53]. The most common recurrent translocation, t(11;18)(q21;q21)/*BIRC3::MALT1,* is specific for EZML and tightly linked to EMZL of the lung, stomach, and intestines, and rarely in other sites [53].

Other translocations in EMZL include t(3;14) (p14;q32) leading to *IGH-FOXP1* rearrangement, frequent in thyroid and ocular adnexal disease, t(1;14) (p22;q32)/*BCL10:IGH*, and t(14;18) (q32;q21)/*IGH:MALT1* (54). The rare translocation t(X;14) (p11;q32)/*IGH::GPR34* occurs exclusively in EMZL of the salivary glands [54]. Sequencing analysis has revealed preferred activation of chromatin remodeling and transcription regulation and mutations in NOTCH, BCR, and NF-κB pathways across MZL entities. *TNFAIP3* deletions and mutations occur mainly in tumors of the ocular adnexa, salivary gland, and thyroid [55]. EMZL has a high occurrence of *NOTCH1, KMT2C, CREBBP, TET2, TBL1XR1, EP300, KMT2D, PRDM1* and *SPEN* mutations [54,55]. The *MYD88 L265P* mutation is found in ~5% of ocular adnexal EMZL cases but is infrequent at other anatomic sites. Deleterious mutations of *TET2, CD274, TNFRSF14,* and *TNFAIP3* are observed in thyroid EMZL [56].

In contrast to EMZL, recurrent translocations are not identified in NMZL [55]. Mutational profiling of NMZL has demonstrated mutations in *KMT2D, TNFRSF14, TET2, PTPRD, KLF2, LRP1B, CARD11, FAS, TNFAIP3, CREBBP, NOTCH2* and *TBL1XR1* [55,57]. *BRAF* and *PTPRD* mutations are nearly exclusive to NMZL [58]. The molecular pathogenesis of pediatric NMZL is not well defined with reported mutations in *MAP2K1, TNFRSF14,* and *IRF8* [59,60]. This suggests that pediatric NMZL and pediatric FL may represent a single entity, pediatric B-cell lymphoma with a broad morphologic spectrum. In SMZL, *KLF2* is the most commonly mutated gene (18%), followed by *NOTCH2* (16%) and *TP53* (12%), occurring at a higher frequency compared to EMZL and NMZL [55,61]. Somatic mutations in *KMT2D, TNFAIP3,* and *NOTCH1* are also frequently identified in SMZL. *KMT2D, TNFRSF14,* and *LRP1B* are more commonly mutated in NMZL than in SMZL. Partial deletion of the long arm of chromosome 7, del(7) (q31), is found exclusively in SMZL and may indicate a more aggressive behavior [55]. Translocation t(2;7) (p12;q21–22) with dysregulation of the *CDK6* occurs in less than 1% of cases. Using a multiplatform approach, Bonfiglio and colleagues [61] identified 2 prominent genetic clusters in SMZL, termed NNK and DMT clusters. NNK-SMZL (58% of cases) express significantly higher levels of genes involved in NF-κB (eg, *TNFAIP3, TRAF3, BIRC3*), NOTCH (eg, *NOTCH2, NOTCH1, SPEN*), and KLF2 signaling pathways that regulate MZL B cell differentiation. DMT (32% of cases) harbored a signature with DNA-damage response (eg, *TP53, ATM*), MAPK (eg, *BRAF*), and TLR genes (eg, *MYD88* modules) indicating dysfunction of TP53 and apoptosis. NNK-SMZLs were enriched in IGHV1-2*04 usage and 7q deletion, whereas, DMT-SMZLs showed depletion of both. The NNK-SMZL demonstrated an inferior prognosis. These subclassifications provide a conceptual edifice for the classification and precision therapies for SMZL. Mutations in *TNFAIP3* and *TP53,* loss of 9p21.3, and gains of 6p are acquired during SMZL transformation, whereas only *TP53* and *TNFAIP3* are identified in NMZL transformation [60].

LYMPHOPLASMACYTIC LYMPHOMA

Waldenström macroglobulinemia (WM) is a distinct type of indolent lymphoplasmacytic lymphoma (LPL) with an immunoglobulin M (IgM) paraprotein. LPL is characterized by bone marrow-predominant infiltration of small lymphocytes, plasma cells, and plasmacytoid lymphocytes [62]. The exact cellular origin of the WM clone remains undetermined. Although the presence of somatic hypermutations in WM patients suggests a memory B cell of origin, a subset of cases lacks CD27 and somatic hypermutations suggesting non-germinal center origin [63]. Recent gene expression profiling of WM clones suggests activated B cells as the cellular origin of the disease [63]. *MYD88* mutations, most frequently *MYD88* L265P, are found in more than 90% of LPL [64]. *MYD88* L265P activates the NF-κB signaling via phosphorylation of Bruton's tyrosine kinase (BTK) in the BCR. Rare cases of MZL, CLL, and MCL can demonstrate *MYD88* mutations, however, multiple myeloma cases are consistently negative [64]. The absence of a *MYD88* mutation is associated with a worse outcome and higher risk of transformation to diffuse large B cell lymphoma (DLBCL) [65]. *MYD88* mutations are also observed in 80% of IgM monoclonal gammopathy of undetermined significance and increase the risk of progression to WM [66]. The next most frequent somatic mutations are *CXCR4* alterations, detected in 40% of patients with *MYD88* mutations [67]. This indicates that *CXCR4* alterations are secondary events. Patients with *CXCR4* mutations have high serum IgM levels, increased hyperviscosity, and resistance to BTK inhibitors [68]. Similarly, *TP53* mutations, though rare in WM, confer an increased risk of progression/transformation and reduced progression-free survival but do not affect BTK inhibitor response [69,70]. Deletions involving chromosome 6q are common in *MYD88*-mutated cases and appear to be exclusive of *CXCR4* in untreated patients [71]. Additional alterations detected in LPL include mutations in *KMT2D, ARID1A, CD79 A* and *B, NOTCH2, PRDM1, BIRC3,* and *TRAF3,* but their impact on prognosis and treatment remains undetermined [69,72].

HAIRY CELL LEUKEMIA AND OTHER SPLENIC B CELL LYMPHOMAS

Hairy cell leukemia (HCL) is an indolent B-cell lymphoma involving the peripheral blood, bone marrow, and spleen. HCL is thought to arise from a post-GCB stage but exhibits heterogeneous somatic hypermutation [73]. The founding genetic lesion in HCL is the activating *BRAF* p.V600 E mutation, present in virtually all cases [74]. *BRAF* V600 E aberrantly activates the oncogenic MEK-ERK pathway, enhancing cell survival and proliferation. The second most common genetic aberration in HCL is heterozygous loss of chromosome 7q, targeting the wild-type *BRAF* in its minimally deleted region [75]. Additional mutations in HCL involve the transcription factor KLF2, the cyclin-dependent kinase inhibitor CDKN1B, and genes implicated in epigenetic regulation, such as *MLL3 (KMT2C), KDM6A, CREBBP, ARID1A* and *ARID1B* (75). Hairy cell leukemia variant, also known as splenic B-cell lymphoma/leukemia with prominent nucleoli (HCL-v), often demonstrates unmutated *IGHV* genes and utilizes VH4-34 rearrangement [75,76]. HCL-v often lacks *BRAF* V600 E mutations, but mutations in *MAP2K1* encoding for the MEK protein are identified in 50% of cases [77]. *TP53* mutations are more common in HCL-v (30% of cases) and are associated with a worse outcome [60]. Other genetic alterations include *KMT2C, U2AF1,* and *CCND3* mutations and 17p and 7q deletions [78]. Splenic diffuse red pulp small B-cell lymphoma (SDRPL) is another splenic lymphoma that can be confused with HCL, especially HCL-v. Similar to HCL-v, SDRPL shows an absence of *BRAF* V600 E with rare *MYD88* L265 mutations. However, sequencing studies have reported mutations in *BCOR* (24%), *CCND3* (26%), *MAP2K1* (7%–10%), and genes involved in the NOTCH pathway (*NOTCH1, NOTCH2, SPEN* (17%)) [60,78].

DISCUSSION AND FUTURE DIRECTIONS

Except for MCL, most small mature B cell lymphomas are indolent. Despite treatment, some cases relapse or transform into diffuse large B-cell lymphoma. Current challenges include identifying molecular predictors of early relapse or histologic transformation and determining better stratification factors for treatment purposes. Molecular analyses may assist in the differential diagnosis of small B cell lymphomas, especially in cases with overlapping features. In cases of diagnostic dilemma between BCL2-R negative FL and follicular colonization of MZL, demonstrating a *BCL6* rearrangement or 1p36 deletion favors FL [49]. *KLF2, NOTCH2,* and *PTPRD* mutations favor MZL, whereas a *STAT6* mutation favors BCL2-R–negative, diffuse, or follicular CD23+ FL. Translocations of *MALT1, FOXP1,* and *BCL10* are specific for EZML lymphomas [79]. Though the *MYD88* L265P mutation is highly suggestive of LPL, it is also found in MZL, creating a diagnostic challenge. Coexisting *CXCR4* mutations further increase the specificity for LPL. Thus, the detection of both *MYD88* and *CXCR4* mutations favors LPL, while mutations involving *NOTCH2, PTPRD,* and *TNFAIP3* favor MZL.

DLBCL has recently been classified into molecular subtypes, allowing for patient selection strategy and candidate treatment targets for future clinical trials [80]. The recent advances obtained via genomic profiling are expanding our understanding of the pathogenesis of small BCL and have opened up potential new avenues for improving diagnosis and treatment. For instance, in FL, the clinicopathologic heterogeneity of neoplasms derived from GCB cells corresponds to distinct molecular subtypes with different biological properties. Notably, several variants, such as duodenal FL and diffuse FL, are associated with localized disease and excellent prognosis. A recent study (Fig. 1A) classified MCL patients into 4 prognostic clusters [38]. Interestingly, the C4 cluster correlates with *TP53* alterations, which have previously shown a poor prognosis. Genomic profiling identified 2 major genetic clusters in SMZL (Fig. 1B), termed NNK and DMT clusters [61]. The former is associated with a worse outcome. This information further substantiates the incorporation of genetic alterations in SBCL diagnosis and classification. EZH2 mutation is predictive of response to EZH2 inhibition in FL. Tazemetostat is FDA-approved for use in patients with EZH2-mutated FL who have received at least 2 prior lines of systemic therapy [79]. Molecular analysis allows the prediction of resistance to targeted therapy. In CLL/SLL, mutations of *BTK, PLCG2,* and *CARD11* are associated with resistance to BTK inhibitors. Similarly, acquired *BCL2* mutations predict resistance to venetoclax in patients with CLL/SLL [81]. Xu and colleagues [82] detected *BTK* mutations with associated *CXCR4* mutations in WM patients with clinical progression on ibrutinib. Understanding both primary and acquired resistance patterns is the key to improving clinical outcomes and defining populations that will benefit from ibrutinib.

In summary, a confident diagnosis of distinct SBCL can be made in the majority of cases based on morphology and immunophenotypic studies. Further analysis with cytogenetic and FISH testing is performed in certain cases. In the absence of helpful translocations, NGS or copy number variation may follow to look for specific alterations, especially in the presence of therapy

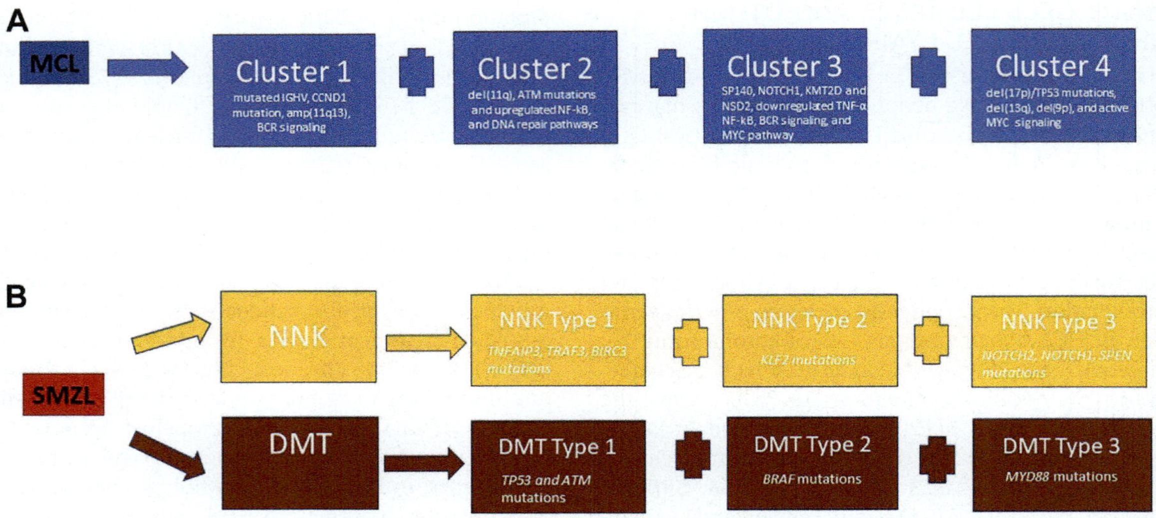

FIG. 1 Molecular classification of mantle cell lymphoma and splenic marginal zone lymphoma. (**A**) In mantle cell lymphoma, 4 different clusters were identified with cluster 4 showing the worst prognosis. (**B**) Splenic marginal zone lymphoma is associated with 2 prominent clusters. The NNK cluster is subdivided into Type 1 (NFkB signaling), Type 2 (NOTCH signaling), and Type 3 (KLF2 signaling) whereas the DMT-SMZL includes Type 1 (DNA damage response), Type 2 (MAPK signaling), and Type 3 (TLR genes).

resistance. Notably, molecular results should not be interpreted in isolation but in the context of clinicopathological findings. Precise molecular features of each patient are helpful in the risk stratification and subsequent treatment of any patient.

CLINICS CARE POINTS

- Gene-expression profiling is used to study the molecular pathogenesis of lymphomas.
- Molecular analyses may assist in the differential diagnosis of small B cell lymphomas particularly in cases that show overlapping of 2 distinct entities.
- Choice of treatment regimen depends on the accurate classification of the defined small B cell lymphoma.
- The presence of certain mutations is predictive of response to certain targeted therapy and resistance to chemoimmunotherapy.

DISCLOSURE

The authors have nothing to disclose.

REFERENCES

[1] Alaggio R, Amador C, Anagnostopoulos I, et al. Correction: "The 5th edition of The World Health Organization Classification of Haematolymphoid Tumours: Lymphoid Neoplasms" Leukemia. 2022 Jul;36(7):1720–1748. Leukemia 2023;37(9):1944–51.

[2] Campo E, Jaffe ES, Cook JR, et al. The International Consensus Classification of Mature Lymphoid Neoplasms: a report from the Clinical Advisory Committee. Blood 2022;140(11):1229–53.

[3] Panda D, Das N, Thakral D, et al. Genomic landscape of mature B-cell non-Hodgkin lymphomas - an appraisal from lymphomagenesis to drug resistance. J Egypt Natl Cancer Inst 2022;34(1):52.

[4] Heise N, De Silva NS, Silva K, et al. Germinal center B cell maintenance and differentiation are controlled by distinct NF-κB transcription factor subunits. J Exp Med 2014;211(10):2103–18.

[5] Caraway NP, Gu J, Lin P, et al. The utility of interphase fluorescence in situ hybridization for the detection of the translocation t(11;14)(q13;q32) in the diagnosis of mantle cell lymphoma on fine-needle aspiration specimens. Cancer 2005;105(2):110–8.

[6] Freedman A, Jacobsen E. Follicular lymphoma: 2020 update on diagnosis and management. Am J Hematol 2020;95(3):316–27.

[7] Baseggio L, Geay M-O, Gazzo S, et al. In non-follicular lymphoproliferative disorders, IGH/BCL2-fusion is not restricted to chronic lymphocytic leukaemia. Br J Haematol 2012;158(4):489–98.

[8] Green MR. Chromatin modifying gene mutations in follicular lymphoma. Blood 2018;131(6):595–604.

[9] Soong D, Kumar P, Jatwani K, et al. Hairy Cell Leukemia Masquerading as CD5+ Lymphoproliferative Disease: The Importance of BRAF V600E Testing in Diagnosis and Treatment. JCO Precision Oncology 2021;(5):1035–9.

[10] Rossi D. Role of MYD88 in lymphoplasmacytic lymphoma diagnosis and pathogenesis. Hematology American Society of Hematology Education Program 2014; 2014(1):113–8.

[11] Scala S, D'Alterio C, Milanesi S, et al. New Insights on the Emerging Genomic Landscape of CXCR4 in Cancer: A Lesson from WHIM. Vaccines 2020;8(2):164.

[12] Bosch F, Dalla-Favera R. Genetics of Chronic Lymphocytic Leukemia. Cancer journal (Sudbury, Mass) 2021; 27(4):259–65.

[13] Foà R, Montserrat E. Introduction Chronic Lymphocytic Leukemia. Where Do We Stand, Where Do We Go. Cancer journal (Sudbury, Mass) 2021;27(4):257–8.

[14] Ten Hacken E, Burger JA. Microenvironment interactions and B-cell receptor signaling in Chronic Lymphocytic Leukemia: Implications for disease pathogenesis and treatment. Biochim Biophys Acta 2016;1863(3):401–13.

[15] Dühren-von Minden M, Übelhart R, Schneider D, et al. Chronic lymphocytic leukaemia is driven by antigen-independent cell-autonomous signalling. Nature 2012; 489(7415):309–12.

[16] Stamatopoulos K, Agathangelidis A, Rosenquist R, et al. Antigen receptor stereotypy in chronic lymphocytic leukemia. Leukemia 2017;31(2):282–91.

[17] Agathangelidis A, Darzentas N, Hadzidimitriou A, et al. Stereotyped B-cell receptors in one-third of chronic lymphocytic leukemia: a molecular classification with implications for targeted therapies. Blood 2012;119(19): 4467–75.

[18] Papakonstantinou N, Ntoufa S, Tsagiopoulou M, et al. Integrated epigenomic and transcriptomic analysis reveals TP63 as a novel player in clinically aggressive chronic lymphocytic leukemia. Int J Cancer 2019; 144(11):2695–706.

[19] Czader M, Amador C, Cook JR, et al. Progression and transformation of chronic lymphocytic leukemia/small lymphocytic lymphoma and B-cell prolymphocytic leukemia: Report from the 2021 SH/EAHP Workshop. Am J Clin Pathol 2023;159(6):554–71.

[20] Hernández JA, Rodríguez AE, González M, et al. A high number of losses in 13q14 chromosome band is associated with a worse outcome and biological differences in patients with B-cell chronic lymphoid leukemia. Haematologica 2009;94(3):364–71.

[21] Quijada-Álamo M, Pérez-Carretero C, Hernández-Sánchez M, et al. Dissecting the role of TP53 alterations in del(11q) chronic lymphocytic leukemia. Clin Transl Med 2021;11(2):e304.

[22] Ouillette P, Saiya-Cork K, Seymour E, et al. Clonal evolution, genomic drivers, and effects of therapy in chronic lymphocytic leukemia. Clin Cancer Res 2013;19(11): 2893–904.

[23] Nadeu F, Delgado J, Royo C, et al. Clinical impact of clonal and subclonal TP53, SF3B1, BIRC3, NOTCH1, and ATM mutations in chronic lymphocytic leukemia. Blood 2016;127(17):2122–30.

[24] Rossi D, Rasi S, Spina V, et al. Integrated mutational and cytogenetic analysis identifies new prognostic subgroups in chronic lymphocytic leukemia. Blood 2013;121(8): 1403–12.

[25] Rossi D, Terzi-di-Bergamo L, De Paoli L, et al. Molecular prediction of durable remission after first-line fludarabine-cyclophosphamide-rituximab in chronic lymphocytic leukemia. Blood 2015;126(16):1921–4.

[26] Allan JN, Furman RR. Current trends in the management of Richter's syndrome. International journal of hematologic oncology 2018;7(4):Ijh09.

[27] Kulis M, Heath S, Bibikova M, et al. Epigenomic analysis detects widespread gene-body DNA hypomethylation in chronic lymphocytic leukemia. Nat Genet 2012;44(11): 1236–42.

[28] Navarro A, Clot G, Royo C, et al. Molecular subsets of mantle cell lymphoma defined by the IGHV mutational status and SOX11 expression have distinct biologic and clinical features. Cancer Res 2012;72(20):5307–16.

[29] Vogt N, Dai B, Erdmann T, et al. The molecular pathogenesis of mantle cell lymphoma. Leuk Lymphoma 2017;58(7):1530–7.

[30] Li JY, Gaillard F, Moreau A, et al. Detection of translocation t(11;14)(q13;q32) in mantle cell lymphoma by fluorescence in situ hybridization. Am J Pathol 1999; 154(5):1449–52.

[31] Salaverria I, Royo C, Carvajal-Cuenca A, et al. CCND2 rearrangements are the most frequent genetic events in cyclin D1(-) mantle cell lymphoma. Blood 2013;121(8): 1394–402.

[32] Lecluse Y, Lebailly P, Roulland S, et al. t(11;14)-positive clones can persist over a long period of time in the peripheral blood of healthy individuals. Leukemia 2009;23(6):1190–3.

[33] Beà S, Amador V. Role of SOX11 and Genetic Events Cooperating with Cyclin D1 in Mantle Cell Lymphoma. Curr Oncol Rep 2017;19(6):43.

[34] Hill HA, Qi X, Jain P, et al. Genetic mutations and features of mantle cell lymphoma: a systematic review and meta-analysis. Blood advances 2020;4(13):2927–38.

[35] Eskelund CW, Dahl C, Hansen JW, et al. TP53 mutations identify younger mantle cell lymphoma patients who do not benefit from intensive chemoimmunotherapy. Blood 2017;130(17):1903–10.

[36] Jain P, Wang ML. Mantle cell lymphoma in 2022—A comprehensive update on molecular pathogenesis, risk stratification, clinical approach, and current and novel treatments. Am J Hematol 2022;97(5):638–56.

[37] Queirós AC, Beekman R, Vilarrasa-Blasi R, et al. Decoding the DNA Methylome of Mantle Cell Lymphoma in the Light of the Entire B Cell Lineage. Cancer Cell 2016;30(5):806–21.

[38] Yi S, Yan Y, Jin M, et al. Genomic and transcriptomic profiling reveals distinct molecular subsets associated with outcomes in mantle cell lymphoma. The Journal of clinical investigation 2022;132(3).

[39] Gagyi E, Balogh Z, Bödör C, et al. Somatic hypermutation of IGVH genes and aberrant somatic hypermutation in follicular lymphoma without BCL-2 gene rearrangement and expression. Haematologica 2008;93(12):1822–8.

[40] Zhou T, Pittaluga S, Jaffe ES. Molecular insights into the pathogenesis of follicular lymphoma. Ann Lymphoma 2021;5(12):1–13.

[41] Xerri L, Dirnhofer S, Quintanilla-Martinez L, et al. The heterogeneity of follicular lymphomas: from early development to transformation. Virchows Arch : an international journal of pathology 2016;468(2):127–39.

[42] Bouska A, Zhang W, Gong Q, et al. Combined copy number and mutation analysis identifies oncogenic pathways associated with transformation of follicular lymphoma. Leukemia 2017;31(1):83–91.

[43] Green MR, Kihira S, Liu CL, et al. Mutations in early follicular lymphoma progenitors are associated with suppressed antigen presentation. Proc Natl Acad Sci USA 2015;112(10):E1116–25.

[44] Nann D, Ramis-Zaldivar JE, Müller I, et al. Follicular lymphoma t(14;18)-negative is genetically a heterogeneous disease. Blood advances 2020;4(22):5652–6.

[45] Huet S, Szafer-Glusman E, Tesson B, et al. BCL2 mutations do not confer adverse prognosis in follicular lymphoma patients treated with rituximab. Am J Hematol 2017;92(6):515–9.

[46] Cucco F, Barrans S, Sha C, et al. Distinct genetic changes reveal evolutionary history and heterogeneous molecular grade of DLBCL with MYC/BCL2 double-hit. Leukemia 2020;34(5):1329–41.

[47] Kridel R, Chan FC, Mottok A, et al. Histological Transformation and Progression in Follicular Lymphoma: A Clonal Evolution Study. PLoS Med 2016;13(12):e1002197.

[48] Schmidt J, Salaverria I, Haake A, et al. Increasing genomic and epigenomic complexity in the clonal evolution from in situ to manifest t(14;18)-positive follicular lymphoma. Leukemia 2014;28(5):1103–12.

[49] Kalmbach S, Grau M, Zapukhlyak M, et al. Novel insights into the pathogenesis of follicular lymphoma by molecular profiling of localized and systemic disease forms. Leukemia 2023;37(10):2058–65.

[50] Xian RR, Xie Y, Haley LM, et al. CREBBP and STAT6 co-mutation and 16p13 and 1p36 loss define the t(14;18)-negative diffuse variant of follicular lymphoma. Blood Cancer J 2020;10(6):69.

[51] Lovisa F, Binatti A, Coppe A, et al. A high definition picture of key genes and pathways mutated in pediatric follicular lymphoma. Haematologica 2019;104(9):e406–9.

[52] Schmidt J, Ramis-Zaldivar JE, Nadeu F, et al. Mutations of MAP2K1 are frequent in pediatric-type follicular lymphoma and result in ERK pathway activation. Blood 2017;130(3):323–7.

[53] Schreuder MI, van den Brand M, Hebeda KM, et al. Novel developments in the pathogenesis and diagnosis of extranodal marginal zone lymphoma. Journal of hematopathology 2017;10(3–4):91–107.

[54] Rodríguez-Sevilla JJ, Salar A. Recent Advances in the Genetic of MALT Lymphomas. Cancers 2021;14(1).

[55] Vela V, Juskevicius D, Dirnhofer S, et al. Mutational landscape of marginal zone B-cell lymphomas of various origin: organotypic alterations and diagnostic potential for assignment of organ origin. Virchows Arch : an international journal of pathology 2022;480(2):403–13.

[56] Wu F, Watanabe N, Tzioni MM, et al. Thyroid MALT lymphoma: self-harm to gain potential T-cell help. Leukemia 2021;35(12):3497–508.

[57] van den Brand M, Rijntjes J, Hebeda KM, et al. Recurrent mutations in genes involved in nuclear factor-κB signalling in nodal marginal zone lymphoma-diagnostic and therapeutic implications. Histopathology 2017;70(2):174–84.

[58] de Leval L, Alizadeh AA, Bergsagel PL, et al. Genomic profiling for clinical decision making in lymphoid neoplasms. Blood 2022;140(21):2193–227.

[59] Lee J, Han JH, Lee CH, et al. Comparison of histological and molecular features of pediatric-type follicular lymphoma and pediatric nodal marginal zone lymphoma. Virchows Arch : an international journal of pathology 2023;482(5):849–58.

[60] Zamò A, van den Brand M, Climent F, et al. The many faces of nodal and splenic marginal zone lymphomas. A report of the 2022 EA4HP/SH lymphoma workshop. Virchows Arch : an international journal of pathology 2023;483(3):317–31.

[61] Bonfiglio F, Bruscaggin A, Guidetti F, et al. Genetic and phenotypic attributes of splenic marginal zone lymphoma. Blood 2022;139(5):732–47.

[62] Owen RG, Treon SP, Al-Katib A, et al. Clinicopathological definition of Waldenstrom's macroglobulinemia: Consensus Panel Recommendations from the Second International Workshop on Waldenstrom's Macroglobulinemia. Semin Oncol 2003;30(2):110–5.

[63] Paiva B, Corchete LA, Vidriales M-B, et al. The cellular origin and malignant transformation of Waldenström macroglobulinemia. Blood 2015;125(15):2370–80.

[64] Willenbacher W, Willenbacher E, Brunner A, et al. Improved accuracy of discrimination between IgM multiple myeloma and Waldenström macroglobulinaemia by testing for MYD88 L265P mutations. Br J Haematol 2013;161(6):902–4.

[65] Zanwar S, Abeykoon JP, Durot E, et al. Impact of MYD88(L265P) mutation status on histological transformation of Waldenström Macroglobulinemia. Am J Hematol 2020;95(3):274–81.

[66] Guerrera ML, Tsakmaklis N, Xu L, et al. MYD88 mutated and wild-type Waldenström's Macroglobulinemia: characterization of chromosome 6q gene losses and their mutual exclusivity with mutations in CXCR4. Haematologica 2018;103(9):e408–11.

[67] Kaiser LM, Hunter ZR, Treon SP, et al. CXCR4 in Waldenström's Macroglobulinema: chances and challenges. Leukemia 2021;35(2):333–45.

[68] Castillo JJ, Moreno DF, Arbelaez MI, et al. CXCR4 mutations affect presentation and outcomes in patients with Waldenström macroglobulinemia: A systematic review. Expert review of hematology 2019;12(10):873–81.

[69] Brunner A, Thalhammer-Thurner GC, Willenbacher W, et al. In-depth molecular analysis of lymphomas with lymphoplasmacytic differentiation may provide more precise diagnosis and rational treatment allocation. Ann Hematol 2023;103(2):553–63.

[70] Wang Y, Gali VL, Xu-Monette ZY, et al. Molecular and genetic biomarkers implemented from next-generation sequencing provide treatment insights in clinical practice for Waldenström macroglobulinemia. Neoplasia 2021; 23(4):361–74.

[71] Treon SP, Xu L, Guerrera ML, et al. Genomic Landscape of Waldenström Macroglobulinemia and Its Impact on Treatment Strategies. J Clin Oncol 2020;38(11):1198–208.

[72] Varettoni M, Zibellini S, Defrancesco I, et al. Pattern of somatic mutations in patients with Waldenström macroglobulinemia or IgM monoclonal gammopathy of undetermined significance. Haematologica 2017;102(12): 2077–85.

[73] Arons E, Roth L, Sapolsky J, et al. Evidence of canonical somatic hypermutation in hairy cell leukemia. Blood 2011;117(18):4844–51.

[74] Tiacci E, Schiavoni G, Martelli MP, et al. Constant activation of the RAF-MEK-ERK pathway as a diagnostic and therapeutic target in hairy cell leukemia. Haematologica 2013;98(4):635–9.

[75] Durham BH, Getta B, Dietrich S, et al. Genomic analysis of hairy cell leukemia identifies novel recurrent genetic alterations. Blood 2017;130(14):1644–8.

[76] Forconi F, Sozzi E, Cencini E, et al. Hairy cell leukemias with unmutated IGHV genes define the minor subset refractory to single-agent cladribine and with more aggressive behavior. Blood 2009;114(21):4696–702.

[77] Mason EF, Brown RD, Szeto DP, et al. Detection of activating MAP2K1 mutations in atypical hairy cell leukemia and hairy cell leukemia variant. Leuk Lymphoma 2017; 58(1):233–6.

[78] Paillassa J, Maitre E, Troussard X. Hairy Cell Leukemia (HCL) and HCL Variant: Updates and Spotlights on Therapeutic Advances. Curr Oncol Rep 2022;24(9): 1133–43.

[79] Deshpande A, Munoz J. Targeted and cellular therapies in lymphoma: Mechanisms of escape and innovative strategies. Frontiers in oncology 2022;12:948513.

[80] Whitehair R, Rosti RO, Obiorah IE. Molecular Classification of Diffuse Large B Cell Lymphoma: Impact on Prognosis and Treatment. Advances in Molecular Pathology 2023;6(1):25–37.

[81] Tausch E, Close W, Dolnik A, et al. Venetoclax resistance and acquired BCL2 mutations in chronic lymphocytic leukemia. Haematologica 2019;104(9):e434–7.

[82] Xu L, Tsakmaklis N, Yang G, et al. Acquired mutations associated with ibrutinib resistance in Waldenström macroglobulinemia. Blood 2017;129(18):2519–25.

Infectious Disease

Advances in Molecular Pathology 7 (2024) 89–97
ADVANCES IN MOLECULAR PATHOLOGY

Advances in Self-collection/Self-testing for Sexually Transmitted Infections and Implications for Health Equity

Meghan W. Starolis, PhD, HCLD(ABB)[a,*], Susan E. Realegeno, PhD, D(ABMM)[b]
[a]Infectious Disease, Quest Diagnostics, Molecular Infectious Disease Department, 14225 Newbrook Drive, Chantilly, VA 20151, USA; [b]Quest Diagnostics, Infectious Disease Department, 33608 Ortega Highway, San Juan Capistrano, CA 92675, USA

KEYWORDS
• Self-collection • Sexually transmitted infections • Health equity

KEY POINTS
- Self-collection is the ability of a patient to collect their own sample for testing from a variety of anatomic sites.
- Samples can be shipped to a laboratory for testing, tested at the point-of-care, or self-tested using over-the-counter devices.
- Specific clinical and analytical studies are required when seeking regulatory claims for self-collection in a health care setting (both observed and unobserved) versus at home or another location.
- Self-collection for direct-to-consumer and over-the-counter testing has the potential to lower barriers to access sexually transmitted infection testing for several key patient populations.

INTRODUCTION

The ways in which patients access medical care are evolving, and laboratory testing must also change in response to these new paradigms. Traditionally, patients would seek in-person medical care at a physician office or hospital, and a trained health care provider would collect specimens required for laboratory testing. New ways of accessing care such as telemedicine and direct-to-consumer (DTC) testing are creating the opportunity to collect specimens differently. Additionally, changing cultural and social norms are creating a push for self-collection, where a patient can collect their own sample from a variety of different anatomic sites using provided instructions. The accuracy of self-collection has been extensively studied and found to accurately correlate with clinician-collected samples for organisms including human papillomavirus (HPV) and various sexually transmitted infections (STIs) in sample types such as vaginal or penile meatal swabs [1,2]. Here, the authors will discuss the growing demand for self-collection, including the different categories and regulatory considerations for self-collection and implications for health equity. At the time of this publication, the regulatory landscape related to laboratory testing is rapidly evolving and thus, the authors will mainly focus the regulatory discussion to Food and Drug Administration (FDA) pathways (Table 1)

The term "self-collection" can be further subdivided to explore the regulatory concerns and the potential patient impact. An assay can be approved by the FDA to allow for patient self-collection, which can be specified in the instructions for use (IFU) as either observed or unobserved by a health care provider. Another category is that of *at home collection*. This is a test that is

*Corresponding author. 8226 Tenbrook Drive, Gainesville, VA 20155. *E-mail address:* Meghan.w.starolis@questdiagnostics.com

https://doi.org/10.1016/j.yamp.2024.07.003 www.advancesinmolecularpathology.com
2589-4080/24/

TABLE 1
Summary of Self-Collection Categories

Type of FDA Claim	Definition	Opportunities	Limitations
Self-collection in a health care setting (observed)	Patient self-collects under supervision of a health care provider	Limits exposure to health care workers for contagious diseases	Not ideal for sexually transmitted infections due to privacy concerns No improvement for health care provider efficiency
Self-collection in a health care setting (unobserved)	Patient self-collects without supervision of a health care provider but must be physically present in a health care setting	Improves health care provider efficiency Improved comfort and convenience for the patient	Patient must seek care and/or arrange to be present at a participating health care location
Self-collection outside of a health care setting (ie, home collection) with laboratory-based testing	Patient self-collects at home or remote location and sample is mailed to a laboratory for testing	Expands capabilities of telemedicine Patient has privacy and convenience Can expand access to testing for those unable to reach a provider in-person Over-the-counter and direct-to-consumer options may be available	Stability of sample during transportation must be assessed Insurance required or out of pocket payment for telehealth or DTC services
Self-collection outside of a health care setting (ie, home collection) self-testing	Patient can collect and test their own samples at home	Tests can be purchased OTC or online Rapid turn-around-time for test results Expands access to testing	Significant regulatory requirements for Food and Drug Administration claims May lack sensitivity and specificity Consumer-friendly cost is optimal No counseling or follow-up with health care provider or public health reporting

self-collected by the patient using a collection device mailed to their home or purchased over-the-counter (OTC), in which the sample can be tested in a laboratory or self-tested by the patient at home. Some assays in this category are DTC, meaning that a health care provider is not required to order the test, whereas others may require a telehealth provider or in-person visit prior to obtaining a self-collection kit. Any test approved for at home collection is a different FDA regulatory category, which is typically specified in the intended use statement. Unless the test is FDA-approved for at home collection, the IFU of the assay may indicate if self-collection (both observed and unobserved) should be performed in a health care setting.

DISCUSSION

Self-Collection in a Health Care Setting

Self-collection in a health care setting has many benefits including increased comfort for patients with privacy concerns and improved efficiency for health care providers [3,4]. Self-collected samples may be sent to an on-site or off-site laboratory for testing, or point-of-care (POC) testing may be performed by the provider for rapid turn-around-time (TAT), such as the Clinical Laboratory Improvement Amendments (CLIA)-waived Visby Medical Sexual Health test that utilizes a POC polymerase chain reaction device to detect the organisms that cause chlamydia, gonorrhea (CT/NG), and trichomoniasis [5]. In both cases, the assay utilized must be validated for self-collection and may specify if a health care provider must observe the collection.

Observed self-collection

If an assay has claims for observed self-collection, then a health care provider must be present to watch the patient collect the specimen. The location to be sampled must be accessible to the patient (eg, anterior nares [nasal] swab vs nasopharyngeal swab). Having an FDA claim for observed self-collection can be useful for contagious respiratory diseases such as severe acute respiratory syndrome coronavirus 2 (SARS-CoV-2) which caused the coronavirus disease 2019 (COVID-19) pandemic. It is safer for the health care provider as the observed collection can be done in an environment less conducive to spread of a contagious disease, such as outdoors or in drive-through pharmacy lines, as was implemented during the COVID-19 pandemic [4].

Unobserved self-collection

Assays approved by the FDA for unobserved self-collection do not require health care provider observation of the collection, but still must be performed in a health care setting unless at home collection claims are obtained. Collection in a health care setting allows for controlled conditions where provider assistance is readily available, if needed. It is important to make the distinction that having an unobserved self-collection claim does not equate to an FDA approval for home collection. Several FDA-cleared or approved assays allow for unobserved self-collection of male and female urine, penile meatal swabs, and vaginal samples, which is preferable to observed self-collection due to the private nature of these specimen types. It is important that the clinician and the laboratory understand and specify which specimen types are validated for self-collection. It is also pertinent that clearly understandable collection instructions are provided to the patient to ensure a proper collection.

Home Self-Collection

Telehealth

Using a telehealth approach, a patient would contact a telehealth provider who would assess the patients' symptoms and risk factors and order appropriate testing. In association with a laboratory that offers testing, a kit would be mailed to the patient's home with instructions for unobserved self-collection. After the patient collects the specimen, it would be shipped to a laboratory for testing. The result is provided to the telehealth provider (and possibly to the patient via a website or virtual portal) and the result can be interpreted by a health care provider. Appropriate treatment, additional testing, or other follow-up can also be administered by a health care provider. This approach can be especially useful when a disease has clear clinical symptoms, a straightforward testing approach, and effective treatment (eg, CT/NG) [6]. Assays requiring a blood-based source such as whole blood, serum, or plasma may currently require the patient to visit a phlebotomy center for blood to be collected. At present, the use of at home blood collection devices (eg, Tasso blood lancet device) is expanding which could open more opportunities in the future for self-collected tests that require a blood-based source [7,8].

Direct-to-consumer

In recent years, a new genre of testing has emerged that offers testing for various conditions without the need for a health care provider order or clinical evaluation [9]. There are now many online sellers who offer DTC testing for STIs, with approximately 95% using Clinical Laboratory Improvement Amendments (CLIA) or College of American Pathologist (CAP)-accredited laboratories for testing [9]. Some vendors provide kits for self-collection in a non-health care setting which must be returned to a laboratory, whereas others require the patient to present to a health care provider for collection. As with most disruptive technologies, there are concerns with oversight and quality for DTC testing that will need to be addressed. For example, a study found that 13 out of 20 online retailers of STI DTC products had misleading information that could promote unneeded testing [9]. However, DTC testing presents opportunities to expand testing to people without easy access to medical care, those who may otherwise not seek care due to personal or privacy concerns, or in the event of epidemics or pandemics where testing is needed on a large scale.

For mail-in self-collection kits, the unobserved self-collected sample is shipped to a laboratory for testing after collection. The assay may be FDA-approved for unobserved self-collected samples and validated for various shipping conditions pursuant to FDA requirements. The assay vendor or the testing laboratory can pursue the required FDA approvals to receive the designation for remote self-collection. Tests may also be approved for at home testing, but options with this format are currently limited. The OTC home tests for SARS-CoV-2 are an example of tests that are self-collected and tested at home. These types of tests require a simple self-collection (eg, nasal swab) and the test itself must be easy to operate using provided instructions, such as a lateral flow device. As of the time of this publication, there are no OTC home testing options for STIs other than the OraQuick In-Home HIV Test, an OTC kit that can be purchased both online and at brick-and-mortar retailers. This assay detects antibodies to human immunodeficiency virus (HIV)-1 and HIV-2 using an oral swab but requires confirmatory testing in a medical setting [6]. Given the increasing demand for at home testing fueled by the COVID-19 pandemic, this may change in the future.

DTC testing modalities are not without challenges. At home tests may lack sensitivity and specificity compared with their in-laboratory comparators and may require confirmatory testing [10,11]. Likewise, follow-up care may be required for preliminary results. For example, if nucleic acid amplification testing (NAAT) for HPV were to be performed using DTC home-collection kits, a follow-up Papanicolaou (pap) smear or colposcopy may be warranted based on the initial results and patients would need to be appropriately linked to care [12]. This can be challenging but could be solved by using a telehealth approach. For OTC testing where there is no health care provider involvement, there are limited opportunities to counsel patients about what clinical scenarios could cause false results, leading to incorrect diagnoses. This could be especially important if the testing modality lacks sensitivity or for diseases that have distinct phases and windows of organism detection (eg, syphilis or genital herpes) [13]. The patient may also not be counseled on the appropriate notification of their sexual partner(s), which can result in further spread of disease. Reporting results of notifiable diseases to public health entities is also problematic with OTC DTC testing. Currently, the various states specify organisms or diseases which require notification to the public health department, but this mandate would not extend to OTC DTC testing or may be difficult to track. This could lead to a lack of epidemiologic data which is critical for the management of outbreaks or disease spread [13].

Advances in Self-Sampling Devices

Certain specimen types are well-suited to patient self-collection, such as urine, vaginal swabs, nasal swabs, saliva, and penile meatal swabs [1,2,4,14,15]. However, this has limited the availability of testing from self-collected samples to assays that can utilize those specific specimen types for testing. To expand the use of self-collected samples, advances are being made in self-sampling devices that can be utilized for downstream testing, including NAATs. These devices allow for collection of samples normally collected by a health care provider, such as blood or cervical samples. As mentioned earlier, devices such as the Tasso blood lancet device and Mitra microsampling device can be used for self-collecting whole blood, or a finger prick can be used to fill a small blood vial or to create a dried blood spot [16,17]. There are also devices that have been designed and optimized for at home self-collection of cervical samples for HPV NAATs. These include the Evalyn Brush and a lower cost version called Viba-Brush which is appropriate for low-income and middle-income countries (both available through Rovers Medical Devices) [18]. Both versions utilize the same collection head and collect a similar yield, but the Viba-Brush has a simpler, more economical design [19]. The Evalyn Brush is reported to cost 3 to 5 times more than other cervical self-collection devices [19]. Qvintip (Aprovix) and Copan Self FLOQSwabs Vaginal collection kit are additional options that have been specifically designed for at home use [18–21]. It is important to note that as of this publication, none of the devices mentioned earlier are currently validated or utilized as part of an FDA-cleared or approved assay for at home collection of STIs. Performance data of these devices are widely available as several countries have implemented self-collection in their HPV screening programs using these devices [19,22,23].

Regulatory Considerations

Self-collection designation for tests can be granted during the FDA approval process and is indicated in the intended use of the assay. Until recently, there were no FDA-approved tests for self-collection outside a health care setting that required the specimen to be shipped back to a clinical laboratory for testing. In late 2023, the FDA approved the first OTC self-collection kit for CT/NG NAAT outside the supervision of a health care provider as a De Novo authorization (LetsGetChecked Simple 2 Test). The product does not require an order from a provider to obtain the specimen collection kit but does include involvement of a health care provider throughout the process. The health care provider evaluates a health suitability questionnaire once the at home kit is activated online. Patients with positive or invalid results will be contacted by a health care provider, and a follow-up consultation is available for any patient. Prior to this approval, regulatory expectations for at home collection and subsequent testing in a clinical laboratory were ambiguous except for certain states who enacted local legislation limiting or prohibiting the use of DTC services, such as New York (NY) and Rhode Island [24]. For example, although DTC testing is limited in NY, the state public health department posted a "Question & Answer" in June 2022 specifically addressing STI self-collection outside of a health care setting [25]. The document outlines specific criteria that need to be met to allow self-collection outside of a health care setting, including involvement of a provider to order the test, complete a health assessment, interpret the results, and link the patient to treatment services. In terms of laboratory testing, the sample submitted for testing must be performed in an NY state-permitted laboratory authorized to perform clinical testing. The test itself should be an FDA-cleared or approved test or a laboratory-developed test (LDT) that has been approved though the NY Clinical Laboratory Evaluation Program (CLEP). If the laboratory is using an FDA-cleared or approved assay without an at home self-collection claim, further validation studies for self-collection outside of a health care setting may need to be submitted and approved by NY CLEP as a test modification. Although this process may be acceptable for NY, additional review from the FDA via a 510(k) may now be expected considering the recent FDA-approval for the first at-home STI collection kit.

The recent FDA-approval for LetsGetChecked has provided a pathway for other entities seeking FDA-approval for STI DTC products through an FDA 510(k) premarket process. Specifically, the approval demonstrates that regulatory bodies are seeking labeling and testing "controls" to ensure safety and effectiveness of specimen collection, testing, and result interpretation [26]. Accuracy in specimen collection and specimen stability during shipping and handling needs to be evaluated in the form of flex and excursion studies. These may include testing the specimen with interfering substances and with extreme temperature fluctuations to mimic various seasonal conditions in different geographic locations. Endogenous specimen adequacy controls (sometimes referred to as "cellularity controls") for NAATs, such as detection of human beta-globin or RNaseP genes, can offer assurance that the sample was properly collected, but may not be required [27]. For example, the Hologic Aptima Combo 2 Assay for detection of CT/NG allows for unobserved self-collection in a health care setting but does not contain an endogenous specimen adequacy control [28]. The laboratory may need to submit data demonstrating that this specific control is not necessary. In addition, "special controls" related to the product's FDA class II (moderate risk) regulatory device classification are required [26]. These special controls include the use of a test that is already approved for an OTC indication (currently there are none for molecular STI tests) or as part of the OTC submission, the submitter should include data demonstrating correct product usability independent of a health care provider.

Extensive details pertaining to clinical indications, analytical testing details, specimen acceptability, and limitations are described in the IFU and package labeling. Although submitters can demonstrate substantial equivalence with an existing FDA-approved device(s), additional design verification and validation studies might be needed. These requirements may differ if the submitter is seeking an OTC claim for a new or existing FDA-cleared or approved test or if seeking clearance for the collection device. In addition, analytical design verification and validation studies for the testing are part of the FDA 510(k) submission. If the assay is already FDA-cleared or approved, then referencing a previous FDA submission may be sufficient for the analytical review. However, for services offering testing using an LDT, validation data would need to be submitted when seeking FDA claims. Having the first FDA-approved at home STI solution may have regulatory consequences for existing programs that offer self-collection testing but have not sought FDA approval and are using an assay outside the intended use.

Considering the lack of regulatory enforcement, several STI mail-in self-collection services are available in most states with varying degrees of transparency and alignment with STI testing and treatment guidelines [9,29]. For instance, in a study examining 20 mail-in programs, a variety of options were available including NAATs for CT/NG, *Trichomonas vaginalis*, *Mycoplasma* spp. (including *Mycoplasma genitalium*), *Ureaplasma* spp., and *Gardnerella* spp. using urine and swabs, as well as dried blood spots for HIV and syphilis serology testing [29]. For certain organisms (CT/NG, *T vaginalis [TV]*), screening in select sexually active individuals may be appropriate based on risk, age, or sexual behaviors [30]. However, other analytes such as *M genitalium* are only recommended in symptomatic individuals, and there are currently no testing recommendations for other *Mycoplasma* spp. or *Ureaplasma* spp [30,31]. Some of these offerings are available only as a fixed order that includes multiple analytes (ie, CT/NG/TV or HIV/Hepatitis C Virus) and there were some offerings that did not specify which analytes were being tested on the website [29]. Another review of mail-in services reported that information posted by the vendor on their websites was often misleading, inaccurate, or inadequate with regards to screening recommendation and the FDA status of the assay(s) [9]. Therefore, some testing services may not be providing appropriate testing options, quality results, or interpretation for proper follow-up care or testing.

In 2021, The American Sexually Transmitted Diseases Association (ASTDA) released a position statement outlining recommendations for DTC STI testing programs or services [13]. These recommendations are focused on reducing risk of harm to the consumer and ensuring quality of testing, clinical management, and public health reporting. In terms of consumer experience, it is recommended that detailed information regarding the entire service process (collection, testing, result reporting, and provider involvement) should be available in a consumer-friendly manner, including up-to-date Frequently Asked Questions (FAQs). Testing menus should include analytes that are consistent with professional recommendations, with limitations or warnings communicated for certain populations (ie, pregnant women). In terms of the laboratory, testing should be performed in an accredited facility where validation data meet regulatory requirements (eg, CAP/CLIA). Once results are available, appropriate clinical management such as interpretation of results, recommendations for additional testing or treatment, and public health reporting is critical. Interfacing with a provider at any point in the process typically involves a telemedicine consultation. Possible solutions to ensure all the recommended components of the testing cycle are fulfilled may include the use of a digital platform to register the kit, receive results/interpretations, communicate with a provider (message, call, or video), and automatic public health reporting. The ASTDA recommendations are in-line with the requirements set forth by the FDA in the approval of the first at home self-collection kit for CT/NG [32]. However, these recommendations do not fully address health equity and access to testing.

Implications for Health Equity

Self-collection, and the associated subcategories of at home collection, home testing, and DTC testing, presents opportunities to bring medical care to previously underserved populations. These populations include, but are not limited to, people who live in medically underserved geographic areas, the transgender community, people living with HIV, people without adequate medical insurance, and those who feel stigmatized or embarrassed by STI testing. It is also pertinent to clarify that the term used by the FDA of "at home collection" does not eliminate people experiencing homelessness or the incarcerated from the eligible patient population who may benefit from self-collection [9,33].

It is important to remember that self-collection can be perceived differently by different patient populations and thus, the freedom of choice and cultural sensitivity is paramount. For example, in the transgender patient population, a meta-analysis showed that transmasculine patients preferred self-collection over clinician-collected samples [3]. Transmasculine patients are under-tested for STIs due to several barriers related to social stigma, distrust of health care providers, and fear of a lack of discretion [34]. Self-collection, especially at home collection, could be particularly effective at lowering some of these barriers to accessing STI testing in this population. Conversely, respondents in several studies preferred clinician-collection for various reasons including body shyness, cultural barriers that prohibit the perception of self-touch of the genital region, or lacking confidence in their ability to self-collect [3,35–37]. Efforts to promote or expand self-collection in these patient populations must aim to create culturally sensitive initiatives, such as instructions that are available with both written instruction as well as appropriate graphic depictions of collection instructions available in a multitude of languages [3].

The current landscape for DTC STI testing primarily consists of online mail-in services with limited OTC options. Online services are thought to increase access to testing by eliminating barriers associated with an in-person health care visit. For example, travel time and accommodations for attending a scheduled appointment, time spent waiting to see a health care provider, and discomfort associated with discussing sexual history with a health care provider can be circumvented with DTC testing [38]. However, studies have suggested that while interventions associated with online DTC testing may alleviate several barriers to access testing, additional barriers still exist. To start, since most services are web-based, this limits access to those with a reliable internet connection and competency navigating the internet. Online follow-up to view results and participate in a virtual consultation with a health care provider may also be required. Although most of the population will have internet at home, it is estimated that 8% of Americans do not have internet in their household [13]. Web-based services that can also be accessed via telephone may be considered as an additional method to ordering mail-in kits. However, according to a study, some online vendors of DTC kits were not easy to contact and may not answer specific customer questions [9].

In addition to internet accessibility, cost of testing may also be a barrier to certain individuals depending on the testing program available [39]. At least 20 DTC programs have been identified as of June 2023. Six provided testing at no cost and others provided testing at a median price of $79 for a single analyte and at lower prices per analyte if multiple analytes are purchased [9,29]. The cost of testing is likely to be out of pocket if obtained through a retailer versus a public health or community program. Five programs were reported to accept insurance for billing [29]. However, DTC testing where a health care provider does not submit the test requisition is often not covered by insurance [13]. State legislation requiring health insurance providers to cover DTC has been proposed in California [40]. Such steps would allow increased access to insured individuals where cost of testing is a barrier. However, there may be additional costs associated with health care provider consultations or for follow-up testing and/or care.

For mail-in services, receiving a kit at home to a fixed mailing address may be a barrier for people experiencing homelessness or those with privacy concerns associated with family or co-habitants. For example, a focus-group-based study examining barriers for DTC testing in youth showed that some individuals preferred the kit to be available in clinics, schools, libraries, or Amazon service lockers [39]. Alternative pick-up locations or widespread retailer availability is important to increase access, including rural areas with few retail stores or shipping/receiving options. One DTC program reported underutilization in a region with unique delivery requirements, such as non-standardized mailboxes [41]. Therefore, it is important to consider various delivery options depending on the targeted population.

SUMMARY

The ability for patients to collect their own samples has tremendous implications for the future of laboratory testing. Self-collection in a health care setting can alleviate discomfort at the health care provider office, especially for those in the transgender community, which can lead to increased willingness to participate in routine STI screening. Going further, self-collection for either at home testing or shipment to a clinical laboratory can bridge gaps in health equity by providing access to people in geographically underserved areas, people without health insurance, or those who feel stigmatized by STI testing. Although the future is promising, there are several hurdles to overcome. Any test developed for at home use must demonstrate adequate performance (ie, clinical sensitivity and specificity) while being easy and safe to use at home. Additionally, there are financial and economic barriers associated with development of these types of assays due to costly clinical studies and regulatory requirements when seeking FDA approval. To solve issues of health equity, the resulting test must also be affordably priced and easy to access by consumers. Meeting all of these design goals and incorporating novel self-sampling collection devices will be the challenge as this area of health care continues to expand.

CLINICS CARE POINTS

- Patients are increasingly accessing medical care through telemedicine which necessitates innovation in how patient samples are collected for laboratory testing.
- Patient self-collection in a health care setting, at home for laboratory-based testing, or at home for home testing is increasing in demand.
- There are significant regulatory requirements for the ability to self-collect, collect at home, and/or test at home when seeking approval from the FDA.
- Self-collection may lower barriers to accessing STI testing and increase patient comfort and likelihood of seeking care.

DISCLOSURES

No funding was received to support the preparation of this article. M.W. Starolis and S.E. Realegeno disclose that they are full-time employees and stockholders of Quest Diagnostics. M.W. Starolis is a council member and chairperson of the Clinical Practice Committee for the Pan American Society for Clinical Virology (PASCV). M.W. Starolis serves on the Clinical Practice Committee for the Association of Molecular Pathology (AMP). This article is intended to be educational. Please seek legal counsel when considering the use of self-collection or home collection.

REFERENCES

[1] Lunny C, Taylor D, Hoang L, et al. Self-collected versus clinician-collected sampling for chlamydia and gonorrhea screening: a systemic review and meta-analysis. PLoS One 2015;10(7):e0132776.

[2] Gennaro GD, Licata F, Trovato A, et al. Does self-sampling for human papilloma virus testing have the potential to increase cervical cancer screening? An updated meta-analysis of observational studies and randomized clinical trials. Front Public Heal 2022;10:1003461.

[3] Camara H, Zhang Y, Lafferty L, et al. Self-collection for HPV-based cervical screening: a qualitative evidence meta-synthesis. BMC Publ Health 2021;21(1):1503.

[4] Cockerill FR, Wohlgemuth JG, Radcliff J, et al. Evolution of specimen self-collection in the COVID-19 era: implications for population health management of infectious disease. Popul Health Manag 2021;24(S1):S-26-S-34.

[5] Renzoni A, Perez F, Nsoga MTN, et al. Analytical evaluation of visby medical RT-PCR portable device for rapid detection of SARS-CoV-2. Diagnostics 2021;11(5):813.

[6] Kersh EN. Advances in sexually transmitted infection testing at home and in nonclinical settings close to the home. Sex Transm Dis 2022;49(11S):S12–4.

[7] Hendelman T, Chaudhary A, LeClair AC, et al. Self-collection of capillary blood using Tasso-SST devices for Anti-SARS-CoV-2 IgG antibody testing. PLoS One 2021;16(9):e0255841.

[8] Cannon CA, Ramchandani MS, Golden MR. Feasibility of a novel self-collection method for blood samples and its acceptability for future home-based PrEP monitoring. BMC Infect Dis 2022;22(1):459.

[9] Manca E. Pol BV der, Exten C, Pinto CN. A review of the scope of direct-to-consumer sexually transmitted infection testing services offered on the internet. Sex Transm Dis 2023;50(6):323–8.

[10] Chu VT, Schwartz NG, Donnelly MAP, et al. Comparison of home antigen testing with RT-PCR and viral culture during the course of SARS-CoV-2 Infection. JAMA Intern Med 2022;182(7):701–9.

[11] Neuman M, Mwinga A, Kapaku K, et al. Sensitivity and specificity of OraQuick® HIV self-test compared to a 4th generation laboratory reference standard algorithm in urban and rural Zambia. BMC Infect Dis 2022; 22(Suppl 1):494.

[12] Bhatla N, Singhal S. Primary HPV screening for cervical cancer. Best Pract Res Clin Obstet Gynaecol 2020;65: 98–108.

[13] Exten C, Pinto CN, Gaynor AM, et al. Direct-to-consumer sexually transmitted infection testing services: a position statement from the american sexually transmitted diseases association. Sex Transm Dis 2021;48(11):e155–9.

[14] Dize L, Barnes P, Barnes M, et al. Performance of self-collected penile-meatal swabs compared to clinician-collected urethral swabs for the detection of Chlamydia trachomatis, Neisseria gonorrhoeae, Trichomonas vaginalis, and Mycoplasma genitalium by nucleic acid amplification assays. Diagn Microbiol Infect Dis 2016;86(2): 131–5.

[15] Estem KS, Catania J, Klausner JD. HIV self-testing: a review of current implementation and fidelity. Curr HIV AIDS Rep 2016;13(2):107–15.

[16] Spielberg F, Critchlow C, Vittinghoff E, et al. Home collection for frequent HIV testing: acceptability of oral fluids, dried blood spots and telephone results. AIDS 2000;14(12):1819–28.

[17] Tucker JD, Bien CH, Peeling RW. Point-of-care testing for sexually transmitted infections. Curr Opin Infect Dis 2013;26(1):73–9.

[18] Clark M, Horton J. Self-sampling devices for HPV Testing: CADTH Horizon Scan. Canadian Agency for Drugs and Technologies in Health. 2021. Available at: https://www.ncbi.nlm.nih.gov/books/NBK594331/. [Accessed 18 April 2024].

[19] Hawkes D, Keung MHT, Huang Y, et al. Self-collection for cervical screening programs: from research to reality. Cancers 2020;12(4):1053.

[20] Sechi I, Muresu N, Puci MV, et al. Preliminary results of feasibility and acceptability of self-collection for cervical screening in italian women. Pathogens 2023;12(9):1169.

[21] Saville M, Hawkes D, Keung M, et al. Analytical performance of HPV assays on vaginal self-collected vs practitioner-collected cervical samples: the SCoPE study. J Clin Virol 2020;127:104375.

[22] Serrano B, Ibáñez R, Robles C, et al. Worldwide use of HPV self-sampling for cervical cancer screening. Prev Med 2022;154:106900.

[23] Latsuzbaia A, Broeck DV, Keer SV, et al. Validation of BD Onclarity HPV assay on vaginal self-samples versus cervical samples using the VALHUDES Protocol. Cancer Epidemiol Biomark Prev 2022;31(12):2177–84.

[24] Survey of direct-to-consumer testing statutes and regulations. 2007. Available at: https://repository.library.georgetown.edu/bitstream/handle/10822/511162/DTCStateLawChart.pdf?sequence=1&isAllowed=y.

[25] STI Self-Collection Outside of a Clinic Setting in New York State - Q & A. 2022. Available at: https://www.health.ny.gov/diseases/communicable/std/docs/self_collection.pdf.

[26] U.S. Food & Drug Administration 10903 New Hampshire Avenue Doc ID # 04017.06.05 Silver Spring, MD 20993. Available at: www.fda.gov.

[27] Brukner I, Resendes A, Eintracht S, et al. Sample Adequacy Control (SAC) Lowers False Negatives and Increases the Quality of Screening: Introduction of "Non-Competitive" SAC for qPCR Assays. Diagnostics 2021; 11(7):1133.

[28] Hologic. Aptima Combo 2 Assay (Panther System) Package Insert. 2023. Available at: https://www.hologic.com/package-inserts/diagnostic-products/aptima-combo-2-assay-ctng. [Accessed 20 May 2024].

[29] Pontes MF, Armington G, Fink R, et al. Landscape review of mail-in self-collection, programs for sexually transmitted infections. Sex Transm Dis 2023;50(6):336–41.

[30] Workowski KA, Bachmann LH, Chan PA, et al. Sexually transmitted infections treatment guidelines, 2021. MMWR Recomm Rep (Morb Mortal Wkly Rep) 2021; 70(4):1–187.

[31] Horner P, Donders G, Cusini M, et al. Should we be testing for urogenital Mycoplasma hominis, Ureaplasma parvum and Ureaplasma urealyticum in men and women? – a position statement from the European STI Guidelines Editorial Board. J Eur Acad Dermatol Venereol 2018;32(11):1845–51.

[32] LetsGetChecked. Simple 2 Test - Package Insert. 2024.

[33] Kersh EN, Shukla M, Raphael BH, et al. At-home specimen self-collection and self-testing for sexually transmitted infection screening demand accelerated by the

COVID-19 pandemic: a review of laboratory implementation issues. J Clin Microbiol 2021;59(11):026466-e2720.

[34] Stewart M, Ryu H, Blaque E, et al. Cisnormativity as a structural barrier to STI testing for trans masculine, two-spirit, and non-binary people who are gay, bisexual, or have sex with men. PLoS One 2022;17(11):e0277315.

[35] Fargnoli V, Petignat P, Burton-Jeangros C. To what extent will women accept HPV self-sampling for cervical cancer screening? A qualitative study conducted in Switzerland. Int J Wom Health 2015;7:883–8.

[36] Teng FF, Mitchell SM, Sekikubo M, et al. Understanding the role of embarrassment in gynaecological screening: a qualitative study from the ASPIRE cervical cancer screening project in Uganda. BMJ Open 2014;4(4):e004783.

[37] Howard M, Lytwyn A, Lohfeld L, et al. Barriers to acceptance of self-sampling for human papillomavirus across ethnolinguistic groups of women. Can J Public Health 2009;100(5):365–9.

[38] Gilbert M, Thomson K, Salway T, et al. Differences in experiences of barriers to STI testing between clients of the internet-based diagnostic testing service GetCheckedOnline.com and an STI clinic in Vancouver, Canada. Sex Transm Infect 2019;95(2):151.

[39] Sao SS, Yu R, Abboud S, et al. Utilizing digital health technology to increase sexual health care access: youth preferences on self-collect, mail-in sexually transmitted infection testing in a high sexually transmitted infection prevalence area. J Adolesc Health 2023;73(6):1002–9.

[40] Doan THP, Adamson PC, Klausner JD. Legislation to increase accessibility to direct-to-consumer tests in California. Sex Transm Dis 2022;49(1):e37.

[41] Rahib D, Delagreverie H, Gabassi A, et al. Online self-sampling kits to screen multipartner MSM for HIV and other STIs: participant characteristics and factors associated with kit use in the first 3 months of the MemoDepistages programme, France, 2018. Sex Transm Infect 2021;97(2):134–40.

Advances in Molecular Pathology 7 (2024) 99–111
ADVANCES IN MOLECULAR PATHOLOGY

Implementation, Optimization, and Stewardship of Advanced Molecular Testing for Infectious Diseases

Vahid Azimi, MD, Rebekah E. Dumm, PhD*
Division of Laboratory and Genomic Medicine, Pathology & Immunology, Washington University School of Medicine, 425 South Euclid Avenue, St Louis, MO 63110, USA

KEYWORDS
• Diagnostic stewardship • Molecular • Infectious disease

KEY POINTS

- Diagnostic stewardship for molecular infectious disease encompasses the implementation of new tests, as well as the stewardship of existing tests through the selection of the right test, specimen, and patient population.
- Appropriate use of syndromic molecular panels can help provide rapid results and guide antimicrobial prescribing.
- Sequencing-based assays can be costly and complex; laboratory input is crucial to guiding selection of the right test, specimen, and patient population.
- The clinical laboratory is well-suited to coordinate diagnostic stewardship efforts for complex molecular infectious disease testing.
- More research on the impact of diagnostic stewardship interventions for molecular infectious disease testing is needed.

BACKGROUND AND GOALS OF DIAGNOSTIC STEWARDSHIP

Technological innovations and health care evolutions drive the increasing complexity and scope of laboratory medicine. Complexity increases as technology advances, especially around advanced molecular testing for the diagnosis of infectious diseases, where both laboratory workflows and test interpretations pose unique challenges [1]. The scope of testing broadens as health care consolidation requires laboratories to make strategic decisions about which testing to maintain in-house for optimal turnaround time (TAT), send to a consolidated or reference laboratories, or offer at the point-of-care [2]. To address the growing complexity of testing options, diagnostic stewardship aims to guide the appropriate selection and interpretation of laboratory testing in the care of an individual patient and support system-wide practices in appropriate utilization of tests. Across laboratory testing, a diagnostic stewardship framework must address (1) new test or technology implementation, (2) existing test and order sets optimization, and (3) approaches to guide send-out tests. We use this framework to discuss common strategies for advanced molecular tests. Specifically, we address multiplex syndromic PCR platforms, which offer an accessible option to diagnose common community-acquired infections and sequencing-based assays, which are often offered by specialized reference laboratories. These frameworks are not mutually exclusive. Syndromic panels which are not offered in-house may be referred elsewhere for testing and sequencing could be performed in-house—both scenarios require

*Corresponding author, *E-mail address:* dumm@wustl.edu

https://doi.org/10.1016/j.yamp.2024.07.004 www.advancesinmolecularpathology.com
2589-4080/24/

stewardship considerations that we will not directly address.

Efforts to steward laboratory testing must be effective and sustainable. Effective interventions incorporate behavioral strategies with systemic support, and are most applicable when crafted with interdisciplinary teams [3]. Given their unique expertise in microbiology, assay technology, and laboratory workflows, the clinical laboratory is well-suited to coordinate stewardship efforts with input from experts in infectious disease, pharmacy and informatics [4–6]. Sustainable interventions, similarly, require support and resources from institutional leaders [3,7]. Traditionally, stewardship is thought of as encompassing the educational efforts and interventions to guide laboratory utilization. Here, we propose that choosing and implementing the appropriate testing methodology for routine use is a critical element of stewarding laboratory testing. Deciding whether a test should be added to the inhouse formulary (ie, a list of approved diagnostic tests with potential additional restrictions based on ordering users or clinical circumstances [8]), maintained as an orderable option, or a by-request-only send-out requires an iterative evaluation process based on clinical need and available resources, efforts which the microbiology laboratory is uniquely positioned to coordinate [9].

Previous reviews of diagnostic stewardship in microbiology testing have focused on blood culture use [10,11], blood culture molecular panels and their impacts on targeted antimicrobial therapy [12,13], *Clostridioides difficile* utilization and algorithms [14,15] and urinary tract infection (UTI) reflex testing [16,17]. While many of these workflows include aspects of molecular testing, we will not address them in this review. Instead, we will focus on a subset of advanced molecular technologies routinely used in clinical microbiology laboratories: multiplexed molecular panels for syndromic testing and sequencing technologies. In contrast to earlier single-target molecular tests which improved sensitivity for pathogen detection but required expensive new instrumentation and involved workflows [18], current multiplexed molecular panels also improve clinical workflows by reducing turnaround time (TAT), and/or increasing laboratory workflow efficiency [1,19,20]. Sequencing-based assays are one step further removed—they are often performed in consolidated, reference or commercial laboratories. Given the limited availability, advanced technical features and unique challenges to result interpretation, sequencing assays may require a different approach to stewardship.

STEWARDSHIP INTERVENTIONS FOR SYNDROMIC MULTIPLEX TESTING

Multiplexed molecular panels for syndromic testing are a fast, often sample-to-answer, accessible strategy to detect many pathogens, and can be used to diagnose both common and complex presentations of disease. Stewardship of these panels can coincide with implemetation of the assay (ie, education or order sets) or can be prompted by reviewing local testing practices retrospectively. These features are encompassed in the traditional definition of diagnostic stewardship. However, we include studies describing assay implementation without traditional stewardship interventions as they provide critical information to target patient populations with highest impact from novel technology. Literature on diagnostic stewardship for syndromic multiplex panel testing can be categorized as: studies that describe the impact of implementing new testing [21–38] (Table 1), and diagnostic stewardship interventions designed to improve ordering practices of preexisting testing [39–49] (Table 2). Very few studies directly address potential benefits of sending these syndromic multiplex panel testing to a referral laboratory, so it will not be addressed in this review.

Implementation-based studies can be categorized based on the syndrome, study design, platform, encounter setting, or outcomes measured. If sorted by syndrome (see Table 1), studies assessing the utility of a respiratory pathogen (RP) panel are most common [21,24,29,32,34–38,50], followed by gastrointestinal (GI) [22,26,31,51], pneumonia (PN) [25,28,30], meningitis-encephalitis (ME) [27,33], and joint infection (JI) [23]. Most studies used a pre-post implementation retrospective analysis framework for assessing the impact of new testing, and few studies used randomized controlled trials [21,24,28,29,32]. Sorted by encounter setting, most studies measured testing of hospitalized inpatients or patients in the emergency department. Only 1 study assessed patients in an intensive care unit [30]. Most studies evaluated testing in adults, with only 2 studies focused on pediatric populations [33,34]. Finally, all but 2 studies exclusively analyzed testing for patients at large, academic referral centers [22,26].

Across implementation studies, measured outcomes included antibiotic or antiviral prescription practices, time to species identification/result, hospital length of stay, hospital admissions, use of isolation facilities, use of other diagnostic procedures (ie, chest radiographs), and financial impact. Generally, most studies reported that implementation of syndromic multiplex panels led to improvements in patient care, including

TABLE 1
Summary of Interventions for Implementation of Syndromic Multiplex Testing

Study	Platform	Design	Setting	Results
Andrews et al, [21] 2017	BioFire FilmArray RP	Quasi-randomized controlled trial	Hospitalized inpatients, tertiary care teaching hospital	• No significant difference in length of stay • 52% reduction in result turnaround time
Brendish et al, [24] 2017	BioFire FilmArray RP	Randomized controlled trial	Emergency Department, teaching hospital	• No significant difference in proportion of patients treated with antibiotics • No significant difference in mean duration of antibiotics • 7% increase in number of patients with only a single dose of antibiotics • 1.1 d median reduction in length of stay • 26.4% increase in patients with appropriate antiviral treatment
Echavarria et al, [29] 2018	BioFire FilmArray RP	Randomized controlled trial	Emergency Department, teaching hospital, adults and pediatric patients	• Increased odds of withholding antibiotics in adults and children (adults: aOR 15.52, children: aOR 12.23) • No significant change in antiviral prescriptions in adults or children • Increased odds of avoiding complementary diagnostic procedures in adults (aOR 9.64) • 92% reduction in result turnaround time
May et al, [32] 2019	BioFire FilmArray RP	Randomized controlled trial	Emergency Department, quaternary care teaching hospital, adults and pediatric patients	• 12% reduction in antibiotic prescriptions • No significant reduction in antiviral use • No significant difference in length of stay, disposition, or 30-d mortality
Nelson et al, [34] 2015	BioFire FilmArray RP	Retrospective analysis	Pediatric Emergency Department, tertiary care hospital	• Savings of $115,556/QALY for children ages 3–36 mo • Savings of $228,000/QALY for children ages 3–18 y

(continued on next page)

TABLE 1
(continued)

Study	Platform	Design	Setting	Results
Rappo et al, [50] 2016	BioFire FilmArray RP	Retrospective analysis	Emergency Department, tertiary care teaching hospital	• 78% reduction in time to influenza diagnosis • Decreased odds of admission, length of stay, duration of antimicrobial use, and number of chest radiographs
Rogers et al, [35] 2014	BioFire FilmArray RP	Retrospective analysis	Hospitalized inpatients, tertiary care hospital	• 66% reduction in result turnaround time • 26 min increase in emergency department length of stay • 0.4 d reduction in antibiotic use • No significant difference in number of patients receiving antibiotics or inpatient length of stay
Subramony et al, [36] 2016	BioFire FilmArray RP	Retrospective analysis	Hospitalized inpatients, tertiary care hospital	• 20% reduction in median antibiotic days • 24% reduction in chest radiographs • 20 h median reduction in isolation hours
Vos et al, [37] 2019	BioFire FilmArray RP	Retrospective analysis	Immunocompromised patients, Emergency Department, tertiary care hospital	• Decreased use of in-hospital isolation facilities (aOR 0.35) • Fewer inappropriate use of antivirals (aOR 0.15) • Greater appropriate use of antivirals (aOR 11.1) • No difference in empirical antibiotic use, hospital admissions, length of stay, or adverse events
Weiss et al, [38] 2019	ePlex RP	Retrospective analysis	Emergency Department, 2 tertiary care teaching hospitals	• 89% reduction in result turnaround time • 24% reduction in antibiotic use • 12% reduction in hospital admissions • No significant different in antimicrobial escalation
Axelrad et al, [22] 2019	BioFire FilmArray GI	Retrospective analysis	Hospitalized inpatients from teaching hospital and outpatients	• 1.2% reduction in endoscopic procedures • 2.3% reduction in use of abdominal radiology • 4.7% reduction in antimicrobial prescriptions

Cybulski et al, [26] 2018	BioFire FilmArray GI	Retrospective analysis	Hospitalized inpatients from teaching hospital and outpatients	• 62% reduction in turnaround time • 3.5% increase in targeted antimicrobial therapy • 16.5% reduction in empiric antimicrobial prescriptions • 64% reduction in time to appropriate antimicrobials
Goldenberg et al, [31] 2015	Luminex xTAG GI	Retrospective analysis	Hospitalized inpatients, teaching hospital	• 34% reduction in time spent in isolation protocol with associated savings of £66,765
Rogers et al, [51] 2020	BioFire FilmArray GI	Retrospective analysis	Hospitalized inpatients, tertiary care hospital	• 12% increase in patients with an infectious diarrheal pathogen identified • No difference in median costs of stool testing per patient
Buchan et al, [25] 2020	BioFire FilmArray PN	Retrospective analysis	Hospitalized inpatients, multiple teaching hospitals	• 6.2 antibiotic days/patient reduction • Appropriate antibiotic de-escalation in 48.2% of patients • Appropriate antibiotic escalation in 4.3% of patients • Inappropriate antibiotic de-escalation in 1.6% of patients • Inappropriate antibiotic escalation in 16.6% of patients
Darie et al, [28] 2022	Unyvero Hospitalized Pneumonia cartridge	Randomized controlled trial	Hospitalized inpatients, 2 tertiary care hospitals	• 45% decrease in duration of antibiotic therapy • 27% reduction in inappropriate antimicrobial therapy
Esplund et al, [30] 2023	BioFire FilmArray PN	Retrospective analysis	ICU inpatients, teaching hospital	• 58% decrease in time to first antibiotic change • Antimicrobial de-escalation in 31% of patients • Antimicrobial escalation in 9% of patients
Dack et al, [27] 2019	BioFire FilmArray ME	Retrospective analysis	Hospitalized inpatients, teaching hospital	• No significant change in duration of antimicrobials • No significant change in length of stay

(continued on next page)

TABLE 1
(continued)

Study	Platform	Design	Setting	Results
Messacar et al [33], 2022	BioFire FilmArray ME	Retrospective analysis	Pediatric inpatients, quaternary care hospital	• 36% reduction in time to optimal antimicrobial treatment • 47% decrease in time to positive CSF results • 33% reduction in IV antimicrobial duration • 50% increase in infectious neurologic diagnoses • No difference in hospital admissions or length of stay
Berinson et al [23], 2023	BioFire FilmArray JI	Retrospective analysis	Hospitalized inpatients, tertiary care teaching hospital	• 49 h median reduction in time to species identification • 99 h median reduction in time to molecular susceptibility data

Abbreviations: d, days; h, hours; RP, respiratory pathogen panel; GI, gastrointestinal pathogen panel; PN, pneumonia panel; ME, meningitis/encephalitis panel; JI, joint infection panel.

TABLE 2
Summary of Interventions for Optimizing Syndromic Multiplex Diagnostic Assays

Study	Platform	Phase	Intervention	Results
Broadhurst et al [40], 2020	BioFire FilmArray ME	Pre-analytic	Restriction of testing to pleocytic CSF samples	• Potential 43% reduction in test utilization with 62% increase in testing yield
Campodonico et al [41], 2023	BD MAX extended enteric bacteria	Pre-analytic	Use of an electronic hard-stop on orders placed for patients hospitalized >3 d	• 86% reduction in tests ordered for patients hospitalized >3 d
Clark et al [42], 2019	BioFire FilmArray GI	Pre-analytic	Restriction of testing to approved clinical criteria (fever, abdominal pain, blood in stool, or immunocompromised condition)	• Potential 32% reduction in test utilization
Hitchcock et al, [43] 2018	BioFire FilmArray GI	Pre-analytic	Restriction of testing to patients hospitalized <72 h	• Potential 18% reduction in test utilization
Marcelin et al, [45] 2019	BioFire FilmArray GI	Pre-analytic	Use of an electronic hard-stop on orders placed for patients hospitalized >3 d	• Potential 30% reduction in overall test utilization • Potential 77% reduction in inappropriate test utilization
O'Neal et al [46], 2020	BioFire FilmArray GI	Pre-analytic	Restriction of testing to approved clinical criteria (diarrheal symptoms, <2 d hospitalization, repeat testing, or laxative use in preceding 48 h)	• Potential 61% reduction in test utilization
Park et al [47], 2017	BioFire FilmArray GI	Pre-analytic	Restriction of repeat tests within 4 wk	• Potential 7% reduction in testing with limited clinical utility of repeat testing
Qavi et al [48], 2020	BioFire FilmArray RP	Pre-analytic	Restriction of testing for patients with previous result within 7 d	• Potential 10% reduction in test utilization • 3336 instances of patients recieving redundant targeted Influenza PCR testing

(continued on next page)

TABLE 2
(continued)

Study	Platform	Phase	Intervention	Results
Schnuriger et al [49], 2022	BioFire FilmArray ME	Pre-analytic	Restriction of testing to pleocytic CSF samples	• Potential 63% reduction in test utilization with 50% increase in testing yield
Bouam et al [39], 2021	BioFire FilmArray ME	Analytical	Use of a dedicated biosafety cabinet combined with preventative measures	• 2.1% decrease in false positive rate
Keske et al [44], 2018	BioFire FilmArray GI	Post-analytic	Implementation of an antimicrobial stewardship program	• 40% reduction in inappropriate antimicrobial use

Abbreviations: d, days; h, hours; wk, weeks; RP, respiratory pathogen panel; GI, gastrointestinal pathogen panel; PN, pneumonia panel; MF, meningitis/encephalitis panel.

increases in appropriate antimicrobial or antiviral de-escalation [22,25,26,28–30,32,33,35–38,50] and/or escalation [25,26,30,36]. Only 1 study demonstrated no significant change in antimicrobial or antiviral prescriptions [27]. All studies that evaluated differences in TAT, isolation facilities, and diagnostic procedures found significant reductions, and 1 study found evidence of cost savings [34]. However, 5 studies found no significant difference in hospital length of stay [21,27,32,33,37] and 3 studies found no difference in the number of hospital admissions [32,33,37]. Of the implementation studies reviewed here, only Messacar and colleagues [33] include a description of the formal education that would be consistent with a traditional definition of diagnostic stewardship. The lack of published educational interventions or guidance for test implementation highlights an important gap in the current literature.

Only 11 studies analyzed the impact of optimizing an existing assay—highlighting the lack of data addressing the direct application of diagnostic stewardship. 7 focused on GI panels [41–47], 3 on ME panels [39,40,49], and 1 on an RP panel [48]. By far the most common diagnostic phase addressed in the identified studies was the pre-analytic phase, and only 1 study addressed each the analytical [39] and post-analytic [44] phases of testing, respectively (see Table 2).

All pre-analytic studies focused on restricting testing to specific clinical scenarios to improve clinical yield and/or reduce test use. Most analyzed test restriction by patient characteristics, while the others used prior testing within a designated timeframe [47,49]. Clinical criteria used to reduce unnecessary GI panels included curbing testing of patients hospitalized greater than 3 days [41,43,45], patients without relevant clinical symptoms [42,46], or patients with recent laxative use [46]. For CSF testing, both studies restricted testing to pleocytic samples (>10 leukocytes/mm^3) [40,49]. Notably, only 2 of the pre-analytic studies analyzed the impact of an intervention [41,45], while the others retrospectively analyzed and reported the potential impact had an intervention been implemented. Of the 2 studies that implemented an intervention, both were "hard stops" built into the electronic health record that prevented providers from placing orders for a GI panel on patients hospitalized for greater than 3 days without obtaining laboratory medical director approval. All studies focused on the pre-analytic phase of testing measured the impact of the intervention (or potential intervention) on test utilization, and all found significant reductions. Of the studies identified, none reported a significant negative impact on yield of identified organisms. 2 studies measured and reported improvements in testing yield (defined as positive predictive value) [40,49]. 1 study optimizing the analytical phase of testing reported a statistically significant decrease in false positive rate on an ME panel through use of a dedicated biosafety cabinet [39]. The sole study using a post-analytic intervention reported a 40% reduction in inappropriate antimicrobial use via implementation of an antimicrobial stewardship program [44].

In summary, most studies evaluating stewardship interventions to optimize the use of syndromic multiplex panels measure and report reductions in antimicrobial or antiviral prescriptions and test TAT. In contrast, few studies measure and report reductions in the use of isolation facilities and ancillary procedures. While some studies report on patient outcome measures, such as hospital length of stay and disposition, the impact of syndromic multiplex panels on these outcomes is mixed, underscoring the difficulty in isolating the contributions of laboratory testing to larger institutional workflows.

STEWARDSHIP INTERVENTIONS FOR SEQUENCING-BASED DIAGNOSTIC ASSAYS

In contrast to syndromic multiplex panels that target specific pathogens, sequencing-based assays can be designed to minimize bias. Some approaches may be able to detect essentially any pathogen's nucleic acid in a single test. Both targeted and shotgun sequencing-based assays from sterile sources are used in clinical and commercial laboratories for the diagnosis of infective endocarditis [52,53], joint infections [54–56], meningitis/encephalitis [57–59] among others which have been previously reviewed [60–63]. Almost all available assays are laboratory developed tests. Implementation of these assays is costly [64], and many laboratories lack the test volume and technical expertise for in-house validation, so most testing is available at consolidated or reference laboratories [65]. Because of the lack of standardization, knowledge of the testing methodology is critical for appropriate testing ordering. For example, assays may target a single group of organisms (ie, bacteria or fungi) or detect only DNA or RNA pathogens, depending on the extraction methodology or library preparation utilized [62,66]. Selection of the best available test requires a clear understanding of the testing methodology. Laboratorians also have unique insight to the quality of the specimen and can provide insight to the optimal sample for testing. For example, specimens with organisms visible on gram stain or histopathology are high-yield for sequencing applications

[61,67]. This is critical in cases where specimen is limited and irretrievable. If there is insufficient specimen to perform all ordered tests, collaboration between laboratories and ordering clinicians can help to select the best specimen and tests based on the differential diagnosis.

The comprehensive nature of sequencing-based detection can result in detection of contaminants or colonizing organisms. If misinterpreted, this can contribute to inappropriate treatment or unnecessary workup [64,68]. Technical caveats such as sampling error or high leukocyte counts could cause false-negatives, further confounding interpretation [64]. Sequencing assays are costly compared to routine microbiology workups and their non-standardized nature leads to variable reimbursement [69]. For these reasons, stewardship can help to target appropriate patient populations, tests, and specimens to maximize clinical utility.

To this end, most published literature evaluates the diagnostic performance and clinical impact for cases where testing was performed. Common measures of impact include positive, negative or no impact on clinical-decision making, antimicrobial therapy prescribing or additional diagnostic workup [61,70–73]. Testing has been recommended for high-yield patient populations such as immunosuppressed individuals [74–77]. Several studies describe the importance of infectious disease experts involvement in guided test ordering and interfacing with primary team around test interpretation [74]. There is a notable lack of literature describing the effects of diagnostic stewardship interventions among assays using sequencing technology, and few measures of pre/post implementation that can be broadly applied. Panel reviews of testing results have been proposed to aid in challenging interpretations, in light of the technical caveats and clinical context [5]. Others have reported scoring methods to identify high-yield specimens as a more standardized approach to stewardship [67]. Scoring methods have the advantage of being accessible to institutions without resources for an active stewardship program. It is likely that many institutions have implemented active or passive stewardship based on their local experience, either via limits on testing indications or restricting ordering to subject matter experts such as infectious diseases. Overall, more data are needed to support informed intervention strategies.

DISCUSSION

Stewardship of diagnostic testing requires attention to technology, methodology, workflow, specimen, patient and clinical context. Since quality testing includes preanalytic, analytical, and post-analytic variables, the efforts to improve quality must similarly address these variables. As the clinical laboratory manages the in-house testing formulary and performs the testing, they have unique insight into the factors influencing the quality of results and are thus centrally poised to coordinate efforts to improve utilization. For advanced molecular tests, these efforts may include decisions around test selection and implementation, optimization of test utilization and coordination of send-out testing in the appropriate clinical context.

Here, we review diagnostic stewardship of advanced molecular tests, including both multiplex molecular panels for syndromic testing and sequencing-based assays for infectious disease. Most studies reported overall improvements when bringing on syndromic panels. Notably, all but 2 studies took place exclusively in large, tertiary care hospitals, and all but 2 focused on adult patients. Thus, an opportunity exists to assess the impact of syndromic multiplex panels in smaller, community hospitals, outpatient, and pediatric care settings. Few studies assess the impact stewardship interventions on an existing test, and of these, even fewer report realized (as opposed to potential) impact. Of studies describing interventions for existing assays, most focused on the pre-analytic phase of testing and reported reductions in test utilization via limiting test ordering to a specific clinical context. Thus, an opportunity exists for additional studies describing the impact of diagnostic stewardship interventions for syndromic multiplex panel testing, especially in the analytical and post-analytic phases. Since sequencing-based assays are primarily available at commercial or reference laboratories, most available studies focus on the utility of these tests in the context of referral testing on a specific patient population. There are opportunities to assess the effect of active or systematic stewardship of these tests in real-world settings, and how these interventions influence patient care.

CLINICS CARE POINTS

- Laboratory testing is increasing in scope and complexity, requiring iterative decision-making around testing to offer internally versus testing to be sent to a referral laboratory.
- Effective and sustainable diagnostic stewardship efforts require multifaceted interventions implemented by interdisciplinary teams.

- Implementing syndromic panels can improve antimicrobial escalation—although generally less frequently antimicrobial de-escalation—as well as reduce turnaround time and additional diagnostic procedures.
- Sequencing-based assays benefit from stewardship due to high technical complexity and potentially challenging interpretation. Active stewardship programs can target high-yield patient populations.

DISCLOSURE

R.E. Dumm has research funding from bioMérieux, France and Pattern Biosciences. V. Azimi has nothing to disclose.

REFERENCES

[1] Miller MB, Atrzadeh, Burnham, et al. Clinical Utility of Advanced Microbiology Testing Tools. J Clin Microbiol 2019;57. https://doi.org/10.1128/jcm.00495-19.

[2] Sautter RL, Thomson RB. Consolidated clinical microbiology laboratories. J Clin Microbiol 2015;53(5):1467–72.

[3] Advani SD, Claeys KC. Behavioral Strategies in Diagnostic Stewardship. Infect Dis Clin 2023;37(4):729–47.

[4] Avdic E, Carroll KC. The Role of the Microbiology Laboratory in Antimicrobial Stewardship Programs. Infect Dis Clin North Am 2014;28(2):215–35.

[5] Patel R, Fang FC. Diagnostic Stewardship: Opportunity for a Laboratory–Infectious Diseases Partnership. Clin Infect Dis 2018;67:799–801.

[6] Hueth KD, Prinzi AM, Timbrook TT. Diagnostic Stewardship as a Team Sport: Interdisciplinary Perspectives on Improved Implementation of Interventions and Effect Measurement. Antibiotics (Basel) 2022;11(2):250.

[7] Fabre V, Davis, Diekema, et al. Principles of diagnostic stewardship: A practical guide from the Society for Healthcare Epidemiology of America Diagnostic Stewardship Task Force. Infect Control Hosp Epidemiol 2023;44(2):178–85.

[8] Jackson BR. Laboratory formularies. Clin Chim Acta 2014;427:151–3.

[9] Samuel LP, Hansen GT, Kraft CS, et al. The Need for Dedicated Microbiology Leadership in the Clinical Microbiology Laboratory. J Clin Microbiol 2021;59(8): e0154919.

[10] Fabre V, Carroll KC, Cosgrove SE. Blood Culture Utilization in the Hospital Setting: a Call for Diagnostic Stewardship. J Clin Microbiol 2022;60(3):e0100521.

[11] Schinkel M, Boerman, Carroll, et al. Impact of Blood Culture Contamination on Antibiotic Use, Resource Utilization, and Clinical Outcomes: A Retrospective Cohort Study in Dutch and US Hospitals. Open Forum Infect Dis 2024;11(2):ofad644.

[12] Banerjee R, Teng, Cunningham, et al. Randomized Trial of Rapid Multiplex Polymerase Chain Reaction–Based Blood Culture Identification and Susceptibility Testing. Clin Infect Dis 2015;61:1071–80.

[13] Juttukonda LJ, Katz S, Gillon J, et al. Impact of a Rapid Blood Culture Diagnostic Test in a Children's Hospital Depends on Gram-Positive versus Gram-Negative Organism and Day versus Night Shift. J Clin Microbiol 2020; 58. https://doi.org/10.1128/jcm.01400-19.

[14] Boly FJ, Reske KA, Kwon JH. The Role of Diagnostic Stewardship in Clostridioides difficile Testing: Challenges and Opportunities. Curr Infect Dis Rep 2020;22(3):7.

[15] Schwenk HT, Pollock NR, Vaughan-Malloy AM. Pediatric Clostridioides difficile Infection: Diagnosis and Diagnostic Stewardship. J Pediatric Infect Dis Soc 2021; 10(Supplement_3):S16–21.

[16] Advani S, Vaughn VM. Quality Improvement Interventions and Implementation Strategies for Urine Culture Stewardship in the Acute Care Setting: Advances and Challenges. Curr Infect Dis Rep 2021;23(10).

[17] Chambliss AB, Van TT. Revisiting approaches to and considerations for urinalysis and urine culture reflexive testing. Crit Rev Clin Lab Sci 2022;59(2):112–24.

[18] Schmitz JE, Stratton CW, Persing DH, et al. Forty Years of Molecular Diagnostics for Infectious Diseases. J Clin Microbiol 2022;60(10):e0244621.

[19] Gaston DC. Clinical Metagenomics for Infectious Diseases: Progress toward Operational Value. J Clin Microbiol 2023;61(2):e0126722.

[20] Miller S, Chiu C, Rodino KG, et al. Point-Counterpoint: Should We Be Performing Metagenomic Next-Generation Sequencing for Infectious Disease Diagnosis in the Clinical Laboratory? J Clin Microbiol 2020;58:e01739-19.

[21] Andrews D, Chetty, Cooper, et al. Multiplex PCR point of care testing versus routine, laboratory-based testing in the treatment of adults with respiratory tract infections: a quasi-randomised study assessing impact on length of stay and antimicrobial use. BMC Infect Dis 2017;17:671.

[22] Axelrad JE, Freedberg, Whittier, et al. Impact of Gastrointestinal Panel Implementation on Health Care Utilization and Outcomes. J Clin Microbiol 2019;57. https://doi.org/10.1128/jcm.01775-18.

[23] Berinson B, Spenke, Krivec, et al. Performance and Hypothetical Impact on Joint Infection Management of the BioFire Joint Infection Panel: a Retrospective Analysis. J Clin Microbiol 2023;61(8):e0059223.

[24] Brendish NJ, Malachira, Armstrong, et al. Routine molecular point-of-care testing for respiratory viruses in adults presenting to hospital with acute respiratory illness (ResPOC): a pragmatic, open-label, randomised controlled trial. Lancet Respir Med 2017;5:401–11.

[25] Buchan BW, Windham, Balada-Llasat, et al. Practical Comparison of the BioFire FilmArray Pneumonia Panel to Routine Diagnostic Methods and Potential Impact on Antimicrobial Stewardship in Adult Hospitalized Patients with Lower Respiratory Tract Infections. J Clin Microbiol 2020;58. https://doi.org/10.1128/jcm.00135-20.

[26] Cybulski RJ, Bateman, Bourassa, et al. Clinical Impact of a Multiplex Gastrointestinal Polymerase Chain Reaction

Panel in Patients With Acute Gastroenteritis. Clin Infect Dis 2018;67:1688–96.

[27] Dack K, Pankow S, Ablah E, et al. Contribution of the BioFire® FilmArray® Meningitis/Encephalitis Panel: Assessing Antimicrobial Duration and Length of Stay. Kans J Med 2019;12:1–3.

[28] Darie AM, Khanna, Jahn, et al. Fast multiplex bacterial PCR of bronchoalveolar lavage for antibiotic stewardship in hospitalised patients with pneumonia at risk of Gram-negative bacterial infection (Flagship II): a multicentre, randomised controlled trial. Lancet Respir Med 2022; 10(9):877–87.

[29] Echavarría M, Marcone DN, Querci M, et al. Clinical impact of rapid molecular detection of respiratory pathogens in patients with acute respiratory infection. J Clin Virol 2018;108:90–5.

[30] Esplund JN, Taylor, Stone, et al. Clinical impact of a multiplex rapid diagnostic pneumonia panel in critically ill patients. Antimicrob Steward Healthc Epidemiol 2023;3(1):e5.

[31] Goldenberg SD, Bacelar M, Brazier P, et al. A cost benefit analysis of the Luminex xTAG Gastrointestinal Pathogen Panel for detection of infectious gastroenteritis in hospitalised patients. J Infect 2015;70:504–11.

[32] May L, Tatro, Poltavskiy, et al. Rapid Multiplex Testing for Upper Respiratory Pathogens in the Emergency Department: A Randomized Controlled Trial. Open Forum Infect Dis 2019;6:ofz481.

[33] Messacar K, Palmer, Gregoire, et al. Clinical and Financial Impact of a Diagnostic Stewardship Program for Children with Suspected Central Nervous System Infection. J Pediatr 2022;244:161.e1.

[34] Nelson RE, Stockmann, Hersh, et al. Economic Analysis of Rapid and Sensitive Polymerase Chain Reaction Testing in the Emergency Department for Influenza Infections in Children. Pediatr Infect Dis J 2015;34(6):577–82.

[35] Rogers BB, Shankar, Jerris, et al. Impact of a Rapid Respiratory Panel Test on Patient Outcomes. Arch Pathol Lab Med 2014;139(5):636–41.

[36] Subramony A, Zachariah P, Krones A, et al. Impact of Multiplex Polymerase Chain Reaction Testing for Respiratory Pathogens on Healthcare Resource Utilization for Pediatric Inpatients. J Pediatr 2016;173:196.e2.

[37] Vos LM, Weehuizen, Hoepelman, et al. More targeted use of oseltamivir and in-hospital isolation facilities after implementation of a multifaceted strategy including a rapid molecular diagnostic panel for respiratory viruses in immunocompromised adult patients. J Clin Virol 2019;116:11–7.

[38] Weiss ZF, Cunha, Chambers, et al. Opportunities Revealed for Antimicrobial Stewardship and Clinical Practice with Implementation of a Rapid Respiratory Multiplex Assay. J Clin Microbiol 2019;57. https://doi.org/10.1128/jcm.00861-19.

[39] Bouam A, Vincent JJ, Drancourt M, et al. Preventing contamination of PCR-based multiplex assays including the use of a dedicated biosafety cabinet. Lett Appl Microbiol 2021;72(1):98–103.

[40] Broadhurst MJ, Dujari, Budvytiene, et al. Utilization, Yield, and Accuracy of the FilmArray Meningitis/Encephalitis Panel with Diagnostic Stewardship and Testing Algorithm. J Clin Microbiol 2020;58. https://doi.org/10.1128/jcm.00311-20.

[41] Campodónico VL, Ann H, Mikula MW, et al. A diagnostic stewardship approach to prevent unnecessary testing of an enteric bacterial molecular panel. Microbiol Spectr 2023;11:e0294523.

[42] Clark SD, Sidlak M, Mathers AJ, et al. Clinical Yield of a Molecular Diagnostic Panel for Enteric Pathogens in Adult Outpatients With Diarrhea and Validation of Guidelines-Based Criteria for Testing. Open Forum Infect Dis 2019;6:ofz162.

[43] Hitchcock MM, Gomez CA, Banaei N. Low Yield of FilmArray GI Panel in Hospitalized Patients with Diarrhea: an Opportunity for Diagnostic Stewardship Intervention. J Clin Microbiol 2018;56. https://doi.org/10.1128/jcm.01558-17.

[44] Keske Ş, Zabun, Aksoy, et al. Rapid Molecular Detection of Gastrointestinal Pathogens and Its Role in Antimicrobial Stewardship. J Clin Microbiol 2018;56. https://doi.org/10.1128/jcm.00148-18.

[45] Marcelin JR, Brewer, Beachy, et al. Hardwiring diagnostic stewardship using electronic ordering restrictions for gastrointestinal pathogen testing. Infect Control Hosp Epidemiol 2019;40:668–73.

[46] O'Neal M, Murray H, Dash S, et al. Evaluating appropriateness and diagnostic stewardship opportunities of multiplex polymerase chain reaction gastrointestinal testing within a hospital system. Ther Adv Infect Dis 2020;7:2049936120959561.

[47] Park S, Hitchcock MM, Gomez CA, et al. Is Follow-Up Testing with the FilmArray Gastrointestinal Multiplex PCR Panel Necessary? J Clin Microbiol 2017;55:1154–61.

[48] Qavi AJ, McMullen A, Burnham C-AD, et al. Repeat Molecular Testing for Respiratory Pathogens: Diagnostic Gain or Diminishing Returns? J Appl Lab Med 2020;5:897–907.

[49] Schnuriger A, Vimont, Godmer, et al. Differential Performance of the FilmArray Meningitis/Encephalitis Assay To Detect Bacterial and Viral Pathogens in Both Pediatric and Adult Populations. Microbiol Spectr 2022;10(2): e0277421.

[50] Rappo U, Schuetz, Jenkins, et al. Impact of Early Detection of Respiratory Viruses by Multiplex PCR Assay on Clinical Outcomes in Adult Patients. J Clin Microbiol 2016;54:2096–103.

[51] Rogers WS, Westblade, Soave, et al. Impact of a Multiplexed Polymerase Chain Reaction Panel on Identifying Diarrheal Pathogens in Hematopoietic Cell Transplant Recipients. Clin Infect Dis 2020;71:1693–700.

[52] Hong H-L, Flurin, Greenwood-Quaintance, et al. 16S rRNA Gene PCR/Sequencing of Heart Valves for Diagnosis of Infective Endocarditis in Routine Clinical Practice. J Clin Microbiol 2023;61(8):e0034123-23.

[53] Miller RJH, Chow B, Pillai D, et al. Development and evaluation of a novel fast broad-range 16S ribosomal

DNA PCR and sequencing assay for diagnosis of bacterial infective endocarditis: multi-year experience in a large Canadian healthcare zone and a literature review. BMC Infect Dis 2016;16:146.

[54] Ivy MI, Thoendel, Jeraldo, et al. Direct Detection and Identification of Prosthetic Joint Infection Pathogens in Synovial Fluid by Metagenomic Shotgun Sequencing. J Clin Microbiol 2018;56:e00402–18.

[55] Kullar R, Chisari, Snyder, et al. Next-Generation Sequencing Supports Targeted Antibiotic Treatment for Culture Negative Orthopedic Infections. Clin Infect Dis 2023;76(2):359–64.

[56] Ramchandar N, Burns, Coufal, et al. Use of Metagenomic Next-Generation Sequencing to Identify Pathogens in Pediatric Osteoarticular Infections. Open Forum Infect Dis 2021;8(7):ofab346.

[57] Rodino KG, Toledano, Norgan, et al. Retrospective Review of Clinical Utility of Shotgun Metagenomic Sequencing Testing of Cerebrospinal Fluid from a U.S. Tertiary Care Medical Center. J Clin Microbiol 2020;58: e01729-20.

[58] Wilson MR, Sample, Zorn, et al. Clinical Metagenomic Sequencing for Diagnosis of Meningitis and Encephalitis. N Engl J Med 2019;380:2327–40.

[59] Graff K, Dominguez SR, Messacar K. Metagenomic Next-Generation Sequencing for Diagnosis of Pediatric Meningitis and Encephalitis: A Review. J Pediatric Infect Dis Soc 2021;10(Supplement_4):S78–87.

[60] Govender KN, Street TL, Sanderson ND, et al. Metagenomic Sequencing as a Pathogen-Agnostic Clinical Diagnostic Tool for Infectious Diseases: a Systematic Review and Meta-analysis of Diagnostic Test Accuracy Studies. J Clin Microbiol 2021;59(9):e0291620.

[61] Kubiak J, Morgan A, Kirmaier A, et al. Universal PCR for bacteria, mycobacteria, and fungi: a 10-year retrospective review of clinical indications and patient outcomes. J Clin Microbiol 2023;61(12):e0095223-23.

[62] Gu W, Miller S, Chiu CY. Clinical Metagenomic Next-Generation Sequencing for Pathogen Detection. Annu Rev Pathol 2019;14:319–38.

[63] Drevinek P, Hollweck R, Lorenz MG, et al. Direct 16S/ 18S rRNA Gene PCR Followed by Sanger Sequencing as a Clinical Diagnostic Tool for Detection of Bacterial and Fungal Infections: a Systematic Review and Meta-Analysis. J Clin Microbiol 2023;61(9):e0033823-23.

[64] Simner PJ, Miller S, Carroll KC. Understanding the Promises and Hurdles of Metagenomic Next-Generation Sequencing as a Diagnostic Tool for Infectious Diseases. Clin Infect Dis 2018;66:778–88.

[65] Rossen JWA, Friedrich AW, Moran-Gilad J. Practical issues in implementing whole-genome-sequencing in routine diagnostic microbiology. Clin Microbiol Infect 2018;24: 355–60.

[66] Goldberg B, Sichtig H, Geyer C, et al. Making the Leap from Research Laboratory to Clinic: Challenges and Opportunities for Next-Generation Sequencing in Infectious Disease Diagnostics. mBio 2015;6:e01888-15.

[67] Dumm RE, Glaser LJ, Rodino KG. Development of a scoring system to identify high-yield specimens for bacterial broad-range 16S rRNA gene PCR with sequencing at a tertiary care medical center. Am J Clin Pathol 2023; 160(5):477–82.

[68] Dulanto Chiang A, Dekker JP. From the Pipeline to the Bedside: Advances and Challenges in Clinical Metagenomics. J Infect Dis 2020;221(Suppl 3):S331–40.

[69] Greninger AL. The challenge of diagnostic metagenomics. Expert Rev Mol Diagn 2018;18:605–15.

[70] Lee RA, Al Dhaheri FA, Pollock NR, et al. Assessment of the Clinical Utility of Plasma Metagenomic Next-Generation Sequencing in a Pediatric Hospital Population. J Clin Microbiol 2020;58.

[71] Hogan CA, Yang, Garner, et al. Clinical Impact of Metagenomic Next-Generation Sequencing of Plasma Cell-Free DNA for the Diagnosis of Infectious Diseases: A Multicenter Retrospective Cohort Study. Clin Infect Dis 2021;72(2):239–45.

[72] Kerkhoff AD, Rutishauser RL, Miller S, et al. Clinical Utility of Universal Broad-Range Polymerase Chain Reaction Amplicon Sequencing for Pathogen Identification: A Retrospective Cohort Study. Clin Infect Dis 2020;71: 1554–7.

[73] Basein T, Gardiner, Andujar Vazquez, et al. Microbial Identification Using DNA Target Amplification and Sequencing: Clinical Utility and Impact on Patient Management. Open Forum Infect Dis 2018;5:ofy257.

[74] Vissichelli NC, Morales, Kolipakkam, et al. Cell-free next-generation sequencing impacts diagnosis and antimicrobial therapy in immunocompromised hosts: A retrospective study. Transpl Infect Dis 2023;25(1):e13954.

[75] Casto AM, Fredricks DN, Hill JA. Diagnosis of infectious diseases in immunocompromised hosts using metagenomic next generation sequencing-based diagnostics. Blood Rev 2022;53:100906.

[76] Azar MM, Schlaberg, Malinis, et al. Added Diagnostic Utility of Clinical Metagenomics for the Diagnosis of Pneumonia in Immunocompromised Adults. Chest 2021;159(4):1356–71.

[77] MacIntyre AT, Hirst, Duttagupta, et al. Budget Impact of Microbial Cell-Free DNA Testing Using the Karius® Test as an Alternative to Invasive Procedures in Immunocompromised Patients with Suspected Invasive Fungal Infections. Appl Health Econ Health Policy 2021;19(2): 231–41.

Informatics

Advances in Molecular Pathology 7 (2024) 113–122
ADVANCES IN MOLECULAR PATHOLOGY

Genomics Clinical Decision Support with Fast Healthcare Interoperability Resources Genomics Operations

Robert H. Dolin, MD[a,*], Bret S.E. Heale, PhD[b], Srikar Chamala, PhD[c,d]
[a]Elimu Informatics, 1709 Julian Court, El Cerrito, CA 94530-2009, USA; [b]Humanized Health Consulting, Salt Lake City, UT, USA; [c]Center for Pathology Informatics and Data Science, Children's Hospital Los Angeles, 4650 Sunset Boulevard, Los Angeles, CA 90027, USA; [d]USC Keck School of Medicine

KEYWORDS
• Genomics • Clinical decision support • Fast Healthcare Interoperability Resources (FHIR)
• Electronic health record (EHR) • Clinical decision support (CDS)

KEY POINTS

- Clinical decision support in genomics is evolving in an uncertain regulatory environment.
- Fast Healthcare Interoperability Resources (FHIR) Genomics Operations encapsulate data complexity, including variant normalization.
- FHIR Genomics Operations encapsulate dynamic variant annotation, enabling real-time decision support that is based on current knowledge.
- FHIR Genomics Operations enable advanced clinical decision support that leverages a person's full genomic data set.

INTRODUCTION

Fast Healthcare Interoperability Resources (FHIR) Genomics Operations [1] have been recently described [2,3]. Referenced articles focus on the ability of operations to *encapsulate data complexity* and *enable dynamic variant annotation (VA),* resulting in a developer-friendly approach to genomics-electronic health record (EHR) integration. Here, the emphasis is on the ability of the Operations to *drive advanced clinical decision support (CDS) that leverages a person's entire genome.*

BACKGROUND

Genomics-Electronic Health Record Integration Challenges

Patients' genomic testing results are commonly integrated into their EHR through custom PDF reports designed by the testing laboratory. These reports include select genomic test findings, interpretation knowledge, and patient care recommendations reflecting the laboratory's most current internal curation process. While state-of-the-art, these textual reports are neither ideal for clinicians nor ideal for CDS [4,5]—they contain only a slice of key variants and a point-in-time snapshot of

*Corresponding author, *E-mail address:* bdolin@elimu.io

https://doi.org/10.1016/j.yamp.2024.07.006 www.advancesinmolecularpathology.com
2589-4080/24/

interpretations; they are difficult and time-consuming to review; clinicians are not assisted in evaluating relevant interactions mentioned in the reports when making decisions; and they do not provide structured data needed for CDS guidance or analytics. To address these limitations, EHR vendors are enhancing their products in anticipation of incorporating structured genomic findings [6], and HL7 Version 2 messaging and HL7 FHIR Genomics reporting standards are maturing [7,8]. Large research projects such as electronic medical records and genomics (eMERGE) [9] and clinical sequencing evidence-generating research (CSER) [10] are exploring the use of FHIR Genomics, and HL7 FHIR is gaining wide traction, as are apps based on the SMART-on-FHIR platform for broader clinical applications [11–13]. But even with FHIR Genomics, EHR integration of genomic data remains challenging for many reasons.

- *Data volume*: Genomic data are voluminous and complex [4,5,14,15]. Next-generation sequencing (NGS) can identify thousands to millions of variants. Significant bioinformatics knowledge and computational resources can be required to interpret the data.
- *Data complexity*: Raw sequencing data formats and EHR data standards differ, with only a limited number of clinical informaticists having a detailed understanding of bioinformatics data specifications. Furthermore, genomic variants can be represented in more than one way, creating a barrier to effective search and aggregation, for such activities as matching a patient's genetic profile with knowledge bases [16].
- *Rapid knowledge evolution*: The implications of genomic data are rapidly changing as our knowledge matures, resulting in these commonly utilized PDF reports quickly becoming outdated. Analysis of data from the National Institutes of Health ClinVar genomic data repository shows that from 2016 to 2018, the number of known pathogenic or likely pathogenic variants in 66 genes of high clinical relevance [17] went from 10,137 to 18,718 [18,19] reflecting over 8000 new or recategorized clinically significant variants over the course of merely 2 years. The amount of variation and complexity considered in clinical interpretation of test results will only increase, especially with the emergence of polygenic risk scores [20].

FHIR Genomics Operations are designed to overcome these challenges.

Clinical Decision Support Standards and Regulations

Clinical decision support standards

CDS standards facilitate CDS scalability, enabling decision support applications written at one institution to be more readily usable by another institution. Primary CDS standards include *Substitutable Medical Applications, Reusable Technologies (SMART)-on-FHIR* [21] and *CDS Hooks* [22], both of which are being extensively tested in genomics-EHR integration approaches (for instance, see references [11,12,23–25]).

SMART-on-FHIR is a standard for integrating third-party applications with EHR systems. Just as mobile phones support the use of compliant apps, available from an app store, the idea behind SMART-on-FHIR is that compliant apps can be written once and run on a variety of EHRs. To date, SMART-on-FHIR app integrations are supported by Allscripts, Cerner, AthenaHealth, Epic, InterSystems, and Meditech. Additionally, third-party platforms support this standard including Apple Health, Google's Cloud Healthcare API, and Microsoft's Azure Health Data Services.

CDS Hooks is a standard that specifies interactions between an EHR and an external CDS server. Defined events (such as clinician order entry or opening a patient's chart) in the EHR trigger a message to the CDS server, which can then gather additional data and execute rules before responding back to the EHR. Of note, the CDS Hooks standard defines a standardized set of application programming interfaces (APIs) that facilitate interactions with the EHR. Data flowing from the EHR to the CDS Hooks server are FHIR-formatted.

Clinical decision support regulations

Emerging CDS regulations are designed to safeguard the use of CDS (including CDS based on artificial intelligence/machine learning) when used for patient care. Primary CDS regulations include

- Office of the National Coordinator for Health Information Technology (ONC) Health Data, Technology, and Interoperability: Certification Program Updates, Algorithm Transparency, and Information Sharing Final Rule (*"ONC HTI-1 Final Rule"* [26,27]);
- United States Core Data for Interoperability (*"USCDI"* [28]);
- Executive order on the Safe, Secure, and Trustworthy Development and Use of Artificial Intelligence (*"Executive Order on AI"* [29]);
- Clinical Decision Support Software—Guidance for Industry and Food and Drug Administration Staff (*"FDA Guidance on CDS Devices"* [30]).

The ONC HTI-1 Final Rule, issued in late 2023, establishes a set of criteria to which EHRs must conform in order to be certified. Included are CDS criteria, mainly for required rule metadata, particularly but not solely for artificial intelligence (AI)-based CDS. These criteria are aligned with Executive Order on AI and United States Food and Drug Administration (FDA) Guidance on CDS Devices to better ensure a consistent approach to CDS transparency. In addition, the ONC HTI-1 Final Rule establishes criteria for a minimal set of clinical data elements, known as USCDI, which must be supported by certified EHRs. This is particularly relevant for interoperable CDS, where SMART-on-FHIR and CDS Hooks applications that use data elements beyond USCDI are likely to encounter increased implementation challenges [31,32].

USCDI and the related FHIR US Core Implementation Guide [33] are important in that, as described earlier, they establish an approximate minimal interoperable CDS bar, especially where CDS is integrated into ONC-certified EHRs.

The Executive Order on AI, issued in late 2023, is focused on ensuring the safe use of AI technology. Section 8 is focused on AI in health care, designed to "help ensure the safe, responsible deployment and use of AI in the healthcare, public-health, and human-services sectors" [29]. Section 8 calls for the establishment of "an HHS AI Task Force that shall, within 365 days of its creation, develop a strategic plan that includes policies and frameworks - possibly including regulatory action, as appropriate - on responsible deployment and use of AI and AI-enabled technologies in the health and human services sector." While the full impact of the Executive Order on AI will be revealed over time, there is no doubt that AI algorithms will find heavy use within genomics CDS applications.

The FDA Guidance on CDS Devices, issued in 2022, attempts to clarify CDS services that are subject to or exempt from FDA regulation. As stated, "The FDA has long regulated software that meets the definition of a device in section 201(h) of the Federal Food, Drug, and Cosmetic Act, including software that is intended to provide decision support for the diagnosis, treatment, prevention, cure, or mitigation of diseases or other conditions (often referred to as clinical decision support software)" [30]. A CDS software function is nondevice (therefore, not subject to FDA regulation) if *all* the following 4 criteria are met:

1. Not intended to acquire, process, or analyze a medical image or a signal from an in vitro diagnostic device or a pattern or signal from a signal acquisition system.
2. Intended for the purpose of displaying, analyzing, or printing medical information about a patient or other medical information (such as peer-reviewed clinical studies and clinical practice guidelines).
3. Intended for the purpose of supporting or providing recommendations to a health care professional about the prevention, diagnosis, or treatment of a disease or condition.
4. Intended for the purpose of enabling such health care professional to independently review the basis for such recommendations that such software presents so that it is not the intent that such health care professional rely primarily on any of such recommendations to make a clinical diagnosis or treatment decision regarding an individual patient.

While industry confusion around the interpretation of these criteria remains, what is clear is that as genomics CDS moves from simply returning VAs to, for example, using AI-based algorithms to predict causal variants or prioritize treatment recommendations, these evolving CDS algorithms may become subject to FDA regulation.

GENOMICS STANDARDS

Fast Healthcare Interoperability Resources Genomics

The HL7 FHIR Genomics standard [8] ("FHIR Genomics") defines FHIR representations for a range of genomic data structures (eg, variants, haplotypes, and variant implications), enabling a standards-based communication of simple and structural variants, germline and somatic variants, pharmacogenomic star alleles, human leukocyte antigen (HLA) typing, and other findings generated from sequencing, chip technology, and cytogenetic analysis.

FHIR Genomics also supports the communication of structured VAs, including diagnostic implications (eg, a patient's variant is known to be associated with a hereditary condition), therapeutic implications (eg, a patient's genotype is known to affect the metabolism of a particular drug, presence of a variant predicts a treatment response to a particular drug), and molecular consequences (eg, presence of a variant predicts loss of function of the containing gene).

At the heart of a typical FHIR Genomics sequencing report are findings (variants, haplotypes, genotypes, and biomarkers) and annotations derived from those findings (diagnostic implications, therapeutic implications, and predicted molecular consequences), as shown in (Fig. 1).

FHIR Genomics Operations are part of the FHIR Genomics standard. As described in later discussion, Operations extend the FHIR Genomics standard and basic FHIR search capabilities in order to simplify developer access to potentially complex and voluminous data structures.

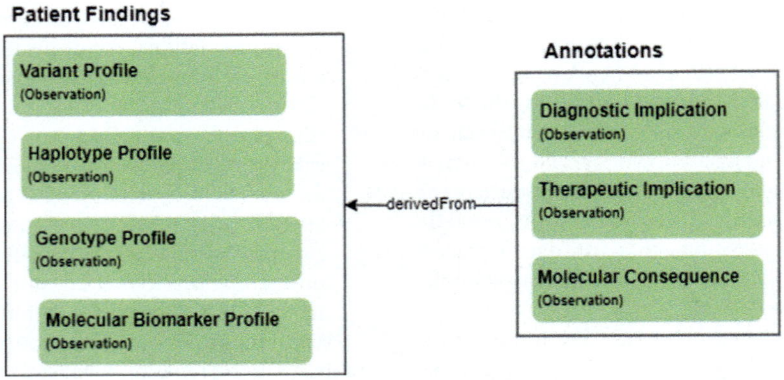

FIG. 1 FHIR genomics supports the communication of structured patient findings and corresponding annotations.

Global Alliance for Genomics and Health

The Global Alliance for Genomics and Health (GA4GH) is an international standards development organization focused on genomic data sharing and interoperability. GA4GH is organized into a set of work streams that bring together users and developers to address real-world needs. Intersecting these work streams are driver projects, real-world genomic data initiatives that help guide development efforts.

Not only is GA4GH the shepherd for core bioinformatics data standards such as the variant call format (VCF) and the binary alignment map, GA4GH is also focused on data security and regulatory issues, standardizing phenotype data, cloud-based data sharing, and more. Driver projects such as the Variant Interpretation for Cancer Consortium and the Clinical Genome Resource are advancing data-sharing initiatives that promise to improve precision medicine and research.

The GA4GH Genomic Knowledge Standards work stream develops standards-based components to enable the exchange of reference genomic information through common APIs, thereby enabling the downstream analysis of genomic data. In particular, the evolving VA standard seeks to establish extensible data models to support representation of diverse kinds of statements made about genetic variation, and the evidence and provenance supporting these statements. The GA4GH VA standard can potentially be used to standardize the contents of genomics knowledge bases such as ClinVar [34], Clinical Interpretation of Variants in Cancer [35], or Pharmacogenomics Knowledge Base [36].

While the boundaries between HL7 and GA4GH can be a bit fuzzy at times, the strategy taken in our ONC Sync for Genes project was to use HL7 FHIR as the format for interacting with EHRs, whereas the GA4GH VA specification was used to standardize knowledge obtained from genomic knowledge bases [3].

FAST HEALTHCARE INTEROPERABILITY RESOURCES GENOMICS OPERATIONS

Introduction

FHIR Genomics Operations [1,2] (Fig. 2) are based on the premise that genomic data, in FHIR format and/or some other format (eg, VCF format), are stored in a repository, either in or alongside an EHR, possibly along with phenotype annotations. The FHIR Genomics Operations essentially wrap the repository, presenting a uniform interface to applications, regardless of internal repository data structures. More importantly, FHIR operations can encapsulate the complexity of data within a repository and normalize redundant data representations. This is particularly relevant in genomics, where a tremendous amount of raw data exists in often-complex non-FHIR formats, and where variability in variant representation is a known barrier to matching a patient's genetic profile against knowledge bases—for example, for clinical trials matching, for prediction of genetic predisposition to disease, for precision medication selection, and for genetic risk calculation.

A common use case driving the Operations is the notion of an application (eg, an SMART-on-FHIR clinical genomics app, a CDS Hooks app, and an EHR screen) needing specific genotype or phenotype information, for a patient or a population. Applications have diverse needs, such as matching a patient with cancer to available clinical trials based on identified

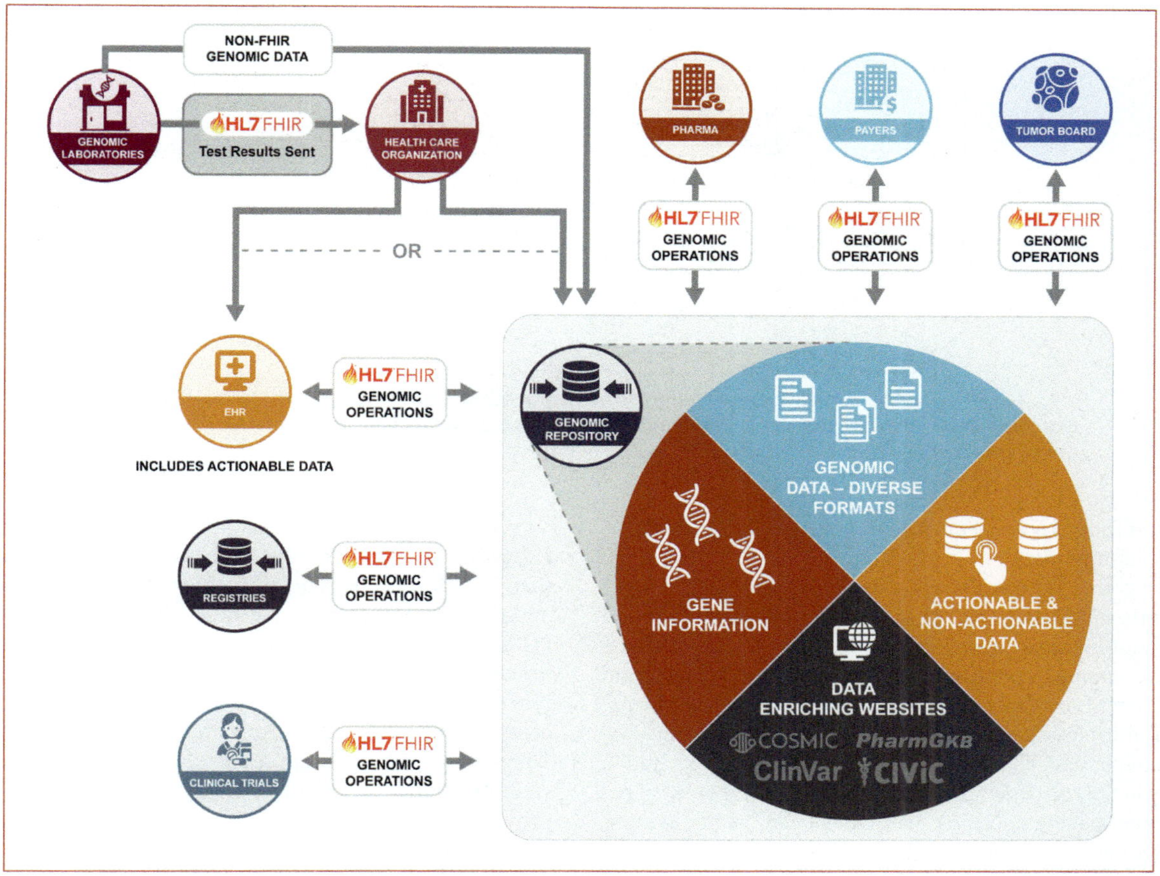

FIG. 2 FHIR Genomics Operations essentially wrap a genomic data repository, presenting a uniform interface to applications. (Image courtesy of HL7 FHIR Accelerator CodeX.)

somatic variants; screening for actionable hereditary conditions; identifying a risk for adverse medication reactions based on pharmacogenomic variants; updating a patient's risk as knowledge of their variants evolves; and more. A goal for FHIR Genomics Operations is to ultimately support any and all of these clinical scenarios.

Returning to the grand genomics-EHR challenges described earlier and how they are addressed by the Operations.

- *Data volume*: A growing number of scenarios (eg, cancer management, rare disease variant discovery, and polygenic risk score calculation) benefit from access to a patient's whole genome. Operations enable access to a patient's complete genomic data set.
- *Data complexity*: Operations are designed to encapsulate normalization, facilitating access to simple and structural variants, copy number changes, and so forth. Experience to date suggests that variant normalization is feasible in real-time and greatly enhances search and annotation.
- *Rapid knowledge evolution*: Operations are designed to encapsulate dynamic annotation (eg, variants annotated on demand, based on current knowledge). As shown in (Fig. 3), an implementation of FHIR Genomics Operations can return previously instantiated, or static, implications (eg, those returned in a laboratory report) and/or dynamically computed implications. Such capabilities were demonstrated in our ONC Sync for Genes project, where we developed a CDS pipeline that dynamically annotates patient's variants through an intersection with current knowledge, encoded in GA4GH format, and serves up the FHIR-encoded variants and annotations (diagnostic and therapeutic implications,

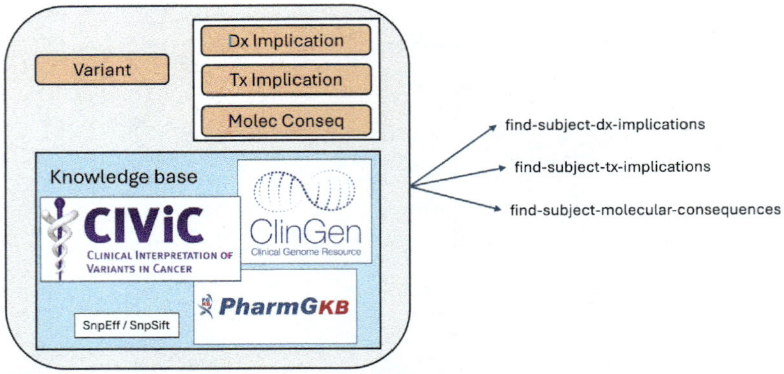

FIG. 3 FHIR Genomics Operations can return previously instantiated implications (eg, those returned in a laboratory report) and/or dynamically computed implications (eg, variants annotated on demand, based on current knowledge).

molecular consequences) via FHIR Genomics Operations [3].

We categorize FHIR Genomics Operations along 2 orthogonal axes (Fig. 4): subject versus population and genotype versus phenotype. For example, the "*find-subject-variants*" operation is categorized as a "subject" and a "genotype" operation, that retrieves genotype information for a single subject, whereas the "*find-population-tx-implications*" is categorized as a "population" and a "phenotype" operation that retrieves a count or list of patients having specific phenotypes (such as being intermediate metabolizers of clopidogrel). The metadata operation retrieves metadata about the genomic studies that generated the data.

While a full technical description of the Operations is beyond the scope of this article, it is worth noting that in addition to encapsulation of normalization and dynamic annotation, a general characteristic of all FHIR Genomics Operations is genomic *region-based searching*. We continue to recognize the clinical significance of variations not only within protein-coding gene exons but also in introns and intergenic regions. To enable a consistent approach to query, whether for variants within or outside a gene, certain operations provide a "ranges" query parameter (eg, to query for variants in the APC gene, one can call the "*find-subject-variants*" operation with a parameter of ranges = "NC_000005.10:112707497-112846239").

	Subject operations	Population operations
Genotype operations	**Retrieve simple/structural variants, haplotypes** •find-subject-variants •find-subject-specific-variants •find-subject-structural-intersecting-variants •find-subject-structural-subsuming-variants •find-subject-haplotypes •find-subject-specific-haplotypes	**Identify cohorts with simple/structural variants, haplotypes** •find-population-specific-variants •find-population-structural-intersecting-variants •find-population-structural-subsuming-variants •find-population-specific-haplotypes
Phenotype operations	**Retrieve variant annotations** •find-subject-tx-implications •find-subject-dx-implications •find-subject-molecular-consequences	**Identify cohorts with various annotations** •find-population-tx-implications •find-population-dx-implications •find-subject-molecular-consequences
Metadata operations	**Retrieve sequencing study metadata** •find-study-metadata	

FIG. 4 FHIR Genomics Operations are organized along 2 orthogonal axes, subject versus population, and genotype versus phenotype. See the official HL7 standard [1] for a detailed description of each API.

Reference Implementation

To make it easier to conceptualize the implementation and use of the Operations, we have developed a full open-sourced reference implementation [37] using synthetic or publicly available and anonymized data. Objectives of the reference implementation project include enabling experimentation with Operations innovations and provision of a functional API to (SMART-on-FHIR, CDS Hooks, and so forth) app developers. Key discoveries from the reference implementation are that (1) clinically relevant slices of genomic data can be extracted from a data-agnostic genomic repository and returned to a client app in real-time; (2) genomic data normalization is feasible in real-time, and greatly enhances search and annotation; and (3) variants can be dynamically intersected with knowledge in real time to provide up to date annotations.

Clinical Scenario

A clinical scenario will serve to help illustrate the use of FHIR Genomics Operations by clinical applications.

Patient Higado Sobreviviente is a synthetic patient loosely derived from the National Cancer Institute (NCI) The Cancer Genome Atlas (TCGA) public case TCGA-DD-A1EH [38], modified for illustrative purposes. Born in April 1998, Mr Sobreviviente is a Hispanic male with a known history of chronic hepatitis B, who was found in June 2021 at the age of 23 to have a liver mass, with biopsy showing hepatocellular carcinoma.

In July 2021, he was started on tenofovir. Clinical staging showed a stage 3, T3 N0 M0 tumor. He underwent a surgical right lobe resection, showing a pathologic stage T3 N0 M0 tumor with inactive chronic hepatitis with fibrosis. In October 2021, he was found to have liver and lung recurrence and was started on sorafenib. By January 2022, his disease was progressing. NGS of his tumor was ordered. Laboratory report showed him to be microsatellite instability (MSI)-stable with a tumor mutational burden (TMB) of 1.3 and showed no FDA Level 1 or Level 2 actionable variants [39].

His clinical team sought to determine clinical trial eligibility. Using a SMART-on-FHIR molecular tumor board (MTB) app, the clinical team discovered 2 *ARID1A* variants (stop-gained variant NC_000001.10:27105549:C:T; frameshift variant NC_000001.10:27106893::T), both of which satisfy screening enrollment criteria for clinical trial NCT05023655 "Phase II Study of Tazemetostat in Solid Tumors Harboring an ARID1A Mutation" [40]. When last seen in follow-up in April 2022, Mr Sobreviviente was enrolled in NCT05023655, with stable disease.

Behind the scenes, the MTB app might leverage a variety of Operations: *find-subject-variants* to screen *ARID1A* for variants; *find-study-metadata* to determine if *ARID1A* was studied (particularly useful where no *ARID1A* variants are identified); *find-subject-molecular-consequences* to determine predicted molecular consequences of identified variants; *find-subject-tx-implications* to cross-check variants against potential treatment (medication, clinical trial) options; *find-population-specific-variants* to identify patients with similar variants. Other Operations of potential use are those that retrieve structural variants (*find-subject-structural-intersecting-variants, find-subject-structural-subsuming-variants*) and *find-subject-dx-implications* to perform secondary American College of Medical Genetics and Genomics (ACMG) screening of germline variants. (Full data set for Higado Sobreviviente is available upon request. All variants are included in the Operations reference implementation.)

FAST HEALTH CARE INTEROPERABILITY RESOURCES GENOMICS OPERATIONS FOR ADVANCED CLINICAL DECISION SUPPORT

Clinical genomics apps such as those for precision cancer care and rare disease variant discovery are data-hungry, benefiting from access to a patient's whole genome.

Cancer is a disease of the genome, with studies showing that a large proportion of tumors harbor potentially actionable oncogenic events [41]. Guidelines from the National Comprehensive Cancer Network, NCI, European Society for Medical Oncology, and other groups cover a growing array of molecular-based cancer treatment guidelines. Many patients who satisfy guideline criteria for molecularly guided therapy are benefiting from precision treatments targeted to their specific germline and somatic genomes, whereas a vast number of patients fall outside established guidelines. Studies reveal the presence of potentially thousands of biomarkers affecting patient outcomes [42], and molecular prediction tools are commonly used to scan large regions of the genome to aid in the identification of potentially oncogenic variants [43], indicating that the determination of advanced therapeutic options for patients with cancer increasingly benefits from a broader view of the patient's genome.

Studies estimate close to 10,000 different rare disorders, the vast majority of which likely have a genetic basis [44]. Clinicians generally apply scenario-based filters to NGS output to help hone in on those variants likely to be most significant [45]. Filters are applied to narrow the scope of genes to consider based on patient phenotype, to limit attention to specific variant types or

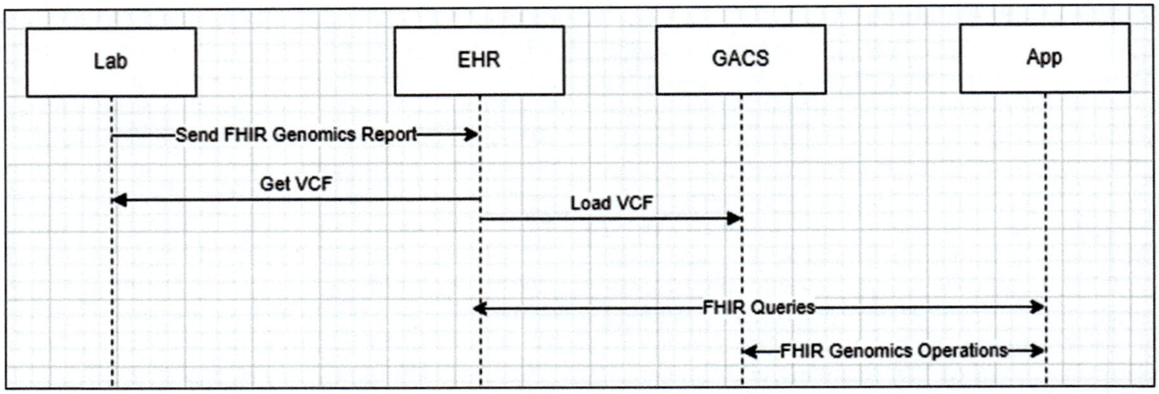

FIG. 5 Standards-based pipeline for automatically gathering a person's full genomic data set and exposing it for advanced CDS.

specific allelic state (eg, only consider homozygous variants), may filter based on annotations (eg, predicted molecular consequences, diagnostic implications, and population allele frequency), and so forth. But different filters may need to be tested, and because of the very nature of rare diseases, systematic exploration of wide swaths of a person's entire genome is often warranted.

Additionally, broad access to a patient's genome may benefit polygenic risk score calculations, where scores can be based on thousands if not millions of variants [46], and even pharmacogenomics, which we generally think of as just needing a handful of a patient's star alleles but may require far broader access, as in the case of ThermoFisher's PharmacoScan, which is a microarray assay of over 4000 markers in over 1000 genes.

A standards-based approach to gathering data and enabling advanced CDS that leverages a person's whole genome is shown in (Fig. 5).

In this approach, (1) A laboratory sends an HL7 Version 2 message or FHIR Genomics diagnostic report to the EHR. Within that report is an explicit reference to the corresponding VCF file (or other raw data file); (2) The EHR uses the explicit VCF link to automatically grab the VCF file, and load it into an Operations-enabled genomic data repository (aka genomic archiving and communication system, GACS); and (3) Apps can now access data stored in an FHIR server using standard FHIR queries and can access a patient's complete genomic data, stored in GACS, using FHIR Genomics Operations. In many cases, GACS also stores variant implication knowledge (eg, that variant NC_000006.11:26091178:C:G is associated with hemochromatosis; that *CYP2C19 *1/*2* is associated with altered clopidogrel metabolism) that can be dynamically associated with a person's variants and returned via Operations.

DISCUSSION

FHIR Genomics Operations are relatively new, where ongoing and future pilots are likely to identify enhancement opportunities that further mature the standard. Several pilots are underway under the sponsorship of the GenomeX "HL7 FHIR Accelerator program" [47]. The FHIR Accelerator program is designed to assist communities and collaborative groups across the global health care spectrum in the creation and adoption of high-quality FHIR Implementation Guides or other standard artifacts to move toward the realization of global health data interoperability. The CodeX FHIR Accelerator is focused on driving advances in cancer care [48,49]. Under the CodeX umbrella, the GenomeX [50] project is driving advances in molecular/precision medicine (not limited to cancer). Feedback from GenomeX-sponsored pilots is channeled to the HL7 Clinical Genomics committee for iterative enhancements to the standard.

Genomics is a rapidly evolving field. Ongoing research is looking to enhance Operations agility (eg, for the structured incorporation of new biomarkers) and Operations dynamic annotation capabilities for more complex categorical [51] or structural variants. Those aspects of a whole genome-enabled CDS pipeline that are subject to FDA regulations will depend heavily on the nature and transparency of the CDS rules.

SUMMARY

FHIR Genomics Operations *encapsulate data complexity*, *enable dynamic VA*, and offer an approach for driving *advanced CDS that leverages a person's entire genome*. Coupled with the tremendous growth and adoption of FHIR along with the growing adoption of SMART-on-FHIR and CDS Hooks across EHRs, FHIR Genomics Operations are poised as a novel enabler of genomics-EHR integration to drive next generation advances in precision care.

CLINICS CARE POINTS

- FHIR Genomics Operations enable advanced CDS leveraging a person's entire genome.
- Many labs consider the VCF file to be 'research-grade'. As a result, the direct use of VCF data in a clinical pipeline may need to be subject to local IRB review.

DISCLOSURE

The authors have nothing to disclose.

REFERENCES

[1] HL7.FHIR.UV.GENOMICS-REPORTING\Operations - FHIR v4.0.1. Available at: http://build.fhir.org/ig/HL7/genomics-reporting/branches/operations/operations.html. [Accessed 24 February 2022].

[2] Dolin RH, Heale BSE, Alterovitz G, et al. Introducing HL7 FHIR Genomics Operations: a developer-friendly approach to genomics-EHR integration. J Am Med Inf Assoc 2023;30(3):485–93.

[3] Dolin R, Heale BSE, Gupta R, et al. Sync for Genes Phase 5: Computable artifacts for sharing dynamically annotated FHIR-formatted genomic variants. Learning Health Systems 2023;7(4):e10385.

[4] Walton NA, Johnson DK, Person TN, et al. Genomic Data in the Electronic Health Record. Advances in Molecular Pathology 2019;2(1):21–33.

[5] Williams MS, Taylor CO, Walton NA, et al. Genomic Information for Clinicians in the Electronic Health Record: Lessons Learned From the Clinical Genome Resource Project and the Electronic Medical Records and Genomics Network. Front Genet 2019;10. https://doi.org/10.3389/fgene.2019.01059.

[6] Sutton J, Wix K, Amusan A. Experiences and Lessons Learned From a New Functionality for Pharmacogenomics CDS in the Electronic Health Record. Available at: https://zerista.s3.amazonaws.com/item_files/1663/attachments/427873/original/amia_summit_2018_poster.pdf. [Accessed 5 November 2020].

[7] HL7 Standards Product Brief - HL7 Version 2.5.1 Implementation Guide: Laboratory Results Interface, Release 1 STU Release 3 - US Realm | HL7 International. Available at: https://www.hl7.org/implement/standards/product_brief.cfm?product_id=279. [Accessed 19 August 2021].

[8] HL7.FHIR.UV.GENOMICS-REPORTING\Home Page - FHIR v4.0.1. Available at: http://build.fhir.org/ig/HL7/genomics-reporting/index.html. [Accessed 18 July 2022].

[9] eMERGE Consortium. Harmonizing Clinical Sequencing and Interpretation for the eMERGE III Network. Am J Hum Genet 2019;105(3):588–605.

[10] Wynn J, Lewis K, Amendola LM, et al. Clinical providers' experiences with returning results from genomic sequencing: an interview study. BMC Med Genomics 2018;11(1):45.

[11] Alterovitz G, Warner J, Zhang P, et al. SMART on FHIR Genomics: facilitating standardized clinico-genomic apps. J Am Med Inform Assoc 2015;22(6):1173–8.

[12] Warner JL, Rioth MJ, Mandl KD, et al. SMART precision cancer medicine: a FHIR-based app to provide genomic information at the point of care. J Am Med Inform Assoc 2016;23(4):701–10.

[13] Mandel JC, Kreda DA, Mandl KD, et al. SMART on FHIR: a standards-based, interoperable apps platform for electronic health records. J Am Med Inform Assoc 2016; 23(5):899–908.

[14] Ohno-Machado L, Kim J, Gabriel RA, et al. Genomics and electronic health record systems. Hum Mol Genet 2018;27(R1):R48–55.

[15] Caraballo PJ, Bielinski SJ, St Sauver JL, et al. Electronic Medical Record-Integrated Pharmacogenomics and Related Clinical Decision Support Concepts. Clin Pharmacol Ther 2017;102(2):254–64.

[16] Holmes JB, Moyer E, Phan L, et al. SPDI: data model for variants and applications at NCBI. Bioinformatics 2020; 36(6):1902–7.

[17] Kalia SS, Adelman K, Bale SJ, et al. Recommendations for reporting of secondary findings in clinical exome and genome sequencing, 2016 update (ACMG SF v2.0): a policy statement of the American College of Medical Genetics and Genomics. Genet Med 2017; 19(2):249–55.

[18] NCBI ClinVar gene-specific summary, 2016 [Internet]. National Institutes of Health (NIH). Available at: ftp://ftp.ncbi.nlm.nih.gov/pub/clinvar/tab_delimited/archive/gene_specific_summary_2016-01.txt.gz. [Accessed 28 April 2020].

[19] NCBI ClinVar gene-specific summary, 2018 [Internet]. National Institutes of Health (NIH). Available at: ftp://ftp.ncbi.nlm.nih.gov/pub/clinvar/tab_delimited/archive/gene_specific_summary_2018-01.txt.gz. [Accessed 28 April 2020].

[20] Topol E. Human genomics vs Clinical genomics. Ground Truths. 2022. Available at: https://erictopol.substack.com/p/human-genomics-vs-clinical-genomics. [Accessed 23 September 2022].

[21] SMART on FHIR (smarthealthit.org). Available at: https://docs.smarthealthit.org/. [Accessed 28 November 2023].

[22] 2.0 - CDS Hooks. Available at: https://cds-hooks.hl7.org/2.0/. [Accessed 14 December 2023].

[23] Dolin RH, Shenvi EC, Alvarez C, et al. PillHarmonics™: An Orchestrated Pharmacogenetics Medication Clinical Decision Support Service. Appl Clin Inform 2024. https://doi.org/10.1055/a-2274-6763.

[24] Dolin RH, Boxwala A, Shalaby J. A Pharmacogenomics Clinical Decision Support Service Based on FHIR and CDS Hooks. Methods Inf Med 2018;57(S 02):e115–23.

[25] Watkins M, Eilbeck K. FHIR Lab Reports: using SMART on FHIR and CDS Hooks to increase the clinical utility of pharmacogenomic laboratory test results. AMIA Jt Summits Transl Sci Proc 2020;2020:683–92.

[26] Health Data. Technology, and Interoperability: Certification Program Updates, Algorithm Transparency, and Information Sharing (HTI-1) Final Rule | HealthIT.gov. Available at: https://www.healthit.gov/topic/laws-regulation-and-policy/health-data-technology-and-interoperability-certification-program. [Accessed 13 December 2023].

[27] HTI-1 Decision Support Interventions Fact Sheet. Accessed December 15, 2023. Available at: https://www.healthit.gov/sites/default/files/page/2023-12/HTI-1_DSI_fact%20sheet_508.pdf.

[28] United States Core Data for Interoperability (USCDI). Official Website of the Office of the National Coordinator for Health Information Technology (ONC). Available at: https://www.healthit.gov/isp/united-states-core-data-interoperability-uscdi. Accessed March 16, 2022.

[29] House TW. Executive Order on the Safe, Secure, and Trustworthy Development and Use of Artificial Intelligence. The White House. Published October 30, 2023. Available at: https://www.whitehouse.gov/briefing-room/presidential-actions/2023/10/30/executive-order-on-the-safe-secure-and-trustworthy-development-and-use-of-artificial-intelligence/. [Accessed 15 December 2023].

[30] FDA. Clinical Decision Support Software - Guidance for Industry and Food and Drug Administration Staff. Published September 22, 2022. Available at: https://www.fda.gov/regulatory-information/search-fda-guidance-documents/clinical-decision-support-software. [Accessed 15 December 2023].

[31] Kukhareva P, Warner P, Rodriguez S, et al. Balancing Functionality versus Portability for SMART on FHIR Applications: Case Study for a Neonatal Bilirubin Management Application. AMIA Annu Symp Proc 2019;2019:562–71.

[32] Gordon WJ, Mandl KD. The 21st Century Cures Act: A Competitive Apps Market and the Risk of Innovation Blocking. J Med Internet Res 2020;22(12):e24824. https://doi.org/10.2196/24824.

[33] HL7 FHIR US Core Implementation Guide v6.1.0. Available at: https://hl7.org/fhir/us/core/STU6.1/. [Accessed 11 January 2024].

[34] Landrum MJ, Chitipiralla S, Brown GR, et al. ClinVar: improvements to accessing data. Nucleic Acids Res 2020; 48(D1):D835–44.

[35] Krysiak K, Danos AM, Saliba J, et al. CIViCdb 2022: evolution of an open-access cancer variant interpretation knowledgebase. Nucleic Acids Res 2023;51(D1): D1230–41.

[36] Gong L, Whirl-Carrillo M, Klein TE. PharmGKB, an Integrated Resource of Pharmacogenomic Knowledge. Curr Protoc 2021;1(8):e226.

[37] HL7 FHIR Genomics Operations - Reference Implementation. Published online May 3, 2022. Available at: https://github.com/FHIR/genomics-operations. [Accessed 18 July 2022].

[38] Patient: TCGA-DD-A1EH. Available at: https://www.cbioportal.org/patient/summary?studyId=lihc_tcga_pan_can_atlas_2018&caseId=TCGA-DD-A1EH#navCaseIds=lihc_tcga_pan_can_atlas_2018:TCGA-DD-A1EH. [Accessed 23 March 2024].

[39] Li MM, Datto M, Duncavage EJ, et al. Standards and Guidelines for the Interpretation and Reporting of Sequence Variants in Cancer. J Mol Diagn 2017;19(1):4–23.

[40] Prisma Health-Upstate. A Phase II Study of Tazemetostat in Solid Tumors Harboring an ARID1A Mutation. clinicaltrials.gov; 2023. Available at: https://clinicaltrials.gov/study/NCT05023655. [Accessed 31 December 2023].

[41] Bailey MH, Tokheim C, Porta-Pardo E, et al. Comprehensive Characterization of Cancer Driver Genes and Mutations. Cell 2018;173(2):371–85.e18.

[42] Smith JC, Sheltzer JM. Genome-wide identification and analysis of prognostic features in human cancers. Cell Rep 2022;38(13):110569.

[43] Masica DL, Douville C, Tokheim C, et al. CRAVAT 4: Cancer-Related Analysis of Variants Toolkit. Cancer Res 2017;77(21):e35–8.

[44] Tisdale A, Cutillo CM, Nathan R, et al. The IDeaS initiative: pilot study to assess the impact of rare diseases on patients and healthcare systems. Orphanet J Rare Dis 2021;16:429.

[45] Austin-Tse CA, Jobanputra V, Perry DL, et al. Best practices for the interpretation and reporting of clinical whole genome sequencing. npj Genom Med 2022;7(1):1–13.

[46] Lambert SA, Gil L, Jupp S, et al. The Polygenic Score Catalog as an open database for reproducibility and systematic evaluation. Nat Genet 2021;53(4):420–5.

[47] HL7 FHIR ACCELERATORTM Program | HL7 International. Available at: https://www.hl7.org/about/fhir-accelerator/. [Accessed 19 July 2022].

[48] Goel AK, Campbell WS, Moldwin R. Structured Data Capture for Oncology. JCO Clinical Cancer Informatics 2021;(5):194–201.

[49] Osterman TJ, Terry M, Miller RS. Improving Cancer Data Interoperability: The Promise of the Minimal Common Oncology Data Elements (mCODE) Initiative. JCO Clin Cancer Inform 2020;4:993–1001.

[50] GenomeX - Genomics Operations - CodeX - Confluence. Available at: https://confluence.hl7.org/display/COD/GenomeX+-+Genomics+Operations. [Accessed 18 July 2022].

[51] Wagner AH, Walsh B, Mayfield G, et al. A harmonized meta-knowledgebase of clinical interpretations of somatic genomic variants in cancer. Nat Genet 2020; 52(4):448–57.

Advances in Molecular Pathology 7 (2024) 123–130
ADVANCES IN MOLECULAR PATHOLOGY

Is Picture Archiving and Communication System a Model for Genomics?

Srikar Chamala, PhD[a,b,*], Robert H. Dolin, MD[c], Nephi Walton, MD, MS[d]
[a]Department of Pathology and Laboratory Medicine, Children's Hospital Los Angeles, CA, USA; [b]Department of Pathology, University of Southern California, CA, USA; [c]Elimu Informatics, El Cerrito, CA, USA; [d]National Human Genome Research Institute, Bethesda, MD, USA

KEYWORDS
• PACS model • Genomics • Genomics data standards • DICOM standards • GACS
• Precision genomics medicine

KEY POINTS

- Reflecting on the picture archiving and communication system (PACS) model offers valuable insights for the potential development of a similar system in genomics, termed genomic archiving and communication system (GACS).
- While the maturity and robust framework of PACS and its Digital Imaging and Communications in Medicine standards have evolved over 40 years, genomic standards are still emerging and have not yet reached widespread adoption.
- Current genomic interoperability efforts, heavily dependent on voluntary contributions, highlight the urgent need for dedicated funding to effectively develop, test, and maintain these standards.
- Furthermore, both public funding agencies and private entities such as electronic health record/pharmacy/health systems are crucial for supporting the development, pilot implementation, and maintenance of genomic standards, which would significantly boost genomic interoperability creation and adoption.
- For GACS to effectively integrate into clinical and research settings, establishing and enforcing policies for adopting genomic data standards is essential.

INTRODUCTION TO PICTURE ARCHIVING AND COMMUNICATION SYSTEM

Picture archiving and communication system (PACS) is a sophisticated medical imaging technology that plays a crucial role in modern health care [1]. Employing both hardware and software, PACS enables hospitals and health care systems to store, retrieve, and share medical images effectively. This technology is integral to managing diagnostic imaging studies and enhances the efficiency of health care services [2].

Historically, medical images were stored and managed using physical film jackets, which required manual filing, retrieval, and physical transportation [3]. This process was not only cumbersome but also time-consuming and prone to errors. In contrast, PACS systems streamline these processes by digitizing images and storing them either online, via cloud storage solutions, or offline on local on-premises servers [4]. The idea to replace film with digital images was first conceptualized in 1970 [5,6], with initial conference on PACS design discussion started in 1982 [5,7]. This digital approach ensures the secure handling and transportation of private patient medical imaging information, safeguarding patient confidentiality.

PACS supports a wide array of medical imaging types, including radiographs, CT scans, MRI scans, and

*Corresponding author, *E-mail address:* schamala@chla.usc.edu

https://doi.org/10.1016/j.yamp.2024.07.007 www.advancesinmolecularpathology.com
2589-4080/24/

ultrasound images. The versatility of PACS allows for comprehensive integration with various imaging modalities, making it an indispensable tool in diagnostic medicine [4]. Additionally, PACS facilitates teleradiology—the remote retrieval and analysis of medical images—which enables radiologists to provide their expertise regardless of their physical location, thereby enhancing the accessibility and delivery of health care [2].

Designed to integrate seamlessly with a hospital's electronic information system, PACS systems are a cornerstone in the digital infrastructure of health care institutions. They are critically evaluated based on their capacity to boost efficiency and productivity while reducing operational costs. The adoption of PACS not only speeds up medical diagnostics but also improves the quality of care, supporting health care providers in delivering timely and accurate treatment decisions [6,7].

THE EVOLUTION OF PICTURE ARCHIVING AND COMMUNICATION SYSTEM IN RADIOLOGY

In the early 1980s, the first experimental PACS were developed, primarily focusing on the digitization of medical images. By the mid-1980s [8], the introduction of the Digital Imaging and Communications in Medicine (DICOM) standard significantly enhanced the interoperability of PACS with various imaging equipment, streamlining processes across health care systems [9,10]. The late 1980s to 1990s saw rapid growth and widespread implementation of PACS in hospitals, accompanied by improvements in network speeds and image compression techniques that further optimized the utility and efficiency of these systems. In the 2000s, PACS technology evolved to integrate with electronic health records (EHRs), benefit from advancements in web-based platforms, and leverage the burgeoning capabilities of cloud storage [8]. Today, the importance of Departmental or Enterprise PACS has become paramount, now crucially enhanced by artificial intelligence to enable more accurate and efficient diagnostics.

THE EVOLUTION OF CLINICAL GENOMICS

The evolution of clinical genomics testing has profoundly transformed modern medicine by enabling personalized treatment approaches, beginning with early genetic mapping techniques following the discovery of DNA's structure in 1953 [11]. The completion of the Human Genome Project in 2003 marked a significant milestone, mapping all human genes and greatly advancing genetic research while reducing sequencing costs. The introduction of next-generation sequencing (NGS) in the mid-2000s revolutionized [12] the field by allowing rapid, cost-effective sequencing of large DNA segments, facilitating the identification of genetic variations associated with diseases [13]. This enabled the integration of genomic testing into routine diagnostics, supporting diverse applications from diagnosing rare genetic disorders to targeted cancer therapies and prenatal testing [13,14]. Despite its successes, clinical genomics data management and reporting both at the laboratory and at EHR faces challenges [15–17]. Overall, clinical genomics testing continues to enhance medical diagnostics and treatment, promising further integration and innovation in health care practices.

CLINICAL GENOMICS DATA

The standard NGS pipeline involves converting raw genomic sequencing reads (FASTQ data) into a binary alignment map (BAM) file by aligning them against the human reference genome. This BAM file is then used to identify genomic variants, resulting in a variant call format (VCF) file. These genetic variants are interpreted further for their impact on patient health, but only clinically actionable variants are typically recorded into the EHR. Throughout this process, the data volume significantly reduces from gigabytes in FASTQ files to only a few kilobytes in the final genomic test reports that enter the EHR, highlighting the impracticality of storing vast and complex genomic data directly in EHR systems [17].

GENOMICS EQUIVALENT OF PICTURE ARCHIVING AND COMMUNICATION SYSTEM

Health care institutions employ PACS to store and manage large medical images, such as those in DICOM format, which are too voluminous to be directly stored in electronic health records (EHRs) or radiology information systems (RIS). In this setup, PACS handle the storage of the images themselves, while EHRs and RIS maintain the final reports and metadata about the images without storing the images. A similar framework could be adapted to manage the substantial data produced by NGS, suggesting a scalable solution for handling extensive genomic data sets in health care settings. The term coined for the genomics counterpart to PACS is known as the genomic archiving and communication system (GACS). Similar to PACS, GACS (Fig. 1 adopted from

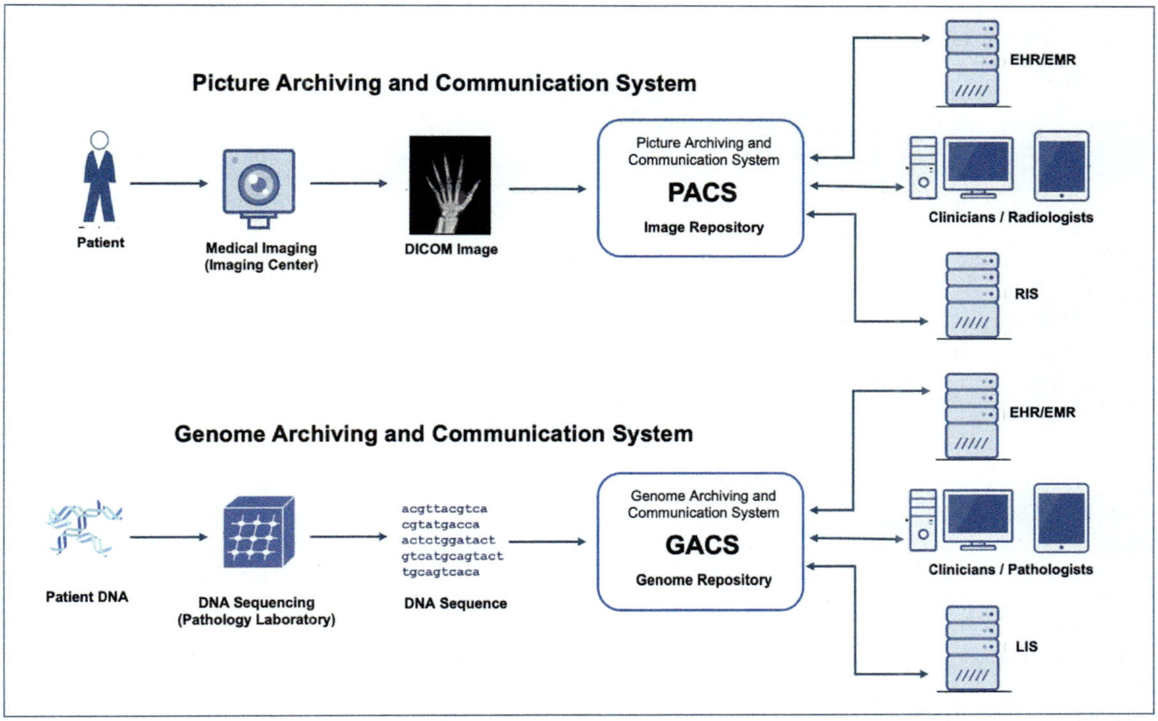

FIG. 1 Depiction of PACS and GACS workflow.

Alterovitz and colleagues [18]) would handle the storage of sequence data generated by sequencing laboratories, accommodating large datasets that are not suitable for direct storage in EHRs [18].

Similarities between the systems for storing imaging and genetic data include the handling of large data volumes that EHRs cannot store or manipulate directly, the reliance on specialist analysis for interpretative reports, the possibility of reporting incidental findings, the requirement for special viewers to interpret the data, the potential for reanalysis to extract additional insights, and the domain-specific expertise needed for an accurate interpretation [17].

However, genetic data systems also present unique challenges compared to PACS. For instance, genetic interpretations may evolve over time as new information emerges, necessitating frequent reanalysis and updates to the EHR. Genetic data retains its value or may even increase in relevance over time, unlike certain medical images. Moreover, the interpretation of genetic data heavily depends on continually updated genetic databases, which can significantly alter diagnostic outcomes. Lastly, unlike imaging data, which had established viewing standards pre-PACS, standardized viewers for genomic data are not yet commonplace [17].

Understanding these nuances is crucial as we develop genetic data storage and access systems, ensuring they are robust enough to handle the complexities of modern genomics.

WORKFLOW SIMILARITIES BETWEEN PICTURE ARCHIVING AND COMMUNICATION SYSTEM AND THE PROPOSED GENOMIC ARCHIVING AND COMMUNICATION SYSTEM MODEL FOR GENOMICS

In both the established PACS used in radiology and the proposed GACS for genomics, there are notable workflow parallels (Fig. 2). Initially, in the radiology workflow, clinic staff utilizes the EHR to register patients and enter imaging examination orders, which are then transmitted to RIS through HL7 standards [19]. The RIS, used by imaging center staff, manages scheduling and tracks radiology technologist workflows. Once an order is queued in the RIS work list, the radiology technologist performs the imaging examination using the appropriate modality (eg, CT and MRI) and the images are acquired and transferred to PACS as DICOM images [20]. PACS components include image management, an image viewer, and a

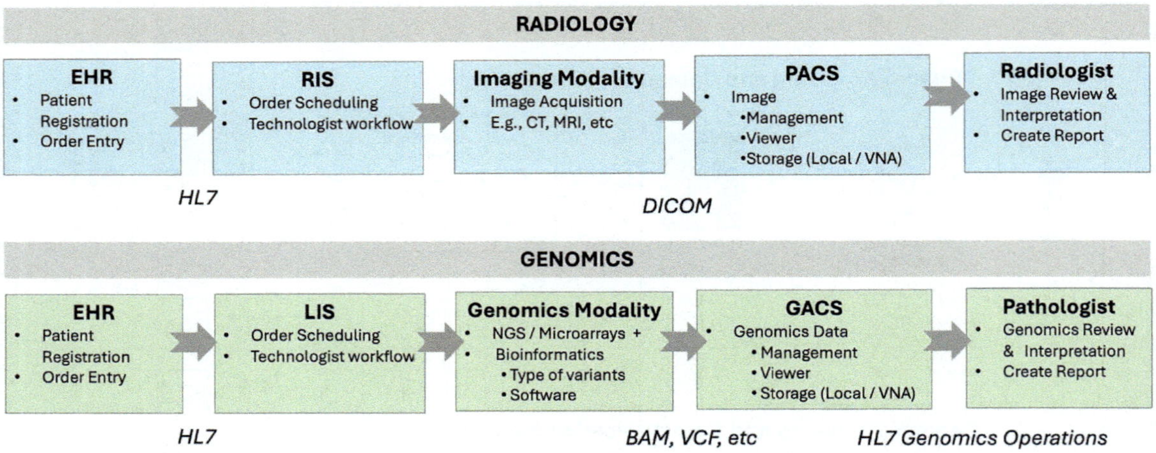

FIG. 2 Workflow illustration of PACS and the proposed GACS model for genomics.

storage server, which can be local or cloud-based. Radiologists use PACS to review, interpret, and annotate images, ultimately creating a final report that is sent back to the EHR via HL7.

Similarly, the genomics workflow starts with clinic staff using the EHR for patient registration and genomic test ordering. These orders are sent to laboratory information systems through HL7 standards. Pathology staff then collects a DNA sample from the patient, processes it, and sequences it to produce raw DNA sequence data. These data are processed through clinical bioinformatics software to generate several types of files, including raw sequence data (FASTQ), alignment files (BAM), and variant files (VCF). Molecular pathologists filter these to identify clinically actionable variants and compile reports [15,17]. A future GACS would store all these files and include applications similar to those in PACS: genomics data management, a genomics data viewer, and a genomic data server. Final reports could be sent back to the EHR as Health Level 7 Fast Healthcare Interoperability Resources (HL7 FHIR) genomics messages or portable document format (PDFs) embedded in HL7, mirroring the PACS process but adapted for genomic data.

DATA STANDARDS MATURITY COMPARISONS IN PICTURE ARCHIVING AND COMMUNICATION SYSTEM AND THE PROPOSED GENOMIC ARCHIVING AND COMMUNICATION SYSTEM MODEL FOR GENOMICS

Data standards in the radiology and genomics fields have evolved significantly, reflecting differing levels of maturity and application. In radiology (Fig. 3), the DICOM standards established by the American College of Radiology (ACR) and the National Electrical Manufacturers Association (NEMA) began in 1983, with the first standard for interoperable image files released in 1985 as ACR-NEMA 300. This evolved into DICOM 3.0 in 1993, which significantly enhanced networked image communication capabilities. Over the years, DICOM standards expanded into other medical disciplines, and by 2004, included advancements such as web access to DICOM objects, spatial registration, and Moving Pictures Expert Group (MPEG2) encoding. In 2010, pathology whole slide imaging was added, with ongoing updates to accommodate new modalities and imaging needs [9,10].

In contrast, genomic standards are still developing (see Fig. 3). Raw outputs like FASTQ for NGS are standardized but vary in quality score encoding, while tabular outputs for microarray are mostly vendor-specific. Bioinformatics alignment outputs, such as sequence alignment map (SAM), BAM, and CRAM [21], are standardized when best practices are followed. While variant file formats like VCF, genomic variant call format (gVCF), and annotated VCF [22] and various forms of VCF are standardized, but these standards are highly extensible and customizable creating variability. Another variant representation format is the Variation Representation Specification [23,24] (VRS, pronounced "verse"), developed by the Global Alliance for Genomics and Health to facilitate accurately representing many classes of genetic variation, which is standardized when best practices are followed. Moreover, data related to quality files, plots, and vendor-specific formats often lack uniformity. Final reports in genomics typically appear in laboratory or vendor-specific PDFs or structured files, although efforts are underway to standardize

RADIOLOGY	GENOMICS
DICOM History • **1983:** ACR and NEMA establish a committee for image format standards. • **1985:** Release of ACR-NEMA 300, the first standard for interoperable image files. • **1993:** Renamed DICOM 3.0, facilitating networked image communication. • **Late 1990s:** DICOM extends into other medical disciplines. • **2004:** Web-access to DICOM objects, spatial registration, MPEG2 encoding. • **2010:** Pathology whole slide imaging added • **Active:** Ongoing updates for new modalities, technologies, imaging needs.	**Raw Outputs** • FASTQ (NGS): standardized but variable quality score encoding • Tabular (Microarray): mostly vendor specific **Bioinformatics Outputs** • BAM / CRAM / SAM: standardized (when best practices are followed) • VCF / VCF Annotation / gVCF: standardized but highly extensible & customizable • VRS: standardized when best practices are followed • Quality Files / Plots: vendor/lab specific • Vendor specific structured formats **Final Report** • PDFs: vendor/lab specific • HL7 V2 / FHIR Genomics: actively working on standards • Lab specific structured formats **Other Data** • Variant Normalization: **VCF** (left justified); **HGVS** (3' justified); **SPDI** (fully justified); **VRS** (fully justified)

FIG. 3 Data standards status in radiology and genomics.

these through HL7 V2 and FHIR Genomics protocols. Even where genomic data has been structured into a standard format, the multiple representations of a variant can hinder search and data retrieval. For example, the same variant may be represented in different ways such as "NM_001195798.2: c.12G>A," "NM_001195803.2: c.12G>A," "NC_000019.9: g.11200236G>A," "NG_009060.1: g.5180G>A," and "NC_000019.10:11089559: G: A," which can impede data search and retrieval.

A GACS server can encapsulate variant normalization, such that one can query using any of these representations, and variants matching any of its synonyms will be returned. This ongoing development highlights a dynamic landscape in genomic data standardization, contrasting with the well-established protocols in radiology, and underscores the continuous efforts required to achieve similar levels of standardization in the genomics field.

KEY EFFORTS IN CURRENT GENOMICS STANDARDIZATION

Current efforts in genomics standardization emphasize enhancing data exchange, accuracy, and collaboration across diverse platforms and organizations. Notable initiatives leading this endeavor include the development of the HL7 FHIR Genomics Reporting Implementation Guide [25] (GRIG) by the Clinical Genomics Work Group of HL7 [26], the GenomeX [27] program within the CodeX FHIR Accelerator [28], and the Global Alliance for Genomics and Health (GA4GH) [28]. These initiatives are instrumental in developing a cohesive framework for managing genomic data.

The HL7 FHIR GRIG and GenomeX play crucial roles in this framework. The genomics data exchange aspect of these standards focuses on the representation and delivery of final FHIR genomic reports, ensuring that these vital documents are accessible and interpretable across different health information systems. The FHIR Genomics Study standard captures essential metadata, such as the instrumentation used, bioinformatics software, and analysis parameters, which are critical for replicating studies and understanding genomic data processing contexts. Moreover, FHIR Genomic Operations [29] standardize how data are retrieved from entities like GACS, promoting consistency and reliability in data pulls that support clinical decisions and research. In fact, the relationship between FHIR Genomics Operations and GACS is analogous to the relationship between DICOM and PACS, offering a standardized interface by which clinical applications can easily access complex genomic findings and annotations.

GA4GH also significantly contributes to genomics standardization by providing specifications and supporting file formats essential for genomic data management. Their VRS [23,24] and Variant Annotation Specification [30] standardize the representation and annotation of genomic variations, promoting uniformity in data analysis. GA4GH also supports various file formats such as SAM, BAM, browser extensible data (BED), compressed reference-oriented alignment map (CRAM), and VCF, which are crucial for the storage and communication of genomic data across platforms. Additionally, tools and frameworks like Phenopackets and Beacon enhance data sharing and interoperability among researchers, fostering a global approach to genomic data handling.

The integration and alignment of standards across different organizations (eg, HL7 GRIG and GA4GH) are critical for the successful implementation of genomic data standards. Cross-collaboration ensures that standards are comprehensive, avoiding duplication of efforts and fostering innovation through shared knowledge and resources. These collaborations also help in addressing the challenges of data privacy, security, and ethical considerations in genomics.

These key efforts in genomics standardization mark significant progress toward a more integrated and accessible global genomic data infrastructure, which is fundamental to advancing personalized medicine and enhancing the understanding of complex genetic information.

ELECTRONIC HEALTH RECORD VIEWING: COMPARING PICTURE ARCHIVING AND COMMUNICATION SYSTEM AND GENOMIC ARCHIVING AND COMMUNICATION SYSTEM IN GENOMICS

In radiology, images are not stored directly in the EHR; instead, only the final report is archived. With PACS, a link to the PACS server is integrated within the EHR radiology examination window, allowing users to view images related to a specific imaging order via the PACS viewer functionality. A similar concept could be applied to genomic data (BAM, VCF files, and so forth) using a proposed GACS viewer integrated within GACS. For an illustration of this integration, refer to Fig. 4. The EHR screens were adopted from Oracle Health Cerner. It is common practice for specialists, such as neurologists, to view the medical images in addition to reading the medical report. This allows them to assess the image in the context of a patient they have personally assessed, a context that the radiologist who generates the report does not have. It is not uncommon for specialists identify additional findings using this context. Similarly, a GACS interface could allow specialists to assess additional genetic variation outside of the clinical report in the context of the patient. The other reason that PACS interfaces are important is the time required to get a radiology report. In urgent situations, physicians look at the images themselves before the report is issued to take an immediate action. This same logic applies to genomic data, where genomic reports that can take weeks to months to be completed.

STORAGE MODELS FOR PICTURE ARCHIVING AND COMMUNICATION SYSTEM AND GENOMIC ARCHIVING AND COMMUNICATION SYSTEM VENDOR NEUTRAL ARCHIVE

A storage model called vendor neutral archive (VNA) is emerging in PACS. This medical imaging technology allows image storage, management, and retrieval in a

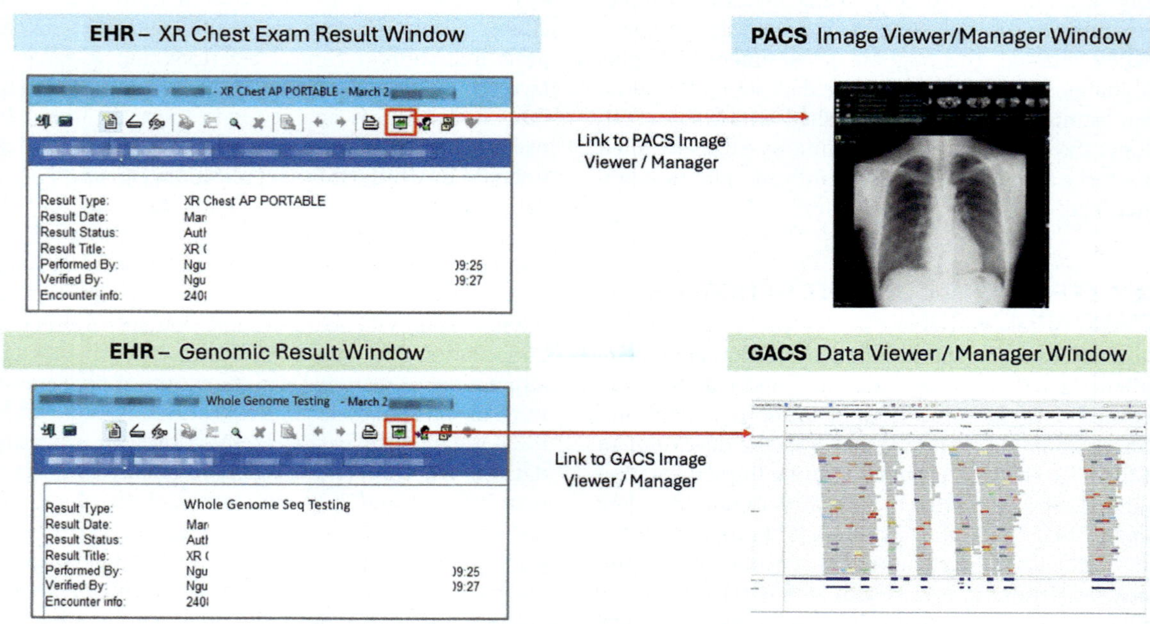

FIG. 4 Depiction of viewing of PACS images vs genomics results or file from EHR.

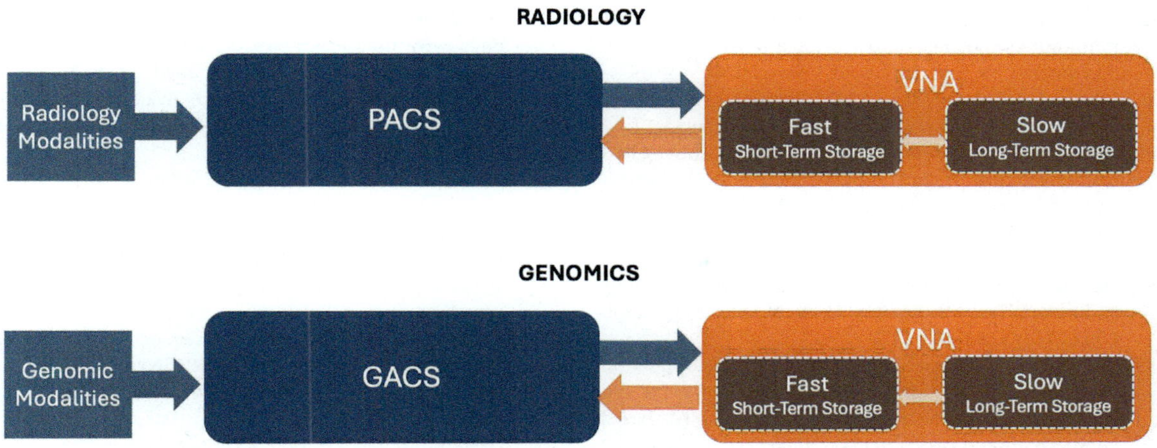

FIG. 5 Depiction of the application of the VNA model as a storage solution for PACS images versus genomics data.

standardized manner, independent of the imaging device manufacturer. VNAs provide a centralized repository for medical images and related data that can be accessed and managed regardless of the original vendor, ensuring interoperability and flexibility [31]. Additionally, different storage tiers are introduced in the PACS model, including short-term storage, which is fast storage used for frequent or rapid access to image files, especially during the image review and sign out process, and long-term storage, which is slower storage used for archiving purposes [32]. VNAs could potentially be adopted by GACS as well, allowing them to expand their capabilities to store genomics data with short-term and long-term storage solutions similar to those adopted by PACS. For an illustration of this comparison, refer to Fig. 5.

SUMMARY

Reflecting on the PACS model offers valuable insights for the potential development of a similar system in genomics, termed GACS. While the maturity and robust framework of PACS and its DICOM standards have evolved over 40 years, genomic standards are still emerging and have not yet reached widespread adoption. Current genomic interoperability efforts, heavily dependent on voluntary contributions, highlight the urgent need for dedicated funding to effectively develop, test, and maintain these standards. Furthermore, both public funding agencies and private entities such as EHR/pharmacy/health systems are crucial for supporting the development, pilot implementation, and maintenance of genomic standards, which would significantly boost genomic interoperability creation and adoption. For GACS to effectively integrate into clinical and research settings, establishing and enforcing policies for adopting genomic data standards is essential. This analysis underscores the transformative potential of a PACS-inspired model in genomic data management, paving the way for enhanced outcomes in precision genomics medicine.

ACKNOWLEDGMENTS

The authors would like to extend our gratitude and acknowledge that some of the insights for the topics discussed here have been enriched by Kevin M. Power (Children's Mercy Kansas City), John David Nolen, MD, PhD (Children's Mercy Kansas City), Alex Wagner, PhD (Nationwide Children's), Matthew Keefer (Children's Hospital Los Angeles), Giustino Paladini (Children's Hospital Los Angeles), and Sectra (https://medical.sectra.com/). Additionally, ChatGPT 4.0 was utilized for grammar checking and to enhance content flow, ensuring clarity and readability of the article.

DISCLOSURE

The authors have nothing to disclose.

REFERENCES

[1] Wikipedia contributors. Picture archiving and communication system — Wikipedia, The Free Encyclopedia. 2024. Available at: https://en.wikipedia.org/w/index.php?title=Picture_archiving_and_communication_system&oldid=1219193662.

[2] Gallardo E. What Is PACS (Picture Archiving and Communications System)?. 2023. Available at: https://builtin.com/articles/pacs. [Accessed 1 May 2024].

[3] Intelerad. What is PACS?. 2022. Available at: https://www.intelerad.com/en/2022/01/24/what-is-pacs/.

[4] Awati R, Charles M, DelVecchio A. Picture archiving and communication system (PACS). Available at: https://www.techtarget.com/searchhealthit/definition/picture-archiving-and-communication-system-PACS. [Accessed 1 May 2024].

[5] Huang H. Some historical remarks on picture archiving and communication systems. Comput Med Imag Graph 2003;27(2–3):93–9.

[6] MacDonald D, Alaghehbandan R, Neville D. Evaluation of picture archiving and communications systems. In: Handbook of eHealth evaluation: an evidence-based approach [internet]. Canada: University of Victoria; 2017. p. 365–82.

[7] Hood MN, Scott H. Introduction to picture archive and communication systems. J Radiol Nurs 2006;25(3): 69–74.

[8] Arora D, Mehta Y. Use of picture archiving and communication system for imaging of radiological films in cardiac surgical intensive care unit. J Anaesthesiol Clin Pharmacol 2014;30(3):447–8.

[9] Dicom. History. Available at: https://www.dicomstandard.org/history. [Accessed 1 May 2024].

[10] Larobina M. Thirty years of the DICOM standard. Tomography 2023;9(5):1829–38.

[11] Pray L. Discovery of DNA structure and function: Watson and Crick. Nat Educ 2008;1(1):100.

[12] Margulies M, Egholm M, Altman WE, et al. Genome sequencing in microfabricated high-density picolitre reactors. Nature 2005;437(7057):376–80.

[13] Cliften P. Base calling, read mapping, and coverage analysis. In: Kulkarni S, Roy S, editors. Clinical genomics. MA, USA: Academic Press; 2015. p. 91–107.

[14] Satam H, Joshi K, Mangrolia U, et al. Next-generation sequencing technology: current trends and advancements. Biology 2023;12(7):997.

[15] Chamala S, Majety S, Mishra SN, et al. Indispensability of clinical bioinformatics for effective implementation of genomic medicine in pathology laboratories. ACI Open 2020;4(02):e167–72.

[16] Dolin RH, Gupta R, Newsom K, et al. Automated HL7v2 LRI informatics framework for streamlining genomics-EHR data integration. J Pathol Inform 2023;14:100330.

[17] Walton NA, Johnson DK, Person TN, et al. Genomic data in the electronic health record. Adv Mol Pathol 2019; 2(1):21–33.

[18] Alterovitz G, Brown J, Chan M, et al. Enabling Clinical Genomics for Precision Medicine Via HL7® Fast Healthcare Interoperability Resources. 2017. Available at: http://www.healthit.gov/sites/default/files/sync_for_genes_report_november_2017.pdf. [Accessed 1 May 2024].

[19] IHE. Scheduled Workflow. 2023. Available at: https://wiki.ihe.net/index.php/Scheduled_Workflow. [Accessed 1 May 2024].

[20] McEnery KW. Coordinating patient care within radiology and across the enterprise. J Am Coll Radiol 2014;11(12): 1217–25.

[21] Caetano-Anolles D. SAM or BAM or CRAM - Mapped sequence data formats. 2023. Available at: https://gatk.broadinstitute.org/hc/en-us/articles/360035890791-SAM-or-BAM-or-CRAM-Mapped-sequence-data-formats: ~:text=SAM%20stands%20for%20Sequence%20Alignment,up%20to%20very%20much%20indeed). Accessed May 1, 2024.

[22] Caetano-Anolles D. VCF - Variant Call Format. 2024. Available at: https://gatk.broadinstitute.org/hc/en-us/articles/360035531692-VCF-Variant-Call-Format. [Accessed 1 May 2024].

[23] Goar W, Babb L, Chamala S, et al. Development and application of a computable genotype model in the GA4GH Variation Representation Specification. World Scientific 2022;383–94.

[24] Wagner AH, Babb L, Alterovitz G, et al. The GA4GH Variation Representation Specification: A computational framework for variation representation and federated identification. Cell Genomics 2021;1(2).

[25] HL7. HL7 FHIR Genomics Reporting Implementation Guide. Available at: https://hl7.org/fhir/uv/genomics-reporting/. [Accessed 1 May 2024].

[26] HL7. Hl7 Clinical Genomics Work Group. 2024. Available at: https://confluence.hl7.org/display/CGW. [Accessed 1 May 2024].

[27] CodeX™. GenomeX. Available at: https://confluence.hl7.org/display/COD/Genomics+-+GenomeX. [Accessed 1 May 2024].

[28] CodeX™. CodeX. Available at: https://codex.hl7.org/. [Accessed 1 May 2024].

[29] Dolin RH, Heale BS, Alterovitz G, et al. Introducing HL7 FHIR Genomics Operations: a developer-friendly approach to genomics-EHR integration. J Am Med Inform Assoc 2023;30(3):485–93.

[30] GA4GH. GA4GH VA-Specification. Available at: https://github.com/ga4gh/va-spec. [Accessed 1 May 2014].

[31] Sirota-Cohen C, Rosipko B, Forsberg D, et al. Implementation and benefits of a vendor-neutral archive and enterprise-imaging management system in an integrated delivery network. J Digit Imaging 2019;32:211–20.

[32] Fennell N, Ralston MD, Coleman RM. PACS and Other Image Management Systems. Practical Imaging Informatics 2021;131–42.

Advances in Molecular Pathology 7 (2024) 131–143

ADVANCES IN MOLECULAR PATHOLOGY

Fast Healthcare Interoperability Resource Genomics and Polygenic Risk Scores

Bret S.E. Heale, PhD

Humanized Health Consulting, 1329 East, 700 South, Salt Lake City, UT, USA

KEYWORDS

• HL7 FHIR • CDS • Polygenic risk scoring • Whole genome sequencing • Precision medicine

KEY POINTS

- Features of reporting polygenic risk scoring for clinical use.
- Health Level 7's (HL7) Fast Healthcare Interoperability Resource (FHIR) can deliver the polygenic risk scoring features computationally.
- Example of polygenic risk scoring in FHIR.
- A critical feature is the genetic similarity between a patient and the underlying population used to develop the score.
- As the clinical expression of polygenic risk scoring evolves, the FHIR representation can evolve.

INTRODUCTION

Polygenic Risk Scoring

While the American College of Medical Geneticists (ACMG) has recently recommended caution [1,2], polygenic risk scoring is becoming a feature in genomic clinical diagnostic reporting. Standardizing the exchange of critical data elements will aid consistency and accessibility in numerous computational applications, such as clinical decision support (CDS), quality control, end-user user interfaces, searching, analysis, and potentially artificial intelligence. Recognizing the importance of polygenic risk scoring, the ACMG has recently published 3 excellent viewpoints on polygenic risk scores (PRSs) [1–3], which, along with other experts [4–10], aid in understanding the crucial elements and offer vital insights. Several features, such as assessing the study population's and the patient's genetic similarity, are indicated. As well as structuring data associated with polygenic risk in a consistent exchange format enable dynamic genomic test reporting paradigms to make test results more useable. Indeed, Brockman and colleagues [4] found in user experience testing that "static genomic test reports that limit one's ability to explore results are not ideal for polygenic risk disclosure." Computable representation lends itself to access through web tools, interactivity, and CDS.

Health Level 7 International

Health Level 7 International (HL7) is an American National Standards Institute (ANSI)-accredited, consensus-driven, nonprofit standards body specializing in computable, standard health care data exchange and retrieval to streamline health services and clinical care [11]. Understanding what being an ANSI standard body means gives insight into HL7. Accredited ANSI standard bodies meet several criteria [12]. The requirements include open-recorded meetings, a consensus-driven

E-mail address: bheale@humanizedhealthconsulting.com

https://doi.org/10.1016/j.yamp.2024.07.008 www.advancesinmolecularpathology.com

2589-4080/24/

approach with a balanced interest among large and small partners, following due process/governance, and continual standard(s) improvement. These features are part of HL7 being a community-driven organization that serves the needs of the national and international health care industry, as well as public and private interests. HL7 membership is drawn from across the globe and health care stakeholders. Members include physicians, nurses, community-based care organizations, nongovernmental organizations, governmental organizations, insurance companies, patient advocates, software engineers, solution architects, data scientists, c-suite leaders, and patients. A significant goal of HL7 members is to devise standards that will streamline and support the ability to interoperate, including across national boundaries.

Interoperability is the ability to share and use data between multiple sources [13]. When data are broken down into discrete pieces, it enables computational systems to share information more explicitly [14]. Consider sending laboratory information as discrete bits of data versus a single picture of the result [15]. The discrete data are more useable by 2 computational systems, allowing them to interoperate. In addition, it is useful to standardize the exchange. This reduces the complexity of the solutions required. Consider that an organization such as a hospital interacts with multiple vendors (perhaps several diagnostic laboratories and community-based organizations), creating unique interfaces for each interaction would require repeating the same resource investment, whereas standardizing the interface code base for the exchange of data between systems can have cost savings [16,17]. HL7 has a unique role in establishing standard specifications of how data should be structured in health care data exchange—reducing the landscape of possible choices implementers/developers might make—aiding in consistency and the ability to repurpose or interoperate [14–19]. Interoperability is believed to be so essential that the US Office of the National Coordinator (ONC) has published in HT-1, the final rule, "The adoption of new and revised standards and criteria in this final rule will facilitate interoperability through standardized health information and functionality, which will lead to better care and health outcomes for patients, while reducing burden and costs" [20].

HL7's Fast Healthcare Interoperability Resource (FHIR) specification has a large implementation and development community [21] (see https://confluence.hl7.org/display/FHIR). FHIR is based on the notion of a resource—the smallest unit in FHIR for exchanging information. Resources, such as patient (https://hl7.org/fhir/R4/patient.html) and organization (https://hl7.org/fhir/R4/organization.html), are independent but can cross-reference each other. To be more readily implementable, FHIR takes advantage of modern web standards, such as JavaScript Object Notation (JSON) and Representational State Transfer (REST) architecture. Additionally, the core FHIR Resource specification can be constrained for specific use cases to produce specialized implementation guidance in computable specifications called implementation guides (IGs). Two notable IGs are the US Core (https://hl7.org/fhir/us/core/) and Clinical Genomics Reporting (https://hl7.org/fhir/uv/genomics-reporting/). To provide an impression of the broad adoption of FHIR, the US ONC, which oversees the electronic health record (EHR) certification process, "adopted the HL7 FHIR US Core Implementation Guide (IG) standard for trial use (STU) version 6.1.0" as the base implementation specification to meet certification requirements for January 2026, this replaces US Core 3.1.1 as the current base. The US Core IG contains US realm use case-specific guidance. For example, to ensure consistent representation of body mass index (BMI) units, the US Core BMI profile (https://hl7.org/fhir/us/core/STU6.1/StructureDefinition-us-core-bmi.html) constrains the valueQuanity.code element to code of kg/m^2. FHIR IGs also provide use case examples and specific narrative implementation guidance to aid implementers. An important facet is that the specification is computable. An IG's computable artifacts can be directly used for validation or in certification, as seen in Touchstone (https://touchstone.aegis.net/touchstone/), Inferno (https://inferno.healthit.gov/and https://inferno.healthit.gov/validator/), the HL7 FHIR validator (https://validator.fhir.org/), or FHIR server implementations (such as https://learn.microsoft.com/en-us/azure/healthcare-apis/fhir/validation-against-profiles).

The Clinical Genomics FHIR IG is a universal realm HL7 IG specific to the exchange of genomic data. Universal in this context means the Clinical Genomics IG is intended to be applicable as a base for all international settings and use cases. The Clinical Genomics working group (WG) has published the STU2 version (https://www.hl7.org/fhir/uv/genomics-reporting/index.html) of the IG and is preparing to publish STU3. The balloted STU3 version (https://hl7.org/fhir/uv/genomics-reporting/2024Jan/) clarifies key areas and adds genomic operations [21]. To help in your implementation efforts or to contribute to the standard, the Clinical Genomics WG weekly call agenda can be found at https://confluence.hl7.org/display/CGW/CG-2024-03-12. Also, there is a zulip chat to interface with experts in FHIR and clinical genomics at https://chat.fhir.org/#narrow/stream/179197-genomics, and an HL7 accelerator (https://confluence.hl7.org/display/COD/Genomics+-+GenomeX).

The Clinical Genomics IG contains many examples of data instances, computable specifications, and narrative guidance on structuring genetic data in FHIR. The authors explore an example of polygenic risk reporting here. With the specifications of the Clinical Genomics WG and other FHIR core Resources, such as the FHIR RiskAssesment Resource, HL7 FHIR has many tools to meet the growing need to communicate the complete data set of polygenic risk reporting elements in a computable manner that takes advantage of existing paradigms of information exchange.

DISCUSSION

Basic Anatomy of Polygenic Risk Scoring and Risk Reporting

While not an exhaustive summative evaluation, the concepts/data elements that follow were derived from a formative survey of the landscape to collect key features in polygenic risk clinical reporting. The sources vary from ACMG points to consider [1–3], including one focused on laboratory reports [3], to a clinical trial of polygenic risk assessment in clinical practice [5], technical requirements for translating scores into risk [7], to standards around reporting new PRSs [9,22], and usability testing [4,6]. Together, these provide access to the experiences and thoughts of a large and diverse cohort of subject matter experts. Table 1 summarizes the sources.

PRS-derived insights in clinical care are newly evolving, and caution is warranted. Yet, PRS has been used as part of screening tools (eg, [24]) for some time. There is an eagerness to improve patient care with the precision promised by PRS (especially with artificial intelligence's explosive evolution). Generally, the sources indicate that the risk calculated from a PRS be treated like a screening tool result as expressed in the laboratory ACMG points to consider, "PRS describes a statistical association, and high risk does not indicate an underlying disease pathology ... whereas PRS is solely considered screening information" [3]. This is an essential conceptual shape to remember when considering the data elements for reporting risk assessments derived from PRS.

The features extracted from the landscape survey are presented in Table 2. Note the granularity in the presentation is variable to keep the list reasonable in length (see Table 2).

Clinical Decision Support Standards Used with Fast Healthcare Interoperability Resource: Substitutable Medical Applications, Reusable Technologies on Fast Healthcare Interoperability Resource and Clinical Decision Support Hooks

Clinical decision support systems aid clinical decision-making by providing patient-specific assessments based on individual patient characteristics [27,28]. They have had successes in streamlining aspects of care such as ordering, timing of screening tests, and providing recommendations [27,28]. With regard to FHIR, 2 critical CDS architectural tools are Substitutable Medical Applications, Reusable Technologies (SMART) on FHIR and CDS Hooks.

SMART on FHIR [29] is a tool for launching external applications from an electronic medical record (EMR). This component of the standard relates to app authentication and launching. The specification initially took advantage of the OAuth 2.0 standard to limit the scope of app access to only what was needed. As of 2021, there appeared to be hundreds of SMART on FHIR apps [28], and in the United States, the 2 largest by market share EMRs (as well as most others) support SMART on FHIR applications. Additionally, SMART on FHIR is part of the US ONCs HT-1 final rule [20] as a system that should be supported, along with CDS Hooks. SMART on FHIR apps can vary in complexity of user interaction. Typically, a button launches the app, and a field of view is populated with the information the app is designed to convey. Once launched SMART on FHIR apps can offer all the options for user interaction and exploration seen in modern web browsing.

CDS Hooks [30] uses triggering events in the clinical interaction with EMRs to call Web services. It is RESTful and uses FHIR expressed in JSON to exchange patient data. Since SMART on FHIR apps are also Web services, CDS Hooks can offer the clinician the opportunity to open a SMART on FHIR app contextually or simply launch the SMART on FHIR app. When the app is opened, CDS Hooks feeds context based on the triggering event to the app. For example, suppose a clinician is opening a chart. In that case, a CDS Hooks might call a polygenic risk reassessment app to quietly look for new PRSs from a catalog of scores and calculate whether there are new traits that the patient has an elevated risk for. When the calculation is finished, a "card" will appear with the result. The "card" can have several features, including an indicator of its importance. A low level of importance might cause the card to wait to be opened. Or, if the card is of high importance, it could interrupt

TABLE 1
Source Articles for Data Elements Discussed

Title	Comment
Patient and provider perspectives on polygenic risk scores: implications for clinical reporting and utilization [6]	User viewpoint (patient and provider)
Design and user experience testing of a polygenic score report: a qualitative study of prospective users [4]	User viewpoint (patient)
The clinical application of polygenic risk scores: A points to consider statement of the American College of Medical Genetics and Genomics (ACMG) [2]	Clinical use (ACMG review/statement)
Clinical utility of polygenic risk scores for embryo selection: A points to consider statement of the American College of Medical Genetics and Genomics (ACMG) [1]	Clinical use (ACMG review/statement)
Laboratory perspectives in the development of polygenic risk scores for disease: A points to consider statement of the American College of Medical Genetics and Genomics (ACMG) [3]	Laboratory clinical reporting (ACMG review/statement)
The need for polygenic score reporting standards in evidence-based practice: lipid genetics use case [8]	Sharing of new PRS (translational)
A tool for translating polygenic scores onto the absolute scale using summary statistics [7]	Technical requirements (risk score)
Development of a clinical polygenic risk score assay and reporting workflow [5]	Laboratory clinical reporting (in practice)
Validation of an Abridged Breast Cancer Risk Prediction Model for the General Population [23]	Risk assessment (mixed PRS and other features)
Breast Cancer Screening in the Precision Medicine Era: Risk-based Screening in a Population-based Trial [24]	Risk assessment (mixed PRS and other features/review) [10]
Polygenic risk scores in pharmacogenomics: opportunities and challenges—a mini review [10]	Laboratory clinical reporting/ clinical use (mini review)
Principles in genetic risk assessment [25]	Risk assessment (genetics general) [9]
Improving reporting standards for polygenic scores in risk prediction studies [9]	Sharing of new PRS (translational)—ClinGen and PRS Catalog
Polygenic risk scores in the clinic: Translating risk into action [26]	Laboratory clinical reporting/ clinical use (recommendations)
The Polygenic Score Catalog as an open database for reproducibility and systematic evaluation [22]	Sharing of new PRS (translational)—PRS Catalog

the current clinical workflow. The card itself can contain a link that launches a SMART on FHIR app, perfect for providing a platform to explore a polygenic risk assessment and scoring results.

Fast Healthcare Interoperability Resource Genetics Brief Anatomy

FHIR is a flexible standard. It can be expressed in JSON and XML and includes a robust RESTful API. FHIR can be thought of as a "platform specification" [31]. REST specifies the typical behaviors you see with Web sites and internet-accessible endpoints. The REST API specifies how to request that an FHIR server search for data. As mentioned, FHIR IGs further adapt the specification to specific use cases. The Clinical Genomics WG has produced and trialed an implementation guide (https://www.hl7.org/fhir/uv/genomics-reporting/index.html) for the exchange of genetic data.

The current Clinical Genomic Reporting IG is written on the FHIR core R4 specification. FHIR uses semantic versioning, so the increment from DSTU3 indicates that

TABLE 2
Features

Feature	More Granular Data Element
Treat like a Clinical Screening Test	
Handling Negative or Low-risk Result	
Accessibility for Exploration	
Limitations/Disclaimers	
Description of Test Performed (methodology)	
References and Citations	
Treatment Recommendations	
Graphical Representations	
Represent Risk in Multiple Ways (stating both 90th percentile and top 10%)	
Recommendation for Posttest Counseling	
Impact on Care	
Guidelines	
Educational Materials Accessible for Patients and Provider	
System for Reanalysis	
Variant	Genetic variation used for calculation (including genome build, coordinates, etc…)
Variant	Imputed (measure of confidence)
Variant	Types of variation (indel, single nucleotide polymorphism [SNP], etc…)
Variant	Platform used for observing variation
Trait	Specific outcome defined
Trait	Method of collection (interviews, self-reported, abstracted, or computed from billing codes)
Trait	Compatible tests for Mendelian gene variation linked to the disorder
Trait	Incidence of disease or outcome
PRS (score)	Analytical validity (including performance metrics)
PRS (score)	Clinical validity
PRS (score)	Clinical utility
PRS (score)	Ancestry adjustment
PRS (score)	Other non-PRS attributes used in scoring and relative impact
PRS (score)	Individual weights
PRS (score)	Threshold needed for action with “gray area”
PRS (study population)	Study population PRS mean and standard deviation
PRS (study population)	Characteristics including text description
PRS (study population)	Similarity to a reference population used to represent the patient

(*continued on next page*)

TABLE 2
(continued)

Feature	More Granular Data Element
PRS (patient population)	Reference population most similar to the patient (principal component analysis has been indicated here with as many as 5000 variants across the genome)
PRS (patient population)	Characteristics including text description
PRS (patient population)	Patient population PRS mean and standard deviation
PRS (risk)	Continuous representation
PRS (risk)	Dichotomous representation
PRS (risk)	Definition of high-risk status
PRS (risk)	Kind (percentile, relative, or absolute risk)
PRS (risk)	Temporal conditions (eg, over 5 y, at the age of 40 y)
PRS (risk)	Percentile
PRS (risk)	Relative risk
PRS (risk)	Threshold needed for action with "gray area"
PRS (risk)	Temporal conditions (eg, over 5 y at the age of 40 y)
PRS (absolute risk)	Underlying disease prevalence/incidence (unlikely to have models for absolute risk)

breaking changes were made. Currently, HL7 is working on R6. With each increment of the FHIR version, the core specification becomes more "normative." In HL7 terms, "normative" means backward compatibility with any future specification updates, and more importantly, the HL7 community (made up of participants and stakeholders in the health care field) has determined that the specification is stable and fit for purpose. The Clinical Genomics WG's IG is on FHIR R4 as that is the maturest version of FHIR to have broad adoption.

The FHIR Resource Observation (https://hl7.org/fhir/R4/observation.html) was chosen by the Clinical Genomic WG as the most consistent way to express genetic findings found in laboratory reporting. Observation Resource is a normative Resource, which means it has had wide adoption and is broadly supported. Additionally, the Observation Resource contains a very flexible tool called "component." The construct of the component is a coded name—value pair. That is, the definition of what data element a particular component represents is conveyed computably within the component through "component.code," a field that communicates a standard coded concept. For example, the Variant Observation Profile (https://hl7.org/fhir/uv/genomics-reporting/StructureDefinition-variant.html) has a component called genomic-source-class (in FHIR speak that would be Observation.component:genomic-source-class). This component has been assigned LOINC code 48002-0. LOINC is a standard terminology organization specializing in concepts for observations, among other things. The entry for LOINC code 48002-0 (https://loinc.org/48002-0) states that the concept is "The genomic class of the specimen being analyzed: Germline for inherited genome, somatic for cancer genome, and prenatal for fetal genome." Looking at the component Observation.component:genomic-source-class, one can see that the component's value has been constrained to a value set of terms that answer the question, "What is the genomic source class?" Constraining Resources (or profiles) are how FHIR can provide a more tightly used case-bound specification. The constraints found in the genomic-source class component make it easier to implement in the specific use case of genomic clinical reporting of genetic variation.

The specification structure is a computable artifact, expressed as JSON on https://hl7.org/fhir/uv/genomics-reporting/StructureDefinition-variant.json. The code field in the component is the data element where the meaning of the component is conveyed. We already have discussed that it has been given a LOINC code to define it. Looking at the component more closely, one will see that the code is composed of 2 parts: system and code. The system tells us computably that the code is a LOINC code and that the concept is found wherever https://loinc.org/ leads. LOINC has a clean URL system that allows the code to be combined with the domain name to retrieve the concept definition.

An essential aspect of identifying the component definition with a codeableConcept is that a server can support searching by component.code concepts. The FHIR REST API (https://hl7.org/fhir/R4/http.html) and Search (https://hl7.org/fhir/R4/http.html#search and https://hl7.org/fhir/R4/search.html) indicate the syntax to perform such a search. The Clinical Genomics Reporting IG has an example query, ": GET/Observation?component-code-value-concept http://loinc.org|48002-0$http://loinc.org|LA6683-2" (https://hl7.org/fhir/uv/genomics-reporting/usecases.html#get-references-to-all-variants-obtained-where-the-analysis-has-b.). The "GET" portion indicates using a RESTful GET interaction. This is nothing more than the base URL of an exposed FHIR server endpoint. So, one can think of it as "https://baseURLOfFHIRserver.com/Observation?component-code-value-concept=http://loinc.org|48002-0$http://loinc.org|LA6683-2." The "Observation?" portion indicates that we are performing a search on FHIR Observation Resource data instances. The portion after the "?" is the parameters of the search. In this case, the syntax is using a combined search parameter of component.code and component.valueCodeableConcept (https://hl7.org/fhir/R4/observation.html#search). The first part "http://loinc.org|48002-0" indicates looking for Observations data instances with a component for genomic-source-class, as defined by component.code having system LOINC and concept code 48002-0. Not all Observations will have the component as the component has cardinality 0 ... 1. This means that there can be 0 to 1 instances of the component.

In addition to components, the Observation Resource has additional fields such as subject (who the observation is about), effective time (clinically relevant period for the observation), and performer (who carried out the observation), a place for a note with attribution (the note field is a coded annotation, see https://hl7.org/fhir/uv/genomics-reporting/StructureDefinition-coded-annotation.html). The codedAnnotation data type allows attribution, time stamp, type of note and the note to be captured, method (like sequencing), device, and so on. These are useful for capturing all the data computably that describes an Observation. The Clinical Genomics IG adds several components to the variant so that the observation instance can capture genomic variation. The variant reporting page (https://hl7.org/fhir/uv/genomics-reporting/sequencing.html) goes into detail on the guidance for implementers to communicate genetic variation observations.

Genetic variation is one of the data elements to represent in Polygenic risk scoring, and the HL7 Clinical Genomic WG uses Observation Resource to do that. However, other resources convey the additional data elements. The FHIR Resource RiskAssesment (https://hl7.org/fhir/R4/riskassessment.html) is a good fit for the concept of assessed polygenic risk, and the Resource narrative definition states that "list of potential health risks based on a patient's genetic analysis" is one of the use cases for the Resource. To tie the RiskAssesment to the observed patient genetic variation used in the calculation of risk, the RiskAssesment.basis field is used. RiskAssesment.basis has the data type Reference (https://hl7.org/fhir/R4/references.html#Reference) with an indicator that data instances of "Any" Resource type can be referenced. The Reference data type can accommodate different types of referencing, as explained on the specification page, for this discussion, we stop at indicating that the reference serves as a pointer to a different data instance. Additionally, RiskAssesment.basis has cardinality 0...*, meaning multiple FHIR Observation Variant Profiles can be referenced.

Terminology

While FHIR does a very excellent job of providing a standard structure, syntactic standard, FHIR core only partially solves the semantic standardization problem. For example, where coded concepts are communicated, there can be differences between systems. Luckily, the Resource profiling constraints inherently provide a mechanism for semantic clarity. For example, the Variant Profile (https://hl7.org/fhir/uv/genomics-reporting/StructureDefinition-variant.html) was constrained in Clinical Genomics Reporting IG. However, in the HL7 FHIR context, it is important that a community determines what terms (coded concepts) will be used and where the definition of those terms will reside. The HL7 Clinical Genomics WG often collaborates with LOINC when new LOINC codes are needed as genomic concepts mature. Additionally, looking at SNOMEDCT, one finds many disease-related concepts. These are often cited in HL7 standards as the coded concepts to use to communicate conditions or problems that a patient might have. The governance and constraining of allowable coded concepts is an open question, but IGs help in constraining to a use-case specific list of concepts, and HL7's Terminology oversight group maintains a large body of sets of concepts grouped for specific purposes (value sets, see https://terminology.hl7.org/) to aid implementers.

Polygenic Risk Score Reporting Risk example

As an example of expressing PRS concepts in FHIR for clinical reporting, 2 key FHIR core Resource instances were populated: the FHIR Risk Assessment Resource and the FHIR Observation Resource.

Fig. 1 shows the FHIR RiskAssessment instance. In English, it reads, "CGPatientExample01 (subject) is predicted (prediction) to have a high risk (qualitativeRisk) with a relative risk of 2.69 (relativeRisk) for developing Diabetes mellitus type 2 (outcome) at age 65 (whenRange). The basis is seven genetic variants and a polygenic score observation (basis). The RiskAssement is related to the polygenic score observation (parent). And there is a disclaimer (note with extension)." If used, the field "mitigation" would guide the steps to take.

It should be noted that a genetic file extension could have been used instead of the 7 observed variants. It is an important discussion item to determine how to handle potentially millions of genetic variants. Luckily, FHIR supports retrieval and relative links. There is a whole set of FHIR Genomic Operations that might be brought to bear here with a preconfigured GET request [21].

Fig. 2 is the polygenic score observation, an FHIR Observation instance. The example shows how components can be used to provide additional data elements. For searching, the Observation.code value is a LOINC code for PRS. This helps make the data instance more discoverable and allows a receiving system to develop specific rules for handling PRS data received in FHIR as part of Genomic Reports. The data instance uses the genomic-risk extension to connect the Observation to the RiskAssesment data instance. It is done through a reference so the RiskAssesment can be accessed appropriately. Additionally, the genomic-artifact extension is being used to provide a citation with study details on the development of the assay, including validation, validity metrics, and descriptions of the development of the score (including population used).

Here, we have taken advantage of FHIR Resource Observation's ability to use "components" to communicate 7 PRS-specific data elements. The components are prs-ancestry-similarityToValidationPopulation, prs-study-dis-mean, prs-study-dis-sd, prs-ancestry-adj-dis-mean, prs-ancestry-adj-dis-sd, prs-ancestry-adj, and prs-percentile. Although these components are not yet in the Clinical Genomics IG and use TBD code, FHIR servers can accept, share, and perform searches on them as they are. However, downstream implementation may lag until the components are widely accepted and part of an FHIR IG. When the broader medical genomics community has determined the features for PRS reporting, they can be added to the IG, perhaps as a profile, and LOINC codes requested. The process takes 6 to 9 months. It should be stressed that FHIR servers, thanks to the FHIR core specification, can accept, share, and search on them as they are, even before they are part of an IG. The FHIR Observation component is a versatile communication tool.

The component "prs-ancestry-similarityToValidationPopulation" shows that the patient is 95% likely to be from the population found in the study that produced the PRS. This is an important metric as it gives confidence in the PRS's applicability to the patient's health. Principal component analysis (PCA) is one tool used when adjusting an individual's score based on genetic ancestry differences from the study population [5]. It is from the PCA that the measure of likelihood can be determined, as well as a tool to adjust scores to account for ancestry. However, PRS clinical reporting has not reached the state where this is considered standard practice. The similarity measure is an essential determinant in a clinician's decision on the meaningfulness of the test result for the clinician's specific patient. In the case of 95%, the score is probably relevant for the patient.

The paired components prs-study-dis-mean and prs-study-dis-sd provide the mean and standard deviation of the distribution of scores for the study population. This allows one to calculate a graphic to show this distribution visually. Also, the paired components prs-ancestry-adj-dis-mean and prs-ancestry-adj-dis-sd provide the means to visualize the adjusted distribution of the population which the patient most matched in the PCA mentioned earlier. These distributions serve as a backdrop to the adjusted score (communicated with the component PRS ancestry adjusted) and the ancestry-adjusted PRS percentile (communicated with the component prs-percentile). The percentile's impact is better understood with some knowledge of the distribution.

Finally, the Observation example in Fig. 2 shares a disclaimer using the note data element. A disclaimer that appropriately indicates that the score has been adjusted for ancestry and the similarity to the study population is an essential caveat in interpreting the result.

The examples show that FHIR standards tools can be used to computationally communicate key concepts and features needed to report and utilize PRS risk. FHIR also contains data elements that capture important metadata such as performers, patient identifiers, and the like. FHIR core offers robust coverage of most data elements in the clinical space.

```
{"resourceType": "RiskAssessment",
  "id": "GenRiskDiabetesT2atAge65",
  "parent": {"reference": "Observation/polyGenicScoreObservation"},
  "status": "final",
  "subject": {"reference": "Patient/CGPatientExample01"},
  "basis": [
    {"reference": "Observation/polyGenicScoreObservation"},
    {"reference": "Observation/VariantExample1"},
    {"reference": "Observation/VariantExample2"},
    {"reference": "Observation/VariantExample3"},
    {"reference": "Observation/VariantExample4"},
    {"reference": "Observation/VariantExample5"},
    {"reference": "Observation/VariantExample6"},
    {"reference": "Observation/VariantExample7"},
    {"reference": "Observation/VariantExample8"},
    {"reference": "Observation/VariantExample9"}
  ],
  "prediction": [
    {
      "outcome": {
        "coding": [{"code": "44054006", "system":
"http://snomed.info/sct", "display": "Diabetes mellitus type 2
(disorder)"}]
      },
      "qualitativeRisk": {
        "coding": [{"code": "high", "system":
"http://terminology.hl7.org/CodeSystem/risk-probability", "display": "High
likelihood"}]
      },
      "relativeRisk": 2.69,
      "whenRange": {"high": {"value": 65, "code": "a", "system":
"http://unitsofmeasure.org", "unit": "years"}}
    }
  ],
  "note": [
    {
      "extension": [
        {"url": "http://hl7.org/fhir/uv/genomics-
reporting/StructureDefinition/annotation-code", "valueCodeableConcept":
{"coding": [{"code": "test-disclaimer",
"system":"http://hl7.org/fhir/uv/genomics-reporting/CodeSystem/coded-
annotation-types-cs"}]}}
      ],
      "text": "PRS provides the relative risk of developing a disease and
should be used as an adjunct tool to determine the likelihood of
developing a specific disorder."
    }
  ]
}
```


FIG. 1 Fast Healthcare Interoperability Resource Risk Assesment Example Data instance showing placement of key polygenic risk score data elements.

```
{"resourceType": "Observation",
  "id": "polyGenicScoreObservation",
  "status": "final",
  "extension": [{"url": "http://hl7.org/fhir/uv/genomics-reporting/StructureDefinition/genomics-artifact","valueRelatedArtifact": {
        "type": "citation",
        "url": "https://paperOnDevelopmentOfScore"}}],
  "category": [{"coding": [{"code": "laboratory","system": "http://terminology.hl7.org/CodeSystem/observation-category"}]}],
  "code": {"coding": [{"code": "102040-3","system": "http://loinc.org",
    "display": "Polygenic risk score (PRS)"}],"text": "Polygenic risk score (PRS)"},
  "subject": {"reference": "Patient/CGPatientExample01"},
  "effectiveDateTime": "2020-07-01",
  "method": {"text": "PRS method"},
  "component": [
    {"code": {"coding": [{"code": "102040-3","system": "http://loinc.org",
      "display": "Polygenic risk score (PRS)"}]},
      "extension": [{"url": "http://hl7.org/fhir/uv/genomics-reporting/StructureDefinition/genomics-risk-assessment",
          "valueReference": {"reference": "RiskAssessment/GenRiskDiabetesT2atAge65","display": "Polygenic Risk Assessment"}}]},
    {"code": {"coding": [{"code": "prs-ancestry-similarityToValidationPopulation","system": "http://hl7.org/fhir/uv/genomics-reporting/CodeSystem/tbd-codes-cs",
        "display": "Similarity of Patient's identified genetic ancestry (population) to the score validation population - as a probability (100% is a perfect match)"}]},
```


FIG. 2 Fast Healthcare Interoperability Resource Observation Example Data instance showing placement of key polygenic risk score data elements.

The examples mentioned earlier demonstrate that when PRS is ready for the clinical audience, FHIR can deliver the data features of PRS computability. FHIR also supports the computation of visual-graphical representations of risk that are easier for clinicians and patients to understand.

The following 2 example flows for FHIR-based PRS reporting provide context for where the example artifacts may be used.

Laboratory reporting flow context

1. Patient physical sample is provided, or patient genetic variation is provided.
   i. Health features required for calculation are also provided
   ii. Sequencing performed if required
2. PRSs are calculated using genomic data and demographic data.
   i. Similarity to study population is evaluated and adjustment is made
3. FHIR Observation instance and RiskAssesment instance similar to the ones exemplified here are produced to be sent.
4. An FHIR DiagnosticReport is packaged up with conclusions and other clinical metadata such as performer and patient identifiers.

Substitutable medical applications, reusable technologies-on-Fast Healthcare Interoperability Resource app flow example context

1. Patient demographic sent as part of CDS Hook

```
      "valueQuantity": {"value": 95,"code": "%","system":
"http://unitsofmeasure.org","unit": "%" }},
    {"code": {"coding": [{"code": "prs-study-dis-mean","system":
"http://hl7.org/fhir/uv/genomics-reporting/CodeSystem/tbd-codes-cs",
        "display": "PRS distribution mean of score validation
population"}]},
      "valueQuantity": {"value": 6.91}},
    {"code": {"coding": [{"code": "prs-study-dis-sd","system":
"http://hl7.org/fhir/uv/genomics-reporting/CodeSystem/tbd-codes-cs",
        "display": "PRS distribution standard deviation of score
validation population"}]},
      "valueQuantity": {"value": 3.75}},
    {"code": {"coding": [{"code": "prs-ancestry-adj-dis-mean","system":
"http://hl7.org/fhir/uv/genomics-reporting/CodeSystem/tbd-codes-cs",
        "display": "PRS distribution mean ancestry adjusted"}]},
      "valueQuantity": {"value": 6.91}},
    {"code": {"coding": [{"code": "prs-ancestry-adj-dis-sd","system":
"http://hl7.org/fhir/uv/genomics-reporting/CodeSystem/tbd-codes-cs",
        "display": "PRS distribution standard deviation ancestry
adjusted"}]},
       "valueQuantity": {"value": 3.75}},
    {"code": {"coding": [{"code": "prs-ancestry-adj","system":
"http://hl7.org/fhir/uv/genomics-reporting/CodeSystem/tbd-codes-cs",
        "display": "PRS ancestry adjusted"}]},
      "valueQuantity": {"value": 14.3}
    },
    {"code": {"coding": [{"code": "prs-percentile","system":
"http://hl7.org/fhir/uv/genomics-reporting/CodeSystem/tbd-codes-cs",
        "display": "PRS percentile ancestry adjusted"}]},
      "valueQuantity": {"value": 95,"code": "%","system":
"http://unitsofmeasure.org","unit": "%"}
    }
  ],
  "note": [{"extension": [{"url": "http://hl7.org/fhir/uv/genomics-
reporting/StructureDefinition annotation-code",
"valueCodeableConcept": {"coding": [{"code": "test-disclaimer", "system":
"http://hl7.org/fhir/uv/genomics-reporting/CodeSystem/coded-annotation-
types-cs"}]}}],"text": "Percentile is adjusted for patient's similarity to
the study population. Check similarity distance to inform clinical
utility"}]}
```


FIG. 2 (*continued*)

2. Endpoint for health data queries (eg, FHIR server)
3. Endpoint of server with genomic data (eg, an FHIR server supporting FHIR Genomics Operations [21])
4. Information is sent to the app server
5. On the app server, Polygenomic Risk scores are calculated using the genomic data and demographic data
   - i. Other patient medical context that is needed is pulled from a Health data server.
   - ii. Similarity to the study population is evaluated and adjustment is made.
   - iii. FHIR Observation instance and RiskAssesment instance similar to the ones exemplified

here are produced to be sent to the front-end app.

6. CDS Hooks/SMART on FHIR app returns RiskAssed Resource with graphical output

Deeper insight into the algorithmic descriptions, such as the population trained on and validation, requires going to the source of the calculation. Definitional FHIR resources such as Measure, ObservationDefinition, and Genomic Study could be explored. However, the FHIR Reference data type has the exquisite ability to provide a URL to make study details accessible.

The final product of the earlier data transmission is a computable artifact supporting calculations, computations, end-user exploration, and communication of clinically critical details.

SUMMARY

HL7 FHIR has tools (specifications) to meet the known and emerging data needs in polygenic risk reporting for clinical decision-making, including supporting representation of continuous risk and ancestry similarity. A question remains regarding the handling of millions of genetic variants that can impact a risk score and finding the balance between delivering care and applying polygenic risk scoring to patients genetically distant from the PRS study population. Currently, the larger corpus of genomic data that fall outside of the few variants disclosed in the clinical report is not available in the clinical environment. How these data are made available to clinicians for generating PRS at the point of care is an open question. The resolution of this question requires engagement with hospitals, laboratories, standards organizations, information technology (IT) specialists, and the relevant regulatory bodies. Trials, such as the GenoVA clinical trial [32], will provide evidence for the critical features required for communication and appropriate application of PRS, but there is work that needs to be done to develop the full stack technical framework for their delivery. The examples here offer a starting point that readily accommodates a technical solution through FHIR's existing tools.

CLINICS CARE POINT

- HL7 FHIR has the tools to enable polygenic risk score reporting.

DISCLOSURES

The authors have nothing to disclose.

REFERENCES

[1] Grebe TA, Khushf G, Greally JM, et al. Clinical utility of polygenic risk scores for embryo selection: A points to consider statement of the American College of Medical Genetics and Genomics (ACMG). Genet Med 2024; 101052. https://doi.org/10.1016/j.gim.2023.101052.

[2] Abu-El-Haija A, Reddi HV, Wand H, et al. The clinical application of polygenic risk scores: A points to consider statement of the American College of Medical Genetics and Genomics (ACMG). Genet Med 2023;25: 100803.

[3] Reddi HV, Wand H, Funke B, et al. Laboratory perspectives in the development of polygenic risk scores for disease: A points to consider statement of the American College of Medical Genetics and Genomics (ACMG). Genet Med 2023;25:100804.

[4] Brockman DG, Petronio L, Dron JS, et al. Design and user experience testing of a polygenic score report: a qualitative study of prospective users. BMC Med Genom 2021;14:238.

[5] Hao L, Kraft P, Berriz GF, et al. Development of a clinical polygenic risk score assay and reporting workflow. Nat Med 2022;28:1006–13.

[6] Lewis ACF, Perez EF, Prince AER, et al. Patient and provider perspectives on polygenic risk scores: implications for clinical reporting and utilization. Genome Med 2022;14:114.

[7] Pain O, Gillett AC, Austin JC, et al. A tool for translating polygenic scores onto the absolute scale using summary statistics. Eur. J. Hum. Genet. EJHG 2022;30:339–48.

[8] Wand H, Knowles JW, Clarke SL. The need for polygenic score reporting standards in evidence-based practice: lipid genetics use case. Curr Opin Lipidol 2021;32: 89–95.

[9] Wand H, Lambert SA, Tamburro C, et al. Improving reporting standards for polygenic scores in risk prediction studies. Nature 2021;591:211–9.

[10] Simona A, Song W, Bates DW, et al. Polygenic risk scores in pharmacogenomics: opportunities and challenges-a mini review. Front Genet 2023;14:1217049.

[11] About Health Level Seven International | HL7 International. Available at: https://www.hl7.org/about/index.cfm.

[12] ANSI Essential Requirements. Available at: https://www.ansi.org/american-national-standards/ans-introduction/essential-requirements.

[13] IEEE Standard Glossary of Software Engineering Terminology. Available at: http://ieeexplore.ieee.org/document/159342/.

[14] Lehne M, Sass J, Essenwanger A, et al. Why digital medicine depends on interoperability. NPJ Digit. Med 2019; 2:79.

[15] Rychert J. In support of interoperability: A laboratory perspective. Int. J. Lab. Hematol 2023;45:436–41.

[16] Simborg DW. Reflections on the history of interoperability in hospitals. J Am Med Inf Assoc 2023;30:2083–5.

[17] Walker J., Pan E., Johnston D., et al., The value of health care information exchange and interoperability. Health Aff (Millwood). 2005;Suppl Web Exclusives:W5-10-W5-18. https://doi.org/10.1377/hlthaff.w5.10.

[18] Ait Abdelouahid R, Debauche O, Mahmoudi S, et al. Literature Review: Clinical Data Interoperability Models. Information 2023;14:364.

[19] Torab-Miandoab A, Samad-Soltani T, Jodati A, et al. Interoperability of heterogeneous health information systems: a systematic literature review. BMC Med Inf Decis Making 2023;23:18.

[20] Federal Register. Health Data, Technology, and Interoperability: Certification Program Updates, Algorithm Transparency, and Information Sharing. Available at: https://www.federalregister.gov/documents/2024/01/09/2023-28857/health-data-technology-and-interoperability-certification-program-updates-algorithm-transparency-and.

[21] Dolin RH, Heale BSE, Alterovitz G, et al. Introducing HL7 FHIR Genomics Operations: a developer-friendly approach to genomics-EHR integration. J. Am. Med. Inform. Assoc. JAMIA 2023;30:485–93.

[22] Lambert SA, Gil L, Jupp S, et al. The Polygenic Score Catalog as an open database for reproducibility and systematic evaluation. Nat Genet 2021;53:420–5.

[23] Spaeth EL, Dite GS, Hopper JL, et al. Validation of an Abridged Breast Cancer Risk Prediction Model for the General Population. Cancer Prev. Res. Phila. Pa 2023; 16:281–91.

[24] Shieh Y, Eklund M, Madlensky L, et al. Breast Cancer Screening in the Precision Medicine Era: Risk-Based Screening in a Population-Based Trial. J Natl Cancer Inst 2017;109.

[25] Baptista PV. Principles in genetic risk assessment. Therapeut Clin Risk Manag 2005;1:15–20.

[26] Lewis ACF, Green RC, Vassy JL. Polygenic risk scores in the clinic: Translating risk into action. Hum. Genet. Genomics Adv 2021;2.

[27] Kawamoto K, Houlihan CA, Balas EA, et al. Improving clinical practice using clinical decision support systems: a systematic review of trials to identify features critical to success. BMJ 2005;330:765.

[28] Strasberg HR, Rhodes B, Del Fiol G, et al. Contemporary clinical decision support standards using Health Level Seven International Fast Healthcare Interoperability Resources. J. Am. Med. Inform. Assoc. JAMIA 2021;28: 1796–806.

[29] Mandel JC, Kreda DA, Mandl KD, et al. SMART on FHIR: a standards-based, interoperable apps platform for electronic health records. J. Am. Med. Inform. Assoc. JAMIA 2016;23:899–908.

[30] CDS Hooks. Available at: https://cds-hooks.hl7.org/.

[31] Conformance-module - FHIR v5.0.0. Available at: https://www.hl7.org/fhir/conformance-module.html#intro.

[32] Vassy J. Pragmatic Randomized Trial of Polygenic Risk Scoring for Common Diseases in Primary Care. 2022. Available at: https://clinicaltrials.gov/study/NCT04331535.

Advances in Molecular Pathology 7 (2024) 145–154
ADVANCES IN MOLECULAR PATHOLOGY

Artificial Intelligence Applications in Genomics

Radha Nagarajan, PhD[a], Chen Wang, PhD[b], Derek Walton, JD[c], Nephi Walton, MD, MS[d,*]
[a]Information Services Department, Children's Hospital of Orange County, 1201 W. La Veta Ave, Orange, CA 92868, USA; [b]Mayo Clinic, 200 First St. SW, Rochester, MN 55905, USA; [c]Walton Legal PLLC, 635 W 5300 S, #204, Murray, UT 84123, USA; [d]National Human Genome Research Institute, National Institutes of Health, BG 6700B RM 3120, 6700B Rockledge Dr 6908, Bethesda, MD 20892-6908, USA

KEYWORDS
• Genomics • Polygenic risk score • Machine learning • Artificial intelligence
• Deep learning and augmented intelligence

KEY POINTS

- The integration of artificial intelligence (AI) and machine learning (ML) in genomics represents a transformative shift in both research and clinical applications.
- As the volume and complexity of genomic data continues to grow, these technologies offer unparalleled opportunities to uncover new insights into the genetic basis of diseases and to personalize medical care.
- AI models are ultilized routinely in the laboratory setting. As we continue to refine AI models and expand their integration into clinical practice, the potential to revolutionize healthcare through genomics-driven AI becomes increasingly attainable, promising to usher in a new era of precision medicine.
- Data privacy, model interpretability, availability of data in clinical settings, and regulatory hurdles are key challenges to fully integrating AI into clinical settings.

INTRODUCTION

Several factors have contributed to the rapid growth of genomic data, including the significant reduction in high-throughput sequencing costs, the availability of scalable and affordable cloud computing infrastructure for efficient storage and processing, increased knowledge of genomic variation leading to clinical utility for diagnosis, and the broader adoption and awareness of genomics, particularly through recreational genomics. These advancements have, in turn, increased the use of genomics for characterizing patient and population profiles, with the potential to support tailored treatment and disease management, ultimately impacting healthcare outcomes. Genomic data growth can also be attributed to national initiatives such as All of Us [1], and the United Kingdom (UK) Biobank [2], as well as academic and commercial partnerships with pharmaceutic industry such as the MyCode program [3] at Geisinger and Heredigene program [4] at Intermountain Healthcare. As the volume of genomic data continues to expand, the application of artificial intelligence (AI) becomes not only more practical but increasingly essential. In this article, we will explore the current applications and technologies of AI in genomics, examine its role in clinical settings, and discuss the challenges that must be addressed to further advance its integration and impact.

STATISTICAL ANALYSIS IN GENOMICS AND POLYGENIC RISK SCORE

Before diving into AI we thought it would be useful to ground the reader in some historic statistical concepts

*Corresponding author, *E-mail address:* nephi.walton@nih.gov

https://doi.org/10.1016/j.yamp.2024.08.001 www.advancesinmolecularpathology.com
2589-4080/24/

in genomics that have helped set the foundation for future AI genomic models. Traditionally, genomic data analyses such as Genome-Wide Association Studies (GWAS) have focused on deciphering genotype-phenotype associations using sophisticated statistical approaches that subscribes to hypothesis testing [5]. GWAS emerged in the early 2000s as a revolutionary approach that allowed researchers to scan the entire genome to identify genetic variations associated with specific diseases or traits. Unlike earlier contributions on linkage analysis within families, GWAS was focused on understanding genetic variants and single nucleotide polymorphisms (SNPs) to disease phenotypes in populations. GWAS is predicated on the common disease-common variant hypothesis, which suggests that common diseases are often influenced by genetic variants that are common in a given population. The approach involves statistical comparison of the genetic variants within a case-control framework with the case and control represented by cohorts with and without a given disease or trait of interest. Over the years, GWAS has been helpful in identifying thousands of genetic associations across a wide range of diseases and traits, including cardiovascular diseases, diabetes, and various forms of cancer. These studies have not only enhanced our understanding of genetic contributions to disease but have also illuminated complex interactions between genes and environmental factors [6–8]. Despite its successes, GWAS has faced translational challenges, more specifically in translating the findings in clinical workflows. Many identified SNPs have small effect sizes, and the biologic mechanisms underlying these associations often remain elusive. Furthermore, the replication of findings across diverse populations has highlighted the need for more inclusive and equitable approaches [9].

Polygenic risk scores (PRSs) aggregate the effects of multiple genetic variants identified from GWAS into a single score that quantifies an individual's genetic predisposition to a disease. PRS represents a significant stride toward precision medicine, offering the potential for individualized disease risk assessment, prevention and disease management strategies [10]. The weights of genetic variants in PRS are proportional to their association to a given disease or traits of interest and the resulting score captured the predisposition or cumulative of an individual to a particular disease phenotype. PRS has shown promise in several areas, notably in predicting the risk of complex diseases such as coronary artery disease [11], breast cancer [12], and type 2 diabetes [13]. It has the potential to inform clinical decision-making by identifying individuals at high genetic risk who may benefit from targeted screening and preventive measures. Moreover, PRS can contribute to understanding the genetic architecture of diseases, distinguishing between individuals with similar clinical profiles but differing genetic risks. This insight is invaluable for tailoring interventions and managing disease in a more personalized manner. The application of PRS in clinical practice is not without challenges. The accuracy of PRS can vary significantly across populations, largely due to the underrepresentation of non-European ancestries in GWAS [9]. Efforts to include more diverse populations in genetic research are critical for improving the applicability and fairness of PRS from an equity standpoint. Additionally, integrating PRS into healthcare requires careful consideration of ethical, legal, and social implications, including privacy concerns and the potential for genetic discrimination.

MACHINE LEARNING, ARTIFICIAL INTELLIGENCE, AND AUGMENTED INTELLIGENCE

More recently there has been interest in using machine learning (ML), deep learning, and AI, especially within an augmented framework (ie, human in the loop) with applications to genomic data, Fig. 1. These approaches mark the shift from classical hypothesis testing to discovery, validation of prior assumptions, and hypothesis generation in a data-driven and evidence-based manner. Their ability to process multimodal data, discovery complex interactions that may not be readily apparent from statistical models with predefined functional forms may be some of the reasons for their increasing adoption in genomics. Harnessing the multimodal data is especially critical as it provides a complete profile of patients and populations with potential to impact clinical decision-making. Multimodal data often reside in enterprise data warehouse and may include genomic data, clinical data, imaging data, clinical notes, demographic data, as well as other characteristics such as social determinants to better accommodate inherent heterogeneity of patients and populations for tailored treatment and disease management. By leveraging the predictive potential of these novel approaches, it might be possible to unravel the complex tapestry of genetic information, paving the way for improved care. More specifically, in shifting the trajectory from predicted outcomes to desired outcomes in a timely and tailored manner.

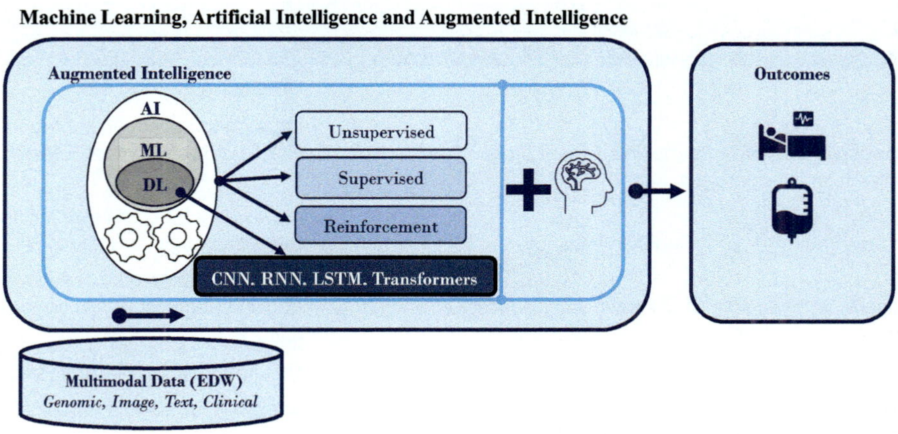

FIG. 1 Impacting healthcare outcomes using multimodal healthcare data in conjunction with machine learning, deep learning, and artificial and augmented intelligence.

MACHINE LEARNING APPLICATIONS IN GENOMICS

Arthur Samuel, 1959, defined ML as the field of study that gives computers the ability to learn without being explicitly programmed. Tom Mitchell, 1980, defined a well-posed learning problem as a computer program that learns from experience with respect to some tasks and performance measure, such that the performance at tasks improves with experience [14]. ML approaches in genomics have traditionally been classified under unsupervised and supervised learning [15]. More recently, reinforcement learning with human feedback has also been added to this repertoire [16]. Unsupervised learning such as clustering have especially proven to be useful exploratory tools for investigating potential grouping of samples such that samples within a group are more similar compared to samples between the groups. Unsupervised learning is especially well-suited to investigating large data sets with minimal a priori information. An example of unsupervised learning would be identifying potential subtypes within a seemingly homogenous disease group from their genomic profiles. In contrast, supervised learning approaches are relatively more involved and include regression and classification models. In regression models, the outputs are continuous whereas in classification models the output variables are stratified into classes or categories. Regression models such as logistic regression and its variants (eg, elastic nets) can in fact be used for classification [17]. Classification problems aim to generate a decision boundary separating the classes by optimizing a chosen objective function as a part of the training phase. Subsequently, performance of the classifier is demonstrated on an independent validation cohort in the testing phase establishing the generalization ability of the classifier. Bias-variance tradeoff is critical in ensuring enhanced generalization ability and performance [17]. High bias is an outcome of underfitting the training data whereas high variance is a result of overfitting the training data. Techniques such as regularization are often used in classification models for minimizing overfitting by penalizing a large number of features and enhance the generalization ability of the classifiers [17].

There have been many successful applications of ML to genomics, some of which are listed in Table 1. One of the primary applications of ML has been for variant classification and prediction. The human genome is replete with variants. While a majority of genetic variation is benign, a growing number of variants have been found to be causative of diseases and/or modifying disease risk. Unsupervised ML approaches have especially proven to be helpful in predicting putative pathogenic variants from multimodal integrated profiles that include genomic sequences, evolutionary conservation scores, and functional assays [18]. On a related note, supervised ML approaches that implicitly incorporate the class labels (benign, pathogenic) in the training phase have been used successfully for variant classification [19]. Tools have also demonstrated the usefulness of ML in deciphering gene function, regulation, and the broader genetic architecture of diseases using network abstractions. Unsupervised ML approaches such as principal component analysis (PCA) may be helpful in dimensionality reduction, feature selection from high-dimensional/high-throughput genomic assays, and population stratification. ML in conjunction with graphical models and community structure detection algorithms have can be helpful in providing preliminary cues into underlying

TABLE 1
Traditional Machine Learning Applications in Genomics

Description	Github
MAGPIE [18] Accurate pathogenic prediction for multiple variant types using machine learning approach	https://github.com/shenlab-genomics/magpie Gradient Boosting Tree Ensemble Classifier
MLVar [19] Classification and Prioritization of Genomic variants	https://github.com/GiovannaNicora/MLVar Penalized Logistic Regression
GENESIS [20] Predict pathogenicity of variants of unknown significance	https://github.com/rachellea/medgenetics Logistic Regression, Multilayer Perceptron
PLINK [21] Principal Component Analysis of Population Genetic Data	https://www.cog-genomics.org/plink/1.9/ Principal Component Analysis
BIGSNPR [22] Principal Component Analysis of Population Genetic Data	https://github.com/privefl/bigsnpr

signaling mechanisms validating known associations while revealing undocumented associations and the putative drug targets. Perhaps the most transformative application of ML in genomics is in the realm of precision health. ML algorithms have been shown to reveal inherent heterogeneity within seemingly clinically homogenous cohorts assisting in tailored treatment and disease management strategies, optimizing therapeutic outcomes and minimizing adverse drug reactions.

DEEP LEARNING/ARTIFICIAL INTELLIGENCE APPLICATIONS IN GENOMICS

Deep learning models are gaining momentum in genomics [23,24] as powerful models that can harness the power of large datasets. Deep learning models are essentially a subset of ML models based primarily on neural networks (eg, DNN: Deep Neural Networks) [25], Fig. 1. These models were inspired by the parallel architecture of the human brain [26]. The term *deep* refers to the significant number of hidden layers accompanying these neural network models and providing greater flexibility in capturing intricate patterns and extracting features from the given data in an automated manner without any constraints on prior knowledge and domain expertise. This is in stark contrast to more classical ML models (ie, shallow learning) where manual feature selection often precedes learning. Several deep learning models have been proposed in the literature [27]. However, unlike classical ML models, DNNs are computationally demanding and may require the use of specialized architectures such as graphics processing units and specialized programming environments that may include those that support high-performance and distributed computing for storage of large data sets and model parameters, as well as processing the data [28]. More recently, there has also been great interest in using pre-trained DNNs for diverse applications under the broad theme Transfer Learning [27]. Operational definition of AI relies on Turing test that emphasizes the ability of machines to exhibit human-level performance on tasks such that an interrogator is unable to discern machines from humans [29]. ML and AI approaches implicitly subscribe to optimization. Therefore, it is not uncommon for these algorithms to converge to a local optimum. Supplementing these algorithms with prior knowledge in a context-specific manner and human intervention in interpreting the results has the potential to improve the overall performance and interpretation. The latter is especially critical when the algorithms encounter scenarios that are not presented adequately in the training data. Augmented intelligence essentially emphasizes the concerted of role of machines and humans working in tandem and subscribes Friedman's fundamental theorem of informatics, which emphasizes that "humans working in partnership with an information resource is better than working unassisted" [30]. Since clinicians have the ability to adapt a large faculty of outside knowledge in arriving at decisions on a given case in contrast to a siloed algorithmic approach that relies on historic data, augmented intelligence perhaps represents the culmination point of AI/ML adoption of genomics in clinical care. The hierarchical relationship between ML, deep learning, AI, and augmented intelligence is shown in Fig. 1. Several DNNs have been proposed in the literature with applications to genomic data, these include Convolutional Neural Networks (CNN), Recurrent Neural Networks (RNN), Long-short Term Memory (LSTM), and Transformers, Fig. 1 [16,31,32]. (Table 2) lists several examples of

TABLE 2
Deep Learning/Artificial Intelligence Applications in Genomics

Description	Deep Learning Approach Implementation
DeepBind [33] Predict sequence specificities for DNA and RNA Binding Proteins	CNN https://github.com/jisraeli/DeepBind
DeepSEA [34] Predict chromatic effects of sequence alterations	CNN http://deepsea.princeton.edu/job/analysis/create/
DeepVariant [35] Variant calling from high-throughput sequencing data	CNN https://github.com/google/deepvariant
Splice2Deep [36] Ensemble approach for the recognition of splice sites in genomic DNA.	https://github.com/SomayahAlbaradei/Splice_Deep CNN
DeepNano [37] Base caller for Oxford Nanopore MINioN	RNN https://github.com/jeammimi/deepnano
DeepMilo [38]	Hybrid: CNN + RNN https://github.com/khuranalab/DeepMILO
DanQ [39]	Hybrid: CNN + RNN https://github.com/uci-cbcl/DanQ
ENNGene [40] GUI driven DNN tool for Genomics	Hybrid: CNN + RNN https://github.com/ML-Bioinfo-CEITEC/ENNGene
DeepClip [41] Predicting the effect of mutations on RNA binding	Bi-directional LSTM http://www.github.com/deepclip
Nucleotide Transformer [42] Molecular phenotype prediction from nucleotide sequences	Transformer https://huggingface.co/InstaDeepAI
Enformer [43] Predicting gene expression from sequence information incorporating long-range interactions	Transformer https://github.com/deepmind/deepmind-research/tree/master/enformer
DNABERT [44]	Transformer https://github.com/jerryji1993/DNABERT
DNABERT2 [45] Multi-species genome foundation model, replacing k-mer tokenization of sequences with Byte Pair Encoding	Transformer https://github.com/MAGICS-LAB/DNABERT_2
HyenaDNA [46] Long-range foundation model in genomics	Transformer https://github.com/HazyResearch/hyena-dna

deep learning applications that have been developed for genomics.

POPULAR DEEP LEARNING ARCHITECTURES

- *CNN*: By processing genomic sequences as 1-dimensional "images," CNNs can identify spatial patterns indicative of gene function, regulatory elements, or pathogenic variants. CNNs are particularly suited for analyzing genetic sequences, identifying patterns and motifs that are indicative of functional elements, such as promoters, enhancers, and splice sites. These models have also been pivotal in variant effect prediction, distinguishing between benign variations and those with potential disease implications.
- *RNN/LSTM*: Specialized in handling sequential data, these networks are adept at modeling the sequential nature of genomics sequences. They can predict the effects of genetic variations over long stretches of sequences, uncovering complex regulatory mechanisms, and gene expression patterns.
- *Transformers*: Transformers and large language models (LLMs) have begun to make significant inroads into

genetics and genomics research, marking a paradigm shift in how complex biologic data is analyzed and interpreted. Originally developed for natural language processing, these models, particularly transformers, excel at handling sequential data, making them well-suited for genomic sequences, which can be viewed as long strings of nucleotide "letters." In genomics, transformers leverage their ability to capture long-range dependencies within sequences, identifying patterns and relationships that span across vast stretches of DNA. This capacity is instrumental in tasks such as predicting the effects of genetic variations, understanding gene regulation mechanisms, and annotating genomic sequences with functional information. LLMs, trained on extensive corpuses of genomic data, can generate predictive models that mimic biologic processes, offering insights into the language of life itself. As these models continue to evolve, their application in genetics and genomics heralds a new era of computational biology, where the lines between biologic sequences and linguistic structures increasingly blur, promising breakthroughs in our understanding of life's genetic blueprint.

ARTIFICIAL INTELLIGENCE IN THE LABORATORY VERSUS CLINICAL CARE SETTINGS

The AI tools mentioned earlier are primarily deployed in research and clinical laboratory settings. In fact, the use of AI for genomics in clinical laboratory settings is commonplace [47], with many commercial vendors offering variant calling workflows that embed AI for variant interpretation. However, AI in clinical care settings has not gained much traction as there are not well-established technical frameworks and this domain and it is subject to more regulatory scrutiny. Despite this, the potential for AI in clinical domains is substantial, particularly with advancements in transformer models. For instance, Delphi-2M, a generative pretrained transformer, shows significant promise in predicting patient's clinical trajectories [48]. Integrating genomic data into such models could be extremely powerful for informing patient health decision and implementation of preventative measures. Combining genomic data with clinical data using AI models has already shown promise in research settings.

CLINICAL GENOMICS DATA ECOSYSTEM

There are currently no data ecosystem for genomics in the healthcare setting that allows for real-time access to large genomic datasets for clinical care. Typically, only PDF reports describing 1 or 2 variants transfer from laboratories to clinical settings, leaving the vast majority of the sequencing data unavailable for patient care. To scale the clinical application of genomics, systems must be developed to provide real-time access to an individual's full genetic sequence at the point of care. Picture Archiving and Communcation System (PACS) like models or Genomics Archiving and Communication System (GACS) systems have been suggested [49] to remedy this problem but such systems are currently only operating in the research domain.

GENOMICS DATA STANDARDS

Data standards in genomics are continuing to evolve, with FHIR (Fast Healthcare Interoperability Resources) standards for genomics just beginning to reach maturity but not yet widely adopted. For instance, the Epic genomics module, one of the more advanced efforts to integrate genomics with electronic health records (EHRs), still relies on an older HL7 2.51 clinical genomics report standard for genetic data messaging [50]. The slow adoption of new standards can be attributed to their relative immaturity and the rapidly changing landscape of genomics and health informatics. However, it is anticipated that FHIR Release 6, will introduce a more granular and stable genomic data model when it is released. This advancement is expected to facilitate the broader and more effective use of genomic data within EHR systems, significantly enhancing the integration of genomics into clinical care.

CLINICAL DECISION SUPPORT

Clinical decision support (CDS) systems powered by AI are an active area of development in medicine, but they still lack maturity. The clinical implementation of these technologies faces 3 major challenges. First, there is a lack of available data, particularly genomic data, due to the aforementioned lack of comprehensive clinical data ecosystems, specifically there is no technical infrastructure to deliver granular genomic data into AI-driven CDS models. Second, even if such data were accessible in clinical settings, questions remain about whether genomic information outside of clinical reports can be utilized for patient care. Third, CDS systems, especially those involving AI and genomics, are hindered by significant regulatory barriers and uncertainties. AI models designed to incorporate complex PRS are likely to be among the first to be used in genomic CDS if these barriers can be overcome. Multimodal AI models combining multiple data types with thousands of genomic data points have the potential to produce highly accurate and meaningful risk assessments to inform CDS systems [51]. However, navigating the regulatory landscape remains one of the biggest challenges for their successful deployment.

THE CURSE OF DIMENSIONALITY

Even with the vast number of genomic datasets currently available, we are still far from having the volume of data necessary to achieve results comparable to those seen with LLMs in other fields [52]. One of the major challenges lies in the sheer complexity of genomic data, which includes over 3 billion base pairs and countless potential outcomes, with thousands of diseases potentially linked to various combinations of genetic variations. While the development of powerful models that could significantly advance gene discovery and our understanding of health are possible with sufficiently large genomic datasets, assembling the required amount of data is a daunting task. It is crucial to balance the need for extensive data with strategies to intelligently reduce the dimensionality of genomic data for AI models. Research aimed at dimensionality reduction could substantially enhance innovation in this field. Additionally, efforts to aggregate large genomic datasets should be encouraged, and even larger national sequencing initiatives than those currently proposed or in place should be considered to support these advancements.

REGULATORY FRAMEWORKS

The clinical deployment of AI faces numerous regulatory challenges, with 2 of the most significant being the lack of clarity in the Food and Drug Administration's (FDA's) regulation of CDS systems and software as a medical device (SaMD) [53], as well as uncertainties from Clinical Laboratory Improvement Amendments (CLIA) regarding the use of entire genome sequences in clinical care beyond what is included in clinical reports. The FDA's current framework does not adequately address adaptive AI approaches, requiring manufacturers to seek additional clearance for significant changes to devices. In January 2021, the FDA introduced the "Artificial Intelligence/Machine Learning (AI/ML)-Based SaMD Action Plan" [54] through the Center for Devices and Radiological Health's Digital Health Center of Excellence. Although this plan proposed a new regulatory framework for AI/ML technologies, no new framework has been implemented to date. Recent FDA guidance on CDS suggests that models used to support, rather than dictate, physician decisions may be exempt from stringent regulations. As these regulatory frameworks continue to evolve, it is crucial to find a balance that ensures patient safety without hindering innovation through overly restrictive regulation of AI technologies.

In the United States, AI regulations are largely still developing, with a focus on balancing innovation with ethical considerations. Key principles include ensuring AI systems are safe, non-discriminatory, and respect privacy. The White House's Office of Science and Technology Policy has also introduced the AI Bill of Rights Blueprint to guide ethical AI practices [55].

In the European Union (EU), AI regulations are more defined and are governed by the comprehensive EU AI Act [56,57], which aims to ensure the safe, transparent, and ethical use of AI. It categorizes AI systems into 4 risk levels—unacceptable, high, limited, and minimal—imposing stricter requirements on higher-risk applications. High-risk AI systems, such as those involving genomic data, must meet stringent standards for data quality, transparency, human oversight, and accountability. The Act also emphasizes compliance with data privacy laws like the general data protection regulation and prohibits certain AI practices, such as social scoring and manipulation, to protect individuals' rights and prevent discrimination. The goal is to balance innovation with the protection of individual rights and prevention of discrimination.

PRIVACY CONCERNS

Using genomic data in AI models presents significant challenges, particularly concerning data privacy and security. Genomic data are highly sensitive because they contain comprehensive information about an individual's genetic makeup, which can reveal predispositions to certain diseases and other personal traits. This makes the data a prime target for misuse if not adequately protected. One of the key challenges is ensuring that AI models are trained on large, diverse datasets without compromising an individual's privacy. This requires robust de-identification techniques, yet even de-identified data can sometimes be re-identified when combined with other datasets. Moreover, as AI models evolve, they might inadvertently retain or infer sensitive information, raising concerns about unintended data breaches. Striking a balance between leveraging genomic data for AI advancements and maintaining strict privacy protections are essential to gain public trust and fully realize the potential of AI in healthcare

MODEL INTERPRETABILITY

The interpretability of AI models in clinical settings is of paramount importance because it directly impacts the trust, safety, and efficacy of AI-driven clinical decisions. In a field where patient outcomes are at stake, clinicians need to understand how and why an AI model arrives at a particular recommendation or diagnosis. This transparency is essential not only for ensuring the model's reliability but also for enabling clinicians to validate and contextualize the AI's findings within the broader clinical picture. Interpretability allows for the identification and correction of potential biases or errors in the model, which is crucial for maintaining patient safety and avoiding harmful outcomes. Moreover, regulatory bodies often require a clear explanation of the AI processes to approve their use in clinical settings, further highlighting the need for interpretable models. As AI continues to evolve in medicine, enhancing the interpretability of these models will be the key to their successful integration into healthcare systems, fostering both clinician and patient confidence in AI-assisted care.

SUMMARY

In conclusion, the integration of AI and ML in genomics represents a transformative shift in both research and clinical applications. As the volume and complexity of genomic data continue to grow, these technologies offer unparalleled opportunities to uncover new insights into the genetic basis of diseases and to personalize medical care. However, the path forward is fraught with challenges, including the need for robust data privacy protections, the development of interpretable and generalizable models, and the establishment of clear regulatory frameworks that support innovation while ensuring patient safety. Addressing these challenges will require concerted efforts from researchers, clinicians, regulatory bodies, and the broader scientific community. As we continue to refine AI models and expand their integration into clinical practice, the potential to revolutionize healthcare through genomics-driven AI becomes increasingly attainable, promising to usher in a new era of precision medicine. As computational power and algorithmic sophistication continue to advance, the role of ML in deciphering the complexities of the genome and transforming healthcare through personalized medicine will only expand, heralding a new era in genetic research and patient care.

CLINICS CARE POINTS

- AI-driven Polygenic Risk Scores offer individualized disease risk assessments for targeted prevention and treatment strategies.
- AI is already being used to classify genetic variants, distinguishing between benign and pathogenic mutations to inform clinical decisions.
- AI models integrating genomic data have the potential to enhance clinical decision-making and patient outcomes.
- AI adoption in clinical genomics faces significant regulatory challenges.
- Real-time access to comprehensive genomic data in clinical settings is crucial for integrating genomics into routine patient care.

REFERENCES

[1] All of Us Research Program Investigators, Denny JC, Rutter JL, et al. The "all of us" research program. N Engl J Med 2019;381(7):668–76.

[2] Sudlow C, Gallacher J, Allen N, et al. UK biobank: an open access resource for identifying the causes of a wide range of complex diseases of middle and old age. PLoS Med 2015;12(3):e1001779.

[3] Carey DJ, Fetterolf SN, Davis FD, et al. The Geisinger MyCode community health initiative: an electronic health record–linked biobank for precision medicine research. Genet Med 2016;18(9):906–13.

[4] Walton NA, Hafen B, Graceffo S, et al. The development of an infrastructure to facilitate the use of whole genome sequencing for population health. J Personalized Med 2022;12(11):1867.

[5] From the editors. Nat Rev Genet 2006;7(10):737.

[6] Sladek R, Rocheleau G, Rung J, et al. A genome-wide association study identifies novel risk loci for type 2 diabetes. Nature 2007;445(7130):881–5.

[7] Scott LJ, Mohlke KL, Bonnycastle LL, et al. A genome-wide association study of type 2 diabetes in finns detects multiple susceptibility variants. Science 2007;316(5829):1341–5.

[8] The Wellcome Trust Case Control Consortium, Management Committee, Burton PR, et al. Genome-wide association study of 14,000 cases of seven common diseases and 3,000 shared controls. Nature 2007;447(7145):661–78.

[9] Graham SE, Clarke SL, Wu KHH, et al. The power of genetic diversity in genome-wide association studies of lipids. Nature 2021;600(7890):675–9.

[10] Dashti HS, Miranda N, Cade BE, et al. Interaction of obesity polygenic score with lifestyle risk factors in an electronic health record biobank. BMC Med 2022;20(1):5.

[11] Naderian M, Hamed ME, Vaseem AA, et al. Effect of disclosing a polygenic risk score for coronary heart disease on adverse cardiovascular events: 10-year follow-up of the MI-GENES randomized clinical trial. medRxiv 2024. https://doi.org/10.1101/2024.07.19.24310709.

[12] Mabey B, Hughes E, Kucera M, et al. Validation of a clinical breast cancer risk assessment tool combining a polygenic score for all ancestries with traditional risk factors. Genet Med 2024;26(7):101128.

[13] Mandla R, Schroeder P, Porneala B, et al. Polygenic scores for longitudinal prediction of incident type 2 diabetes in an ancestrally and medically diverse primary care physician network: a patient cohort study. Genome Med 2024;16(1):63.

[14] Mitchell TM. Machine learning. Dubuque, IA: McGraw-Hill; 1997.

[15] Libbrecht MW, Noble WS. Machine learning applications in genetics and genomics. Nat Rev Genet 2015;16(6):321–32.

[16] Vaswani A, Shazeer N, Parmar N, et al. Attention is all you need. In: Advances in Neural Information Processing Systems. vol. 30. 2017.

[17] Hastie T, Tibshirani R, Friedman JH. The elements of statistical learning: data mining, inference, and prediction. 2nd edition. New York, NY: Springer; 2009.

[18] Liu Y, Zhang T, You N, et al. MAGPIE: accurate pathogenic prediction for multiple variant types using machine learning approach. Genome Med 2024;16(1):3.

[19] Nicora G, Zucca S, Limongelli I, et al. A machine learning approach based on ACMG/AMP guidelines for genomic variant classification and prioritization. Sci Rep 2022;12(1):2517.

[20] Draelos RL, Ezekian JE, Zhuang F, et al. GENESIS: gene-specific machine learning models for variants of uncertain significance found in catecholaminergic polymorphic ventricular tachycardia and long QT syndrome-associated genes. Circ Arrhythm Electrophysiol 2022;15(4):e010326.

[21] Purcell S, Neale B, Todd-Brown K, et al. PLINK: a tool set for whole-genome association and population-based linkage analyses. Am J Hum Genet 2007;81(3):559–75.

[22] Privé F, Luu K, Blum MGB, et al. Efficient toolkit implementing best practices for principal component analysis of population genetic data. Bioinformatics 2020;36(16):4449–57.

[23] Vatsyayan A, Kumar M, Saikia BJ, et al. WilsonGenAI a deep learning approach to classify pathogenic variants in Wilson Disease. PLoS One 2024;19:e0303787.

[24] Penzar D, Nogina D, Noskova E, et al. LegNet: a best-in-class deep learning model for short DNA regulatory regions. Bioinformatics 2023;39(8):btad457.

[25] LeCun Y, Bengio Y, Hinton G. Deep learning. Nature 2015;521(7553):436–44.

[26] Sejnowski TJ. The unreasonable effectiveness of deep learning in artificial intelligence. Proc Natl Acad Sci U S A 2020;117(48):30033–8.

[27] Yue T, Wang H. Deep learning for genomics: a concise overview. 2018. Available at: http://arxiv.org/abs/1802.00810. Accessed July 8, 2022.

[28] Ananthaswamy A. In AI, is bigger always better? Nature 2023;615(7951):202–5.

[29] Russell SJ, Norvig P. Artificial intelligence: a modern approach. 4th edition. Hoboken, NJ: Pearson; 2021.

[30] Friedman CP. A "fundamental theorem" of biomedical informatics. J Am Med Inform Assoc JAMIA 2009;16(2):169–70.

[31] Goodfellow I, Bengio Y, Courville A. Deep learning. Cambridge, MA: The MIT Press; 2016.

[32] Hochreiter S, Schmidhuber J. Long short-term memory. Neural Comput 1997;9(8):1735–80.

[33] Alipanahi B, Delong A, Weirauch MT, et al. Predicting the sequence specificities of DNA- and RNA-binding proteins by deep learning. Nat Biotechnol 2015;33(8):831–8.

[34] Zhou J, Troyanskaya OG. Predicting effects of noncoding variants with deep learning–based sequence model. Nat Methods 2015;12(10):931–4.

[35] Poplin R, Chang PC, Alexander D, et al. A universal SNP and small-indel variant caller using deep neural networks. Nat Biotechnol 2018;36(10):983–7.

[36] Albaradei S, Magana-Mora A, Thafar M, et al. Splice2-Deep: an ensemble of deep convolutional neural networks for improved splice site prediction in genomic DNA. Gene 2020;763:100035.

[37] Boža V, Brejová B, Vinař T. DeepNano: deep recurrent neural networks for base calling in MinION nanopore reads. PLoS One 2017;12(6):e0178751.

[38] Trieu T, Martinez-Fundichely A, Khurana E. DeepMILO: a deep learning approach to predict the impact of non-coding sequence variants on 3D chromatin structure. Genome Biol 2020;21(1):79.

[39] Quang D, Xie X. DanQ: a hybrid convolutional and recurrent deep neural network for quantifying the function of DNA sequences. Nucleic Acids Res 2015. https://doi.org/10.1101/032821.

[40] Chalupová E, Vaculík O, Poláček J, et al. ENNGene: an easy neural network model building tool for genomics. BMC Genom 2022;23(1):248.

[41] Grønning AGB, Doktor TK, Larsen SJ, et al. DeepCLIP: predicting the effect of mutations on protein–RNA binding with deep learning. Nucleic Acids Res 2020. https://doi.org/10.1093/nar/gkaa530 gkaa530.

[42] Dalla-Torre H, Gonzalez L, Mendoza-Revilla J, et al. The nucleotide transformer: building and evaluating robust foundation. Models for Human Genomics 2023. https://doi.org/10.1101/2023.01.11.523679.

[43] Avsec Ž, Agarwal V, Visentin D, et al. Effective gene expression prediction from sequence by integrating long-range interactions. Nat Methods 2021;18(10):1196–203.

[44] Ji Y, Zhou Z, Liu H, et al. DNABERT: pre-trained bidirectional encoder representations from transformers model for DNA-language in genome. Bioinforma Oxf Engl 2021;37(15):2112–20.

[45] Zhou Z, Ji Y, Li W, et al. DNABERT-2: efficient foundation model and benchmark for multi-species genome. arxiv 2023. https://doi.org/10.48550/ARXIV.2306.15006.

[46] Nguyen E, Poli M, Faizi M, et al. HyenaDNA: long-range genomic sequence modeling at single nucleotide resolution. ArXiv 2023 arXiv:2306.15794v2.

[47] Aradhya S, Facio FM, Metz H, et al. Applications of artificial intelligence in clinical laboratory genomics. Am J Med Genet C Semin Med Genet 2023;193(3): e32057.

[48] Shmatko, Artem, et al. "Learning the natural history of human disease with generative transformers." medRxiv (2024): 2024-06.

[49] Walton NA, Johnson DK, Person TN, et al. Genomic data in the electronic health record. Adv Mol Pathol 2019; 2(1):21–33.

[50] Chamala S, Majety S, Mishra SN, et al. Indispensability of clinical bioinformatics for effective implementation of genomic medicine in pathology laboratories. ACI Open 2020;04(02):e167–72.

[51] Zhou Y, Cosentino J, Yun T, et al. Utilizing multimodal AI to improve genetic analyses of cardiovascular traits. medRrxiv 2024. https://doi.org/10.1101/2024.03.19.24304547.

[52] Koumakis L. Deep learning models in genomics; are we there yet? Comput Struct Biotechnol J 2020;18:1466–73.

[53] FDA releases guidance on AI-driven clinical decision support tools. HealthIT analytics. Available at: https://healthitanalytics.com/news/fda-releases-guidance-on-ai-driven-clinical-decision-support-tools. Accessed December 10, 2022.

[54] Artificial intelligence/machine learning (AI/ML)-Based software as a medical device (SaMD) action plan. 2021. Available at: https://www.fda.gov/media/145022/download. Accessed December 12, 2022.

[55] The white House. Blueprint for an AI Bill of rights. Available at: https://www.whitehouse.gov/ostp/ai-bill-of-rights/. Accessed August 1, 2024.

[56] European Commission. AI Act. Available at: https://digital-strategy.ec.europa.eu/en/policies/regulatory-framework-ai.

[57] European Parliament and the Council of the European Union. Regulation (EU) 2024/1689 of the European Parliament and of the Council of 13 June 2024 laying down harmonised rules on artificial intelligence and amending regulations. Official Journal of the European Union. Available at: https://eur-lex.europa.eu/eli/reg/2024/1689/oj.

Hot Topics

Advances in Molecular Pathology 7 (2024) 155–164
ADVANCES IN MOLECULAR PATHOLOGY

A Concise Overview of Circulating Tumor DNA Detection for Solid Tumors

Eric Goold, MD[a,b,1], Evan Raps, MD[a,b,1], Valarie McMurtry, MD, PhD[a,b,*]
[a]Department of Pathology, University of Utah, Salt Lake City, UT, USA; [b]ARUP Laboratories, Salt Lake City, UT, USA

KEYWORDS
• ctDNA • cfDNA • Solid tumor • ctDNA testing • Circulating tumor • Tumor DNA

KEY POINTS

- Current circulating tumor DNA (ctDNA) assays take varied approaches and methods; selection of testing is dependent on the goal of the study or clinical care.
- Many solid tumor recommendations incorporate ctDNA testing; however, if results are negative, tissue biopsy is recommended.
- ctDNA detection sensitivity is dependent on the assay deployed and care should be taken to understand the role of false negatives.

INTRODUCTION

Molecular analysis is now an important component of almost any cancer diagnosis. Since the advent of mutation-specific, targeted drugs, this testing has been achieved on tumor tissue, including large surgical specimens, small biopsies, and even cytology specimens for solid tumors. However, there is an unmet need for accurate monitoring of disease following definitive therapy, and its response to treatment. Currently, clinical examination and radiologic imaging are used to monitor for recurrence and/or progression; these methods have room for improvement in accuracy, sensitivity, and specificity. Minimal residual disease (MRD), or measurable residual disease, is commonly tested in patients with hematologic malignancies; a small number of cancer cells that are not detected by microscopy are identified by sensitive molecular techniques. MRD for solid tumors has not progressed at the same rate and remains a challenge.

Liquid biopsy is a broad term that encompasses detection of circulating tumor cells, cell-free DNA (cfDNA), circulating tumor DNA (ctDNA), circulating tumor RNA, or other biologic components of the tumor in the patient's body fluids. cfDNA was first described in 1948—Mandel and Métais understood that nucleic acid concentration was related to leukocytes in the blood but were interested in investigating nucleic acids in blood plasma from normal subjects [1]. The majority of cfDNA is contributed by hematopoietic cells [2], but the main areas of interest for cfDNA are fragments contributed by a fetus, solid organ transplant, or tumor (Fig. 1A).

cfDNA is composed of extracellular fragments of double-stranded DNA and often DNA-associated proteins that are found in various body fluids including

[1] Present address: 2000 Circle of Hope, RM 3100, Salt Lake City, UT 84112.

*Corresponding author. 2000 Circle of Hope, RM 3100, Salt Lake City, UT 84112. *E-mail address:* valarie.mcmurtry@aruplab.com

https://doi.org/10.1016/j.yamp.2024.06.005
www.advancesinmolecularpathology.com
2589-4080/24/

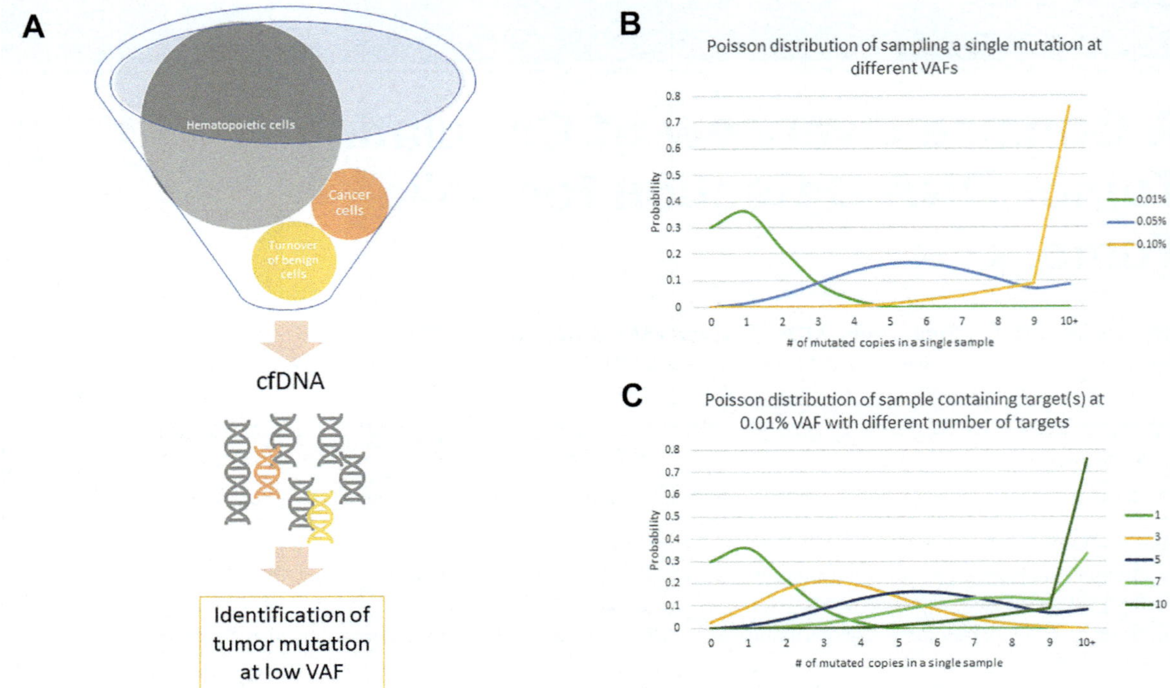

FIG. 1 **(A)** Composition of cfDNA. cfDNA is largely composed of DNA from hematopoietic cells with cancer cells and benign cells contributing a small amount. Variant allele frequency (VAFs) for ctDNA is often 0.01% or lower. **(B)** Poisson distribution of sampling a single mutation at different VAFs. The probability of a sample containing 0 or 1 copy of a mutated target from the tumor at a VAF of 0.01% is high while the probability of a sample containing 10 or more copies of a mutated target is high at a VAF of 0.1%. **(C)** Poisson distribution of a sample containing a mutated copy of a target at 0.01% VAF depending on the number of targets per sample. Methods using lower number of targets have higher chances of a sample containing 1 to 6 targets, and methods using greater than 7 targets have much higher chances of a sample containing greater than 10 targets.

serum, plasma, cerebrospinal fluid, cyst contents, and so forth [3]. However, due to the ease of venipuncture for sampling, the body of literature for cfDNA focuses largely on the cfDNA in the plasma. The concentration of cfDNA in the plasma of normal individuals is usually low, rarely above 30 ng/mL. In patients with a malignancy, this can increase to levels of 1000 ng/mL [4]. ctDNA represents only a portion of cfDNA (between 0.1% and 23%) and can be extremely variable; levels can be associated with stage, metabolic tumor volume, and tumor histology, reflecting the multiple biologic factors that influence the levels present in the plasma [4–6]. ctDNA is composed of fragments of the tumor's DNA and DNA-associated proteins, and thus contains the genetic alterations in nucleotides, methylation profiles, fusions, gene expression, tumor mutational burden, and microsatellite status. In addition, ctDNA theoretically represents the entire tumor burden [7]. These factors make ctDNA an attractive biomarker: monitoring for residual/recurrent disease, possibly even MRD, guide therapy by identifying actionable mutations and resistance mutations, and inform staging and prognosis.

In this review, we will cover the basics of ctDNA, new and emerging technologies, and briefly discuss implications in 2 common solid tumor types: breast cancer and non-small cell lung cancer (NSCLC).

SCARCITY OF A VALUABLE RESOURCE

A 10 mL blood tube (4 mL plasma) from patients with early stage cancer typically yields an average of 20 ng of cfDNA [8]. Looking at ctDNA mutation detection as a mathematical calculation: 4 mL of plasma containing 6000 genome equivalents within the cfDNA would contain approximately 12×10^3 DNA fragments per loci from all sources. Assuming an average 0.1% variant allele frequency (VAF) of a ctDNA, there is an average of approximately 12 ctDNA fragments per loci per tube with the mutational burden present at a lower VAF. This presents the challenge of stochastic sampling variation as lower ctDNA VAFs have lower probability of being sampled within 4 mL of plasma—the probability of a mutated copy from ctDNA (VAF 0.01%) not being present in a sample is approximately 30% using Poisson distribution (Fig. 1B). Improvements can be made by increasing the volume of plasma obtained to increase the amount of input ctDNA; however, this is not clinically feasible. Many methods focus on analytical and postanalytical factors, but preanalytical factors should not be ignored. Timing of sample collection, collection tubes, storage, temperature, centrifugation, and extraction protocols are known to influence ctDNA levels and fraction. In-depth reviews of preanalytical factors include Bronkhorst and colleagues [9] and Chen and Zhou [10].

cfDNA generally has a bimodal distribution with average lengths of 161 and 317 base pairs (bp) with a half-life of minutes to hours [2,11]. The length of cfDNA is related to the nucleosome, the basic structural unit of the chromosome. ctDNA tends to have a shorter fragment length than the cfDNA from healthy cells (132–145 bp), but longer fragments do occur and may be unrecognized [11,12]. ctDNA can be found in the plasma of patients with cancer due to the near continuous turnover of cancer cells by apoptosis and necrosis as well as secretion of DNA [13]. Fragment length can also play an important role in distinguishing somatic from germline cfDNA. As such, shorter fragment length has been incorporated into some assays [14]. However, in some methods, size selection disproportionately favored certain variants and decreased the sensitivity when used in a tumor-independent model, but improved sensitivity in some personalized panels but not others [5,12]. The short half-life of ctDNA can be seen as a benefit as it provides a precise time point for evaluation.

Beyond the low yield, clonal hematopoiesis (CH) and the mutations associated with it are a major hurdle for ctDNA assays. CH is an age-related phenomenon of acquired somatic alterations in hematopoietic stems cells that have a selective advantage, thus overlapping with many cancer-related mutations in the aging population. The prevalence of CH varies depending on the sequencing method used (eg, the more sensitive the sequencing method, the higher prevalence of CH), thus methods deployed for the detection of ctDNA often find an increased prevalence of CH [15]. Because hematopoietic cells contribute the most DNA to the plasma cfDNA, the majority of variants identified in cfDNA can be attributed to CH [5,14].

METHODOLOGY AND TECHNIQUES

ctDNA detection methods can be classified by technique, such as amplicon-based sequencing, hybridization capture-based sequencing, and whole genome sequencing, and whether these technologies use a patient's a priori tumor information for personalized or tumor-informed panels. ctDNA was integrated through these personalized approaches or relied on the detection of driver mutations using polymerase chain reaction (PCR) methods until massively parallel sequencing (MPS) became widely available at affordable cost.

Digital droplet PCR (ddPCR) is one of the simplest approaches to detecting ctDNA. The sensitivity of assays using ddPCR is high, as they can detect a VAF of 0.01% and some go down to a VAF of 0.001% [16]; however, the target must be known, and the designed probes should be highly specific for a single alteration. ddPCR serves as a detection technique for hot spot mutations in hematologic malignancies: *IDH1*, *IDH2*, *BRAF*, and *NPM1* among others. It is cheaper and less time-consuming than MPS techniques [17]. Tarazona and colleagues used personalized ddPCR panels of 2 hotspot mutations to show detection, after surgical management in localized colon cancer, is associated with decreased disease-free survival. Interestingly, the detection of ctDNA preceded radiologic evidence of recurrence by approximately 11.5 months [18].

Tumor-informed (also known as tumor-guided) approaches increase both sensitivity and specificity by tracking patient-specific mutations that were identified by sequencing diagnostic material. The tumor sequencing data are compared to a germline sample to identify alterations only found in the tumor, and these alterations can then be tracked during treatment and follow-up. Multiple targets are generally identified that can be leveraged to increase sample level sensitivity as the ability to detect ctDNA in the MRD setting is highly correlated with the number of informative loci (illustrated in Fig. 1C) [8]. The targets can be patient-specific or broad with only a select few that are applicable to the individual patient. These techniques often use unique molecular identifiers (UMIs), which are a type of sequencing barcode that provides error correction to increase accuracy during sequencing as well as allow for sample pooling. UMIs are ligated to sample DNA prior to PCR so that duplicate reads and PCR errors can be removed easily by tracking uniquely labeled reads. Development of a personalized ctDNA approach by the detection of multiple mutations (increasing sample level sensitivity) and patient-specific mutations (overcome limits of sampling and improve limit of detection) improves the analytical performance of ctDNA detection and quantification at all stages of treatment. However, this method may not be possible for many laboratories as the patient-specific mutations may not be known, and identifying these mutations through sequencing of the original tumor and the patient in combination is likely cost prohibitive [8]. However, some institutions have the resources necessary as McDonald and colleagues describe a 3 to 4 week turnaround time from the receipt of surgical specimen to the development of a patient-specific assay [8]. Another factor to consider with tumor-guided approaches is that the clonal evolution of the tumor may not be readily identified and resistance mutations may be masked [12]. Tumor-informed approaches are not suited for screening or primary diagnosis.

Bioinformatic pipelines used for tumor-informed approaches are aimed at decreasing errors and increasing sensitivity. Targeted digital sequencing (TARDIS) is a target capture method that preserves the target DNA length and uses that information to group sequencing reads and decrease background errors [8]. TARDIS is highly personalized, requiring tumor and germline whole exome sequencing and selection of an average of 30 mutations/patient to detect ctDNA in stages I to III breast cancer throughout neoadjuvant therapy. Targeted error correction sequencing is another target capture method combined with deep sequencing; the panel has 58 genes sequenced to a depth of 30,000× [19]. This method identified positive ctDNA in 59% to 71% of stage I or II patients with colorectal, lung, ovarian, or breast cancer. Another method, the integration of variant reads (INVAR) pipeline, uses hundreds to thousands of mutations identified by tumor genotyping to detect ctDNA [12]. To reduce errors, INVAR uses UMIs and the process of blacklisting (bioinformatically masking) loci that showed increased error signals in control samples or had a background error rate of greater than 1%. INVAR does not require personalized sequencing panels so long as the data from the diagnostic material are available [12]. MRDetect (minimal residual disease detection) uses breadth of sequencing to overcome barriers in ctDNA levels, employing whole genome sequencing with relatively low depth to integrate mutations as well as amplification/deletion status [20]. This approach appears better suited for broad cancer detection since there is limited sensitivity for individual alterations; however, its current form uses the patient's prior tumor information to inform the ctDNA testing [20].

Most of the earlier methods utilize multiple markers, but even using a single alteration to assess ctDNA has been shown to be useful. For example, Safe-Sequencing system uses a single mutation identified in the tumor as the ctDNA marker, and in a study of stage III colon cancer as well as those with resectable colorectal liver metastases, postsurgical ctDNA presence was associated with an inferior recurrence-free survival [21,22].

Tumor-independent methods do not need a priori knowledge of tumor mutations but use concurrent germline sequencing data or general knowledge of tumor genetics. Memorial Sloan Kettering—Analysis of circulating cfDNA to examine somatic status utilizes 129 key cancer-associated genes and raw coverage of approximately 20,000× [14]. The process uses plasma for the cfDNA component and genomic DNA from leukocytes to serve as a germline control; they reported that 95% of mutations identified were called de novo without the need for paired tumor genomics [14]. Cancer personalized profiling by deep sequencing (CAPP-Seq) uses hybrid affinity capture with deep sequencing to detect ctDNA in a panel specific to a tumor type without knowledge of the patient's germline or somatic mutations [23]. The NSCLC panel integrates 139 recurrently mutated genes. Additional bioinformatic analysis to decrease recurrent background errors (integrated digital error suppression [iDES], "polishing") combined with molecular barcoding suppressed stereotypical and stochastic backgrounds, respectively. These methods were tested using longitudinal ctDNA samples from patients with NSCLC and showed a positive predictive value of 72% for detected hotspot single nucleotide variants (SNVs) confirmed by tumor biopsy as well as a sensitivity of 94% for activating mutations in *EGFR*, 91% for subclonal p.Thr790Met resistance mutations [24]. Chabon and colleagues investigated CAPP-Seq as a potential screening tool for NSCLC; machine learning was used to provide the likelihood of NSCLC (lung cancer likelihood in plasma), which was 98% specific with a sensitivity of 41%, 54%, and 67% in stage I, II, and III patients, respectively [5].

Developed to be a pan-cancer screening tool, methylation profiling of cfDNA has the potential to overcome some of the difficulties of MPS [25]. A targeted methylation panel that uses over 1 million cytosine-guanine dinucleotides does not appear to have interference from CH. In this method, tissue from the patient's tumor is not necessary as the assay uses a large database of methylation patterns to identify cancer ctDNA and match to a particular cancer type.

Studies using this assay were able to achieve a specificity of 99.3% and sensitivity of 67.3% in 12 common cancer types; overall, sensitivity was 18% in all cancer types [26]. The initial findings were achieved using 2 tubes of plasma per participant, but were reduced to 1 tube of plasma in the validation study [26,27]. Global methylation profiling of ctDNA in the central nervous system (CNS) is an emerging field that may have significant utility. Profiling of ctDNA from CNS lesions introduces an additional variable in the form of the blood–brain barrier. Even with this barrier, advancing technologies are allowing researchers to make strides in the analysis of blood samples from patients with glioma for methylation profiling of CNS neoplasms [28–35].

Standardization of ctDNA assays is certainly lacking and a one-size-fits-all model is unlikely to work for all solid tumors. A joint consensus recommendation from the Association for Molecular Pathology (AMP) and the College of American Pathologists (CAP) set 13 best practices for validating, reporting, and publishing clinical ctDNA assays [36]. Interestingly, in the authors' literature review, the analytical sensitivity, analytical specificity, and limit of detection were only reported in 47%, 30%, and 41% of ctDNA studies limiting their applicability for meta-analysis or clinical consideration [36].

SOLID TUMOR APPLICATIONS: NON-SMALL CELL LUNG CANCER AND BREAST CANCER

In many studies across different tumor types, if ctDNA is detected after definitive therapy, it is associated with recurrence. A meta-analysis including rectal, breast, gastric, and bladder cancer, reported the positive predictive value (PPV) and negative predictive value (NPV) of detectable ctDNA for residual disease after neoadjuvant therapy to be 82% to 100% and 11% to 79%, respectively [37]. Two hypothetical patient timelines and the potential benefits of using ctDNA monitoring are shown in Fig. 2. Guidelines for many tumor types include ctDNA; however, most guidelines recommend reflexing to tissue based testing when ctDNA testing yields a negative result due to the varying degrees of sensitivity. Here, we will focus on 2 of the more common tumor types: NSCLC and breast cancer.

NSCLC served as one of the first solid tumors where ctDNA was shown to have utility. The Cobas *EGFR* mutation test was the first liquid biopsy test approved by the United States Food and Drug Administration in 2016. Since that time, advances in NSCLC have been dramatic, owing largely to the development of therapy targeted to driver mutations and the inevitable development of resistance mutations. Studies have shown that undetectable ctDNA after neoadjuvant treatment was significantly associated with progression-free survival and overall survival and was shown to outperform radiologic assessments [38]. The addition of ctDNA resulted in a 42% to 65% increase in actionable mutation detection including many patients who did not have adequate tissue for testing [39–41]. A consensus statement from the International Association for the Study of Lung Cancer (IASLC) supports plasma ctDNA as a source for genotyping in newly diagnosed patients and recommends using an MPS platform if available due to the growing number of guideline-recommended oncogene targets to be assessed [42]. In addition, progression after targeted therapy should use ctDNA prior to tissue biopsy for the detection of resistance alterations per IASLC; however, CAP and AMP recommendations are much more narrow and advocate the use of ctDNA when tissue is limited or hard to obtain for *EGFR* mutations [42,43]. ctDNA could also play a role in stratifying patients for selected treatments. Moding and colleagues reported that NSCLC patients with undetectable ctDNA after chemoradiation had excellent outcomes regardless of the use of a checkpoint inhibitor [44].

In a meta-analyses of ctDNA in breast cancer, elevated ctDNA was associated with a high risk of relapse in both early-stage and metastatic/locally advanced groups [45–47]. In patients with high-risk early breast cancer, lack of ctDNA clearance was a predictor of poor response and metastatic recurrence. Conversely, clearance of ctDNA was associated with improved survival even in patients who did not achieve pathologic complete response after neoadjuvant therapy [48]. However, complete pathologic response in breast cancer was not always associated with complete clearance of ctDNA [8,47]. In patients with detectable metastatic or recurrent breast cancer, the detection of ctDNA by ddPCR and sequencing wasused to both identify mutations in *PIK3CA*, *ESR1*, *ErbB2* (HER2), and *AKT1* and select patients for targeted therapy according to identified mutations [49]. The majority of these mutations were not confirmed with concurrent tumor biopsy, but those that were showed high concordance, and the targeted therapies were comparable to other studies using tumor tissue [49]. The American Society of Clinical Oncology guidelines in metastatic breast cancer for biomarkers supports the use of ctDNA to detect *PIK3CA* mutations; however, biopsy should be pursued if no mutation is identified. In addition, the committee found insufficient data to recommend routine use of ctDNA as of 2022 [50].

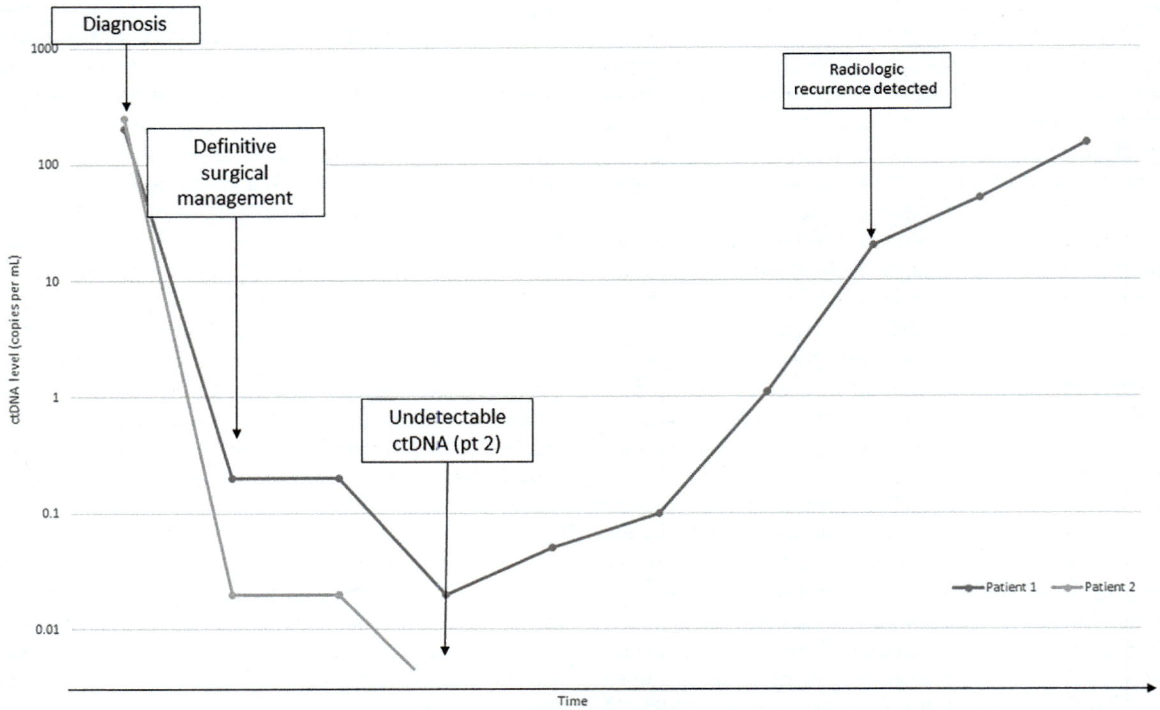

FIG. 2 Theoretical ctDNA levels over time for a patient with recurrence and without recurrence. ctDNA levels at diagnosis are typically high; however, after definitive surgery and during therapy, ctDNA levels are very low. Undetectable ctDNA in patient 2 could lead to treatment de-escalation while rising ctDNA in patient 1 could lead to alternative therapies prior to radiologic detection of recurrence. Depending on the limit of detection of the ctDNA assay, both patients may have undetectable ctDNA at certain time points.

One of the benefits of ctDNA is that the tumor, clones and subclones, and metastatic lesions are represented in the ctDNA. This has been leveraged for measuring tumor heterogeneity as well as amplified markers. Interestingly, tumor heterogeneity is increasingly being monitored by ctDNA; patients with breast cancer with high tumor heterogeneity in ctDNA had significantly worse progression free survival than those with low heterogeneity [51]. HER2-amplification in breast tumors treated with chemotherapy has been shown to be discordant between primary tumor and metastases in up to a quarter of cases resulting in testing the primary tumor and any metastatic or recurrent lesions [52]. Dynamic monitoring of HER2 status using ctDNA may aid therapeutic response monitoring as the concordance rate between ctDNA and tumor is greater than 80% [53]. In HER2-positive solid tumors (nonbreast, nongastric), HER2 amplification was detected from ctDNA analysis of baseline plasma samples in 85% of patients and the copy number from ctDNA analysis was concordant with results from tissue sequencing in 89% [54]. Many nonbreast tumors display tumor heterogeneity with HER2 immunohistochemistry (IHC) and fluorescence in situ hybridization results, raising the question of whether ctDNA may be the better suited assay for HER2 heterogenous tumors as there may be less sampling bias.

DISCUSSION

In an ideal situation, ctDNA would be sensitive enough to detect alterations in tumor cells related to therapy and prognosis without the need for invasive biopsies. As of this writing, many techniques can be utilized to achieve this desired outcome with considerations summarized in Fig. 3. In MRD testing, ctDNA could provide considerable lead time over imaging or biochemical markers. However, an important consideration for solid tumors is whether the detection of disease by ctDNA and early treatment initiation based on ctDNA results improves patient outcomes in prospective trials. Avoidance of overtreatment is challenging as an abnormal result is

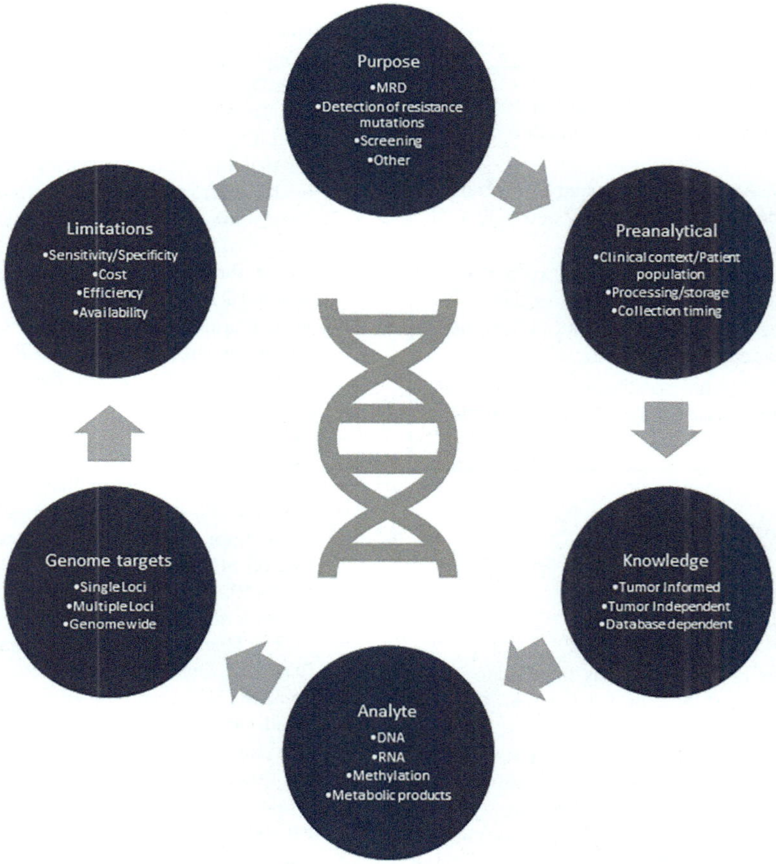

FIG. 3 Considerations and options for ctDNA testing. The purpose, preanalytical factors, methods, analytes, targets, and limitations are the main considerations when planning and utilizing a ctDNA assay.

often the trigger to procedures, increased follow-up, and more testing. Cancer screening is another area in which ctDNA could become a potential solution, but the area has much growth to be seen in the future.

False-negative and false-positive results are reported in most studies [8,37,54–56]. Patients who harbor detectable ctDNA, but do not recur in the study time frame may represent false-positive results due to sequencing errors, overcalling of a clonal process, or a small subset of tumor cells that do not form a detectable recurrence within the study time frame. There is evidence that in situ lesions contribute to positive ctDNA results; however, this area of ctDNA detection requires more study [8]. False-negative results are seen when the patient has no detectable ctDNA, but overt metastatic lesions are present. Generally, the level of ctDNA is high in patients with large tumors or metastatic disease, but lower in patients with early-stage disease. For tumor-informed methods, the knowledge of many specific alterations leads to increased sensitivity whereas tumor-independent methods increase sensitivity with depth of sequencing or targets. The cause of these false negatives can be lack of assay sensitivity, tumor heterogeneity, or stochastic sampling.

SUMMARY

The impact of ctDNA is being realized by many clinicians and pathologists. The field continues to make improvements, and ctDNA monitoring is being incorporated into many clinical trials. Choosing the appropriate testing for the patient in question is critical, and molecular tumor boards are indispensable in assisting the clinician with appropriate interpretation of results as the limitations of ctDNA testing may not be readily apparent [57,58]. It is no longer a question of ctDNA feasibility, but a question of the methods and necessary sensitivity.

CLINICS CARE POINTS

- Circulating tumor (ctDNA) is composed of fragments of a tumor's DNA at varying levels within the cell-free DNA fraction.
- Detection of ctDNA may provide valuable lead time over the development of radiologically detectable lesions.
- Tumor-informed ctDNA detection methods are more sensitive, however, tumor-independent ctDNA methods may detect the development of new mutations including resistance mutations.
- Although most assays are specific, many lack sensitivity and false negatives remain an area of concern.

DISCLOSURE

The authors have nothing to disclose.

REFERENCES

[1] Mandel P, Metais P. [Nuclear Acids In Human Blood Plasma]. C R Seances Soc Biol Fil 1948;142(3–4):241–3.

[2] Snyder MW, Kircher M, Hill AJ, et al. Cell-free DNA Comprises an In Vivo Nucleosome Footprint that Informs Its Tissues-Of-Origin. Cell 2016;164(1–2):57–68.

[3] Kim J, Hong SP, Lee S, et al. Multidimensional fragmentomic profiling of cell-free DNA released from patient-derived organoids. Hum Genomics 2023;17(1):96.

[4] Jahr S, Hentze H, Englisch S, et al. DNA fragments in the blood plasma of cancer patients: quantitations and evidence for their origin from apoptotic and necrotic cells. Cancer Res 2001;61(4):1659–65.

[5] Chabon JJ, Hamilton EG, Kurtz DM, et al. Integrating genomic features for non-invasive early lung cancer detection. Nature 2020;580(7802):245–51.

[6] Volik S, Alcaide M, Morin RD, et al. Cell-free DNA (cfDNA): Clinical Significance and Utility in Cancer Shaped By Emerging Technologies. Mol Cancer Res MCR 2016;14(10):898–908.

[7] Heitzer E, Haque IS, Roberts CES, et al. Current and future perspectives of liquid biopsies in genomics-driven oncology. Nat Rev Genet 2019;20(2):71–88.

[8] McDonald BR, Contente-Cuomo T, Sammut SJ, et al. Personalized circulating tumor DNA analysis to detect residual disease after neoadjuvant therapy in breast cancer. Sci Transl Med 2019;11(504):eaax7392.

[9] Bronkhorst AJ, Aucamp J, Pretorius PJ. Cell-free DNA: Preanalytical variables. Clin Chim Acta 2015;450:243–53.

[10] Chen H, Zhou Q. Detecting liquid remnants of solid tumors treated with curative intent: Circulating tumor DNA as a biomarker of minimal residual disease (Review). Oncol Rep 2023;49(5):106.

[11] Jiang P, Lo YMD. The Long and Short of Circulating Cell-Free DNA and the Ins and Outs of Molecular Diagnostics. Trends Genet 2016;32(6):360–71.

[12] Wan JCM, Heider K, Gale D, et al. ctDNA monitoring using patient-specific sequencing and integration of variant reads. Sci Transl Med 2020;12(548):eaaz8084.

[13] Openshaw MR, Page K, Fernandez-Garcia D, et al. The role of ctDNA detection and the potential of the liquid biopsy for breast cancer monitoring. Expert Rev Mol Diagn 2016;16(7):751–5.

[14] Rose Brannon A, Jayakumaran G, Diosdado M, et al. Enhanced specificity of clinical high-sensitivity tumor mutation profiling in cell-free DNA via paired normal sequencing using MSK-ACCESS. Nat Commun 2021;12(1):3770.

[15] Jaiswal S, Ebert BL. Clonal hematopoiesis in human aging and disease. Science 2019;366(6465):eaan4673.

[16] Hindson BJ, Ness KD, Masquelier DA, et al. High-throughput droplet digital PCR system for absolute quantitation of DNA copy number. Anal Chem 2011;83(22):8604–10.

[17] Galimberti S, Balducci S, Guerrini F, et al. Digital Droplet PCR in Hematologic Malignancies: A New Useful Molecular Tool. Diagn Basel Switz 2022;12(6):1305.

[18] Tarazona N, Gimeno-Valiente F, Gambardella V, et al. Targeted next-generation sequencing of circulating-tumor DNA for tracking minimal residual disease in localized colon cancer. Ann Oncol 2019;30(11):1804–12.

[19] Phallen J, Sausen M, Adleff V, et al. Direct detection of early-stage cancers using circulating tumor DNA. Sci Transl Med 2017;9(403):eaan2415.

[20] Zviran A, Schulman RC, Shah M, et al. Genome-wide cell-free DNA mutational integration enables ultra-sensitive cancer monitoring. Nat Med 2020;26(7):1114–24.

[21] Tie J, Cohen JD, Wang Y, et al. Circulating Tumor DNA Analyses as Markers of Recurrence Risk and Benefit of Adjuvant Therapy for Stage III Colon Cancer. JAMA Oncol 2019;5(12):1710–7.

[22] Tie J, Wang Y, Cohen J, et al. Circulating tumor DNA dynamics and recurrence risk in patients undergoing curative intent resection of colorectal cancer liver metastases: A prospective cohort study. PLoS Med 2021;18(5):e1003620.

[23] Newman AM, Bratman SV, To J, et al. An ultrasensitive method for quantitating circulating tumor DNA with broad patient coverage. Nat Med 2014;20(5):548–54.

[24] Newman AM, Lovejoy AF, Klass DM, et al. Integrated digital error suppression for improved detection of circulating tumor DNA. Nat Biotechnol 2016;34(5):547–55.

[25] Jamshidi A, Liu MC, Klein EA, et al. Evaluation of cell-free DNA approaches for multi-cancer early detection. Cancer Cell 2022;40(12):1537–49.e12.

[26] Liu MC, Oxnard GR, Klein EA, et al. Sensitive and specific multi-cancer detection and localization using methylation signatures in cell-free DNA. Ann Oncol Off J Eur Soc Med Oncol 2020;31(6):745–59.

[27] Klein EA, Richards D, Cohn A, et al. Clinical validation of a targeted methylation-based multi-cancer early detection test using an independent validation set. Ann Oncol Off J Eur Soc Med Oncol 2021;32(9):1167–77.
[28] Trivedi R, Bhat KP. Liquid biopsy: creating opportunities in brain space. Br J Cancer 2023;129(11):1727–46.
[29] Soffietti R, Bettegowda C, Mellinghoff IK, et al. Liquid biopsy in gliomas: A RANO review and proposals for clinical applications. Neuro Oncol 2022;24(6):855–71.
[30] Lo YMD, Han DSC, Jiang P, et al. Epigenetics, fragmentomics, and topology of cell-free DNA in liquid biopsies. Science 2021;372(6538):eaaw3616.
[31] Dolgin E. Blood Test Catches Cancers That Shed Little DNA. Cancer Discov 2020;10(9):1246–7.
[32] Nassiri F, Chakravarthy A, Feng S, et al. Detection and discrimination of intracranial tumors using plasma cell-free DNA methylomes. Nat Med 2020;26(7):1044–7.
[33] Johnson KC, Verhaak RGW. Serum cell-free DNA epigenetic biomarkers aid glioma diagnostics and monitoring. Neuro Oncol 2021;23(9):1423–4.
[34] Shen SY, Singhania R, Fehringer G, et al. Sensitive tumour detection and classification using plasma cell-free DNA methylomes. Nature 2018;563(7732):579–83.
[35] Sabedot TS, Malta TM, Snyder J, et al. A serum-based DNA methylation assay provides accurate detection of glioma. Neuro Oncol 2021;23(9):1494–508.
[36] Lockwood CM, Borsu L, Cankovic M, et al. Recommendations for Cell-Free DNA Assay Validations. J Mol Diagn 2023;25(12):876–97.
[37] Gögenur M, Hadi NAH, Qvortrup C, et al. ctDNA for Risk of Recurrence Assessment in Patients Treated with Neoadjuvant Treatment: A Systematic Review and Meta-analysis. Ann Surg Oncol 2022;29(13):8666–74.
[38] Provencio M, Serna-Blasco R, Nadal E, et al. Overall Survival and Biomarker Analysis of Neoadjuvant Nivolumab Plus Chemotherapy in Operable Stage IIIA Non-Small-Cell Lung Cancer (NADIM phase II trial). J Clin Oncol 2022;40(25):2924–33.
[39] Mack PC, Banks KC, Espenschied CR, et al. Spectrum of driver mutations and clinical impact of circulating tumor DNA analysis in non–small cell lung cancer: Analysis of over 8000 cases. Cancer 2020;126(14):3219–28.
[40] Page RD, Drusbosky LM, Dada H, et al. Clinical Outcomes for Plasma-Based Comprehensive Genomic Profiling Versus Standard-of-Care Tissue Testing in Advanced Non-Small Cell Lung Cancer. Clin Lung Cancer 2022;23(1):72–81.
[41] Wang HY, Ho CC, Lin YT, et al. Comprehensive Genomic Analysis of Patients With Non-Small-Cell Lung Cancer Using Blood-Based Circulating Tumor DNA Assay: Findings From the BFAST Database of a Single Center in Taiwan. JCO Precis Oncol 2024;8:e2300314.
[42] Rolfo C, Mack P, Scagliotti GV, et al. Liquid Biopsy for Advanced NSCLC: A Consensus Statement From the International Association for the Study of Lung Cancer. J Thorac Oncol 2021;16(10):1647–62.
[43] Lindeman NI, Cagle PT, Aisner DL, et al. Updated Molecular Testing Guideline for the Selection of Lung Cancer Patients for Treatment With Targeted Tyrosine Kinase Inhibitors: Guideline From the College of American Pathologists, the International Association for the Study of Lung Cancer, and the Association for Molecular Pathology. Arch Pathol Lab Med 2018;142(3):321–46.
[44] Moding EJ, Liu Y, Nabet BY, et al. Circulating Tumor DNA Dynamics Predict Benefit from Consolidation Immunotherapy in Locally Advanced Non-Small Cell Lung Cancer. Nat Cancer 2020;1(2):176–83.
[45] Cullinane C, Fleming C, O'Leary DP, et al. Association of Circulating Tumor DNA With Disease-Free Survival in Breast Cancer: A Systematic Review and Meta-analysis. JAMA Netw Open 2020;3(11):e2026921.
[46] Lee JH, Jeong H, Choi JW, et al. Liquid biopsy prediction of axillary lymph node metastasis, cancer recurrence, and patient survival in breast cancer: A meta-analysis. Medicine (Baltimore) 2018;97(42):e12862.
[47] Papakonstantinou A, Gonzalez NS, Pimentel I, et al. Prognostic value of ctDNA detection in patients with early breast cancer undergoing neoadjuvant therapy: A systematic review and meta-analysis. Cancer Treat Rev 2022;104:102362.
[48] Magbanua MJM, Swigart LB, Wu HT, et al. Circulating tumor DNA in neoadjuvant-treated breast cancer reflects response and survival. Ann Oncol Off J Eur Soc Med Oncol 2021;32(2):229–39.
[49] Turner NC, Kingston B, Kilburn LS, et al. Circulating tumour DNA analysis to direct therapy in advanced breast cancer (plasmaMATCH): a multicentre, multicohort, phase 2a, platform trial. Lancet Oncol 2020; 21(10):1296–308.
[50] Henry NL, Somerfield MR, Dayao Z, et al. Biomarkers for Systemic Therapy in Metastatic Breast Cancer: ASCO Guideline Update. J Clin Oncol 2022;40(27):3205–21.
[51] Ma F, Guan Y, Yi Z, et al. Assessing tumor heterogeneity using ctDNA to predict and monitor therapeutic response in metastatic breast cancer. Int J Cancer 2020; 146(5):1359–68.
[52] Niikura N, Liu J, Hayashi N, et al. Loss of human epidermal growth factor receptor 2 (HER2) expression in metastatic sites of HER2-overexpressing primary breast tumors. J Clin Oncol 2012;30(6):593–9.
[53] Guan X, Liu B, Niu Y, et al. Longitudinal HER2 amplification tracked in circulating tumor DNA for therapeutic effect monitoring and prognostic evaluation in patients with breast cancer. Breast Edinb Scotl 2020;49:261–6.
[54] Hyung J, Lee JY, Kim JE, et al. Safety and efficacy of trastuzumab biosimilar plus irinotecan or gemcitabine in patients with previously treated HER2 (ERBB2)-positive non-breast/non-gastric solid tumors: a phase II basket trial with circulating tumor DNA analysis. ESMO Open 2023;8(3):101583.
[55] Turner NC, Swift C, Jenkins B, et al. Results of the c-TRAK TN trial: a clinical trial utilising ctDNA mutation tracking to detect molecular residual disease and

trigger intervention in patients with moderate- and high-risk early-stage triple-negative breast cancer. Ann Oncol Off J Eur Soc Med Oncol 2023;34(2): 200–11.

[56] Chiu J, Su F, Joshi M, et al. Potential value of ctDNA monitoring in metastatic HR +/HER2 - breast cancer: longitudinal ctDNA analysis in the phase Ib MONALEESASIA trial. BMC Med 2023;21(1):306.

[57] Rolfo C, Manca P, Salgado R, et al. Multidisciplinary molecular tumour board: a tool to improve clinical practice and selection accrual for clinical trials in patients with cancer. ESMO Open 2018;3(5):e000398.

[58] Kato S, Kim KH, Lim HJ, et al. Real-world data from a molecular tumor board demonstrates improved outcomes with a precision N-of-One strategy. Nat Commun 2020;11(1):4965.

Advances in Molecular Pathology 7 (2024) 165–173
ADVANCES IN MOLECULAR PATHOLOGY

Detection of Germline Structural Variants Using Short-Read Whole-Genome Sequencing

Lucilla Pizzo, MS, PhD[a,b], Erica F. Andersen, PhD[b,c], Hunter Best, PhD[a,b,*]
[a]Department of Pathology, University of Utah School of Medicine, Salt Lake City, UT, USA; [b]ARUP Laboratories, 500 Chipeta Way, MS #115, Salt Lake City, UT 84108, USA; [c]Cytogenetics and Genomic Microarray, Department of Pathology, University of Utah School of Medicine, Salt Lake City, UT, USA

KEYWORDS
• Structural variant • SV • Copy-number variant • CNV • Read signatures

KEY POINTS

- Structural variants (SVs) are associated with a wide variety of human genetic conditions, and polymerase chain reaction-free based whole-genome sequencing has the potential to identify clinically relevant SVs.
- Distinctive read patterns or "signatures" are diagnostic of different SV types; however, no single method consistently performs best across different SV types and sizes.
- Best practices outlined by expert groups emphasize rigorous validation, standardization protocols, and the incorporation of diverse reference samples to ensure accurate and reliable SV detection in clinical practice.
- Clinical laboratories should establish policies concerning confirmation using orthogonal methods, consider visualization using "digital karyogram" plots, and cytogenetic characterization of certain SV types.

INTRODUCTION

Structural variants (SVs) constitute a diverse category of genetic variation, generally exceeding 50 base pairs in size and extending to several megabase pairs. SVs include unbalanced copy-number variants (CNVs), such as deletions, duplications, and insertions, as well as balanced rearrangements including inversions, insertions, and translocations. The definition of SVs has evolved over time to encompass smaller events, as well as complex genomic rearrangements such as mobile element insertions, multiallelic CNVs, segmental duplications, and events involving combinations of the aforementioned variants.

SVs affect more base pairs of the genome than any other class of genomic variant [1,2]. In fact, whole-genome differences in sequence among individuals conferred by SVs have been estimated to be 3 to 10 times higher than that of single-nucleotide variants (SNVs) [3–5], thus explaining the vast diversity of genomes. Moreover, SVs are associated with a wide variety of human genetic conditions, including neurodevelopmental disorders [6,7] and cancer [8,9], underscoring the importance of their accurate identification in clinical genetics.

Genomic microarrays (GMAs) have been instrumental in the discovery of unbalanced genomic SVs, beginning with array-comparative genomic hybridization, which relies on the hybridization of differentially labeled test and reference samples to a set of hybridization targets. This method resulted in the discovery of approximately 300 regions of variable copy number in the genomes of individuals from the general

*Corresponding author. 500 Chipeta Way, MS #115, Salt Lake City, UT 84108. *E-mail address:* hunter.best@aruplab.com

https://doi.org/10.1016/j.yamp.2024.06.006 www.advancesinmolecularpathology.com
2589-4080/24/

population [10,11]. The evolution of array platforms from the use of bacterial artificial chromosome (BAC)-based to oligonucleotide probes, including simultaneous single-nucleotide polymorphism (SNP) interrogation, further improved sensitivity in detecting CNVs down to 10s to 100s of kb in size, significantly increasing estimates of CNV burden per genome [12,13], and leading the discovery of recurrent CNVs associated with neurodevelopmental disorders [6,7].

In 2007, the first report on the application of next-generation sequencing (NGS) technologies for the discovery of SVs was published [14]. Since then, the continuous decline in the cost of short-read sequencing approaches has broadened the application of this technology in research and contributed to the discovery of numerous methods for SV identification. Compared to catalogs solely constructed based on GMA data, the advent of NGS technologies has enabled the identification of SVs at higher resolution, along with the discovery of balanced SVs and novel insertions not previously cataloged in reference genomes, significantly advancing SV discovery over the past decade [15].

Various NGS-based applications in clinical genetics, including targeted gene panels, exome sequencing (ES), and whole-genome sequencing (WGS), have demonstrated different capacities in detecting balanced and unbalanced SVs. For instance, the detection of CNVs using high-depth-coverage gene panels has shown high sensitivity, but it is limited to those genes selected for targeting, and typically to exonic regions, thereby limiting resolution of CNV sizing and breakpoint determination [16–18]. Capture of coding regions of the genome using ES enables the detection of larger CNVs; nevertheless, its focus on coding regions also restricts precise breakpoint identification in intragenic or intergenic CNVs. Moreover, the capture-based methodology employed in both approaches results in variable sequencing coverage across genomic regions, thereby introducing additional challenges in copy-number detection.

WGS offers enhanced accuracy in breakpoints definition for unbalanced events and holds the potential to detect balanced structural rearrangements. However, technical aspects of short-read wet laboratory processes can also bias identification of CNVs. Trost and colleagues demonstrated that employing as low as 6 to 8 polymerase chain reaction (PCR) cycles could introduce bias in coverage, resulting in decreased uniformity of read depth and systemic PCR biases, potentially leading to false-positive CNVs [19]. PCR-free sequencing strategies mitigate enrichment bias in coverage, thereby minimizing technical artifacts that could result in false-positive events. Additional factors that may introduce bias in sequence coverage and limit SV detection and resolution are related to the complexity of the genome, repetitive sequences, homopolymeric regions, highly homologous regions, and regions with high GC content. In contrast to the relatively straightforward identification of SNVs during the discovery phase of NGS data analysis, the inherent attributes of SVs (ie, extended multiread span and alterations in genomic architecture) require more sophisticated bioinformatic analysis to achieve precise detection.

FOUR READ SIGNATURES CONTRIBUTE TO STRUCTURAL VARIANT DISCOVERY USING NEXT-GENERATION SEQUENCING DATA

The identification of SVs using NGS relies on mapping the sequence reads to a reference genome and identifying read patterns or "signatures" distinctive or diagnostic of different types of SVs.

The first strategy for the detection of SVs by NGS involves changes in read depth (Fig. 1A). This method was initially applied in the identification of gene rearrangements in cancer and segmental duplications in human genomes [2,20]. This method is based on the observation that NGS read depth is expected to follow a random Poisson or extended Poisson distribution [21–23]. Deviations from this distribution enable the identification of unbalanced events, with duplications expected to exhibit increased read depth and deletions to display reduced depth compared to the diploid reference genome. Read counts are usually computed in "analytical" bins, which refers to nonoverlapping regions of the genome, where the depth of sequencing is compared between the sequenced sample and reference samples or the whole genome. A deviation from the anticipated read depth in adjacent bins is usually a requisite to identify the presence of a CNV. The bin size may vary depending on the SV detection algorithm, thus it is directly related to the resolution of detected deletions and duplications. Many of the initial NGS SV algorithms were based on read depth, including CNVnator [24], CNV-seq [25], CoNIFER [26], and ERDS [27].

Another NGS-based SV calling method exploits the occurrence of split reads (see Fig. 1B). Split reads refer to sequences of reads that demonstrate characteristic splitting. For example, the observation of a read sequence aligning to 2 nonsequential regions relative to the reference genome may serve as evidence of the presence of a deletion involving the flanking sequence. Similarly, split reads can aid in identifying direct or inverted tandem duplications, and small insertions.

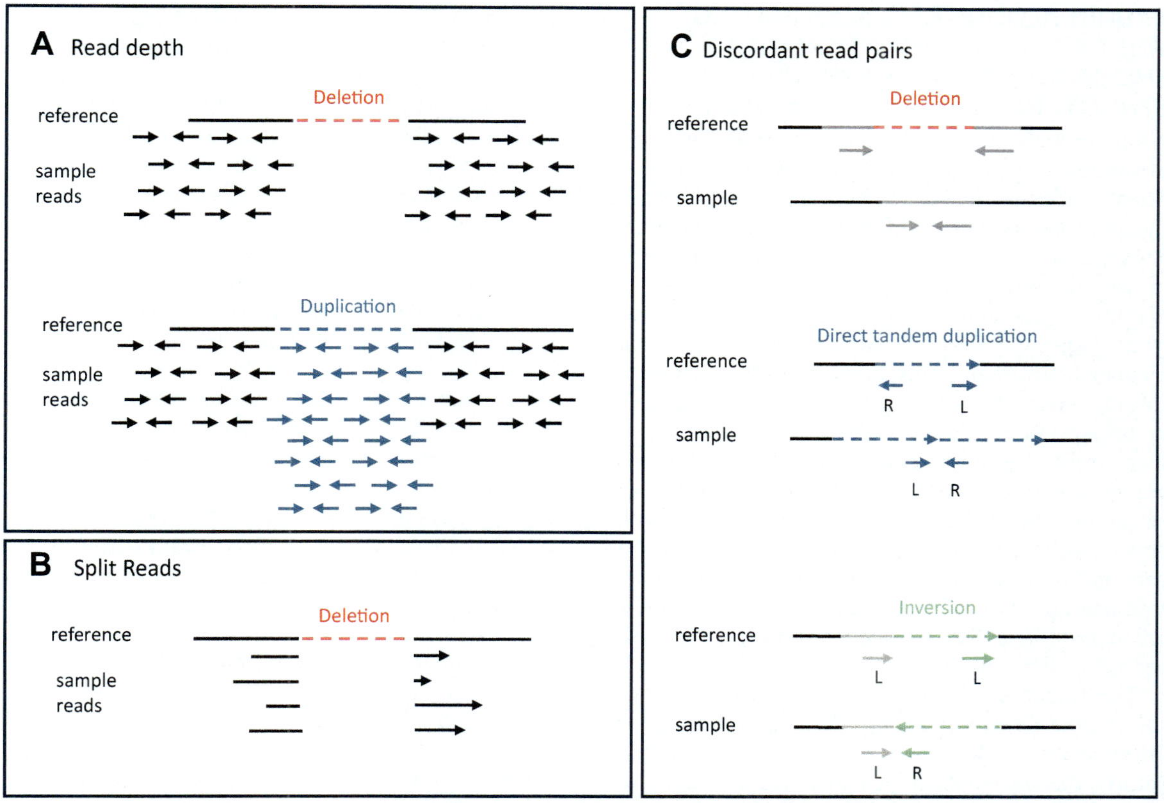

FIG. 1 Read signatures to identify SVs using short-read WGS data. (**A**) Read depth. Decreased or increased coverage is indicative of a deletion or duplication, respectively. (**B**) Split reads. Read sequence aligned to 2 regions of the reference genome can be indicative of a deletion of the genomic region flanked by the split reads. (**C**) Discordant read pairs. For each SV type: top panel shows sample reads aligned to reference genome; bottom panel represents sample reads showing expected orientation and distance. Aberrant distance and/or orientation of read pairs to a reference genome can be indicative of different SVs. Deletions represented in red, duplications in blue, inversions in green, flanking regions to SVs in gray. L, left-oriented read; R, right-oriented read.

This read signature holds the potential for single-base pair resolution and has been demonstrated to be highly useful in defining breakpoints of SVs. SV algorithms exclusively utilizing split-read features include Pindel [28] and SVseq2 [29].

SV detection approaches based on discordant read pairs (see Fig. 1C) assess both the distance and the orientation of paired-end reads, clustering pairs in which their distance and/or orientation deviates from what is expected in the reference genome [30]. For instance, read pairs mapping too far apart compared to the anticipated distance in the reference genome are a signature of deletions. Additionally, observing right-to-left orientation of read pairs in contrast to the expected left-to-right orientation can be indicative of tandem direct duplications. Similarly, pairs in right-to-right or left-to-left orientation might signify inversions. This method not only enhances confidence in SV prediction but also aids in more accurately delineating breakpoints and event size. BreakDancer [31] and PEMer [32] are examples of algorithms that solely rely on discordant read pairs for SV detection.

A fourth approach to SV detection involves the de novo assembly method [33], where read information is consolidated into contigs that are then aligned either to another assembly or a reference genome. SVs are subsequently identified through systematic comparisons to detect variations between the sequences. This approach has primarily been utilized in a research context to discover novel SV sequences within the human genome.

HYBRID ALGORITHMS INTEGRATING MULTIPLE READ SIGNATURES AND ENSEMBLE METHODS IMPROVE STRUCTURAL VARIANT DETECTION

While recognizing a read signature can raise suspicion of various SV types, a single feature is usually not sufficient to identify an SV with high specificity. Each read signature approach has different strengths and weaknesses, depending on the variant type or the properties of the underlying sequence at the SV locus. For example, read-depth-based methods excel in identifying large CNVs, such as segmental-duplication-mediated recurrent CNVs or aneuploidies. However, coverage-based algorithms often exhibit low accuracy in breakpoint resolution. Conversely, balanced SVs, such as inversions, or smaller CNVs (<5 kbp) may not be identified by read-depth approaches but can be successfully identified with high accuracy in breakpoint resolution using split-read or discordant read pair approaches. Of note, split-read and discordant read pair approaches have limited utility in identifying unbalanced large SV and perform poorly in repetitive regions of the genome.

The limitation of individual read signature methods spurred the development of hybrid algorithms, which integrate and combine evidence from multiple read signatures, thereby enhancing the identification and precision of SV calls. Examples of hybrid SV algorithms include DELLY [34], Manta [35], and LUMPY [36]. Another approach to enhance sensitivity and specificity in SV calling involved applying multiple independent algorithms and integrating and combining their variant calls as part of the unique output of an "ensemble algorithm." With this approach, it becomes possible to maximize the strengths of each of the callers, and the results are combined and integrated using different principles, such as assessing the confidence interval of the breakpoints or prioritization of calls identified by different read signatures.

A recently described ensemble algorithm, Parliament2 [37], employs any combination of 6 SV calling programs, including single-feature callers (Breakdancer [31] and CNVnator [24]), hybrid callers (DELLY [34], LUMPY [36], and Manta [35]) as well as Breakseq, an algorithm based on aligning raw reads directly onto SV breakpoint junctions of nonreference alleles from a library containing previously-identified SVs [38]. SVs identified by each caller are consolidated into a unified set and genotyped. Based on the performance by each individual caller to identify established SVs in the HG002 (also known as NA24385) reference genome, Parliament2 assigns quality values of each SV call coming from different algorithms, which are displayed as Phred quality scores to the user. Similarly, MetaSV [39], another ensemble algorithm, incorporates and merges calls from Breakseq [38], Breakdancer [31], CNVnator [24], and Pindel [28], and includes soft-clip analysis. MetaSV prioritizes read signatures with higher resolution in its output (eg, split reads over discordant read pairs), and designates SV calls as either high or low confidence based on their overlap detection by different SV algorithms. High-confidence calls then undergo breakpoint resolution refinement through local assembly.

Another method for enhancing precision and recall of SVs involves the implementation of artificial intelligence (AI)-based tools in short-read WGS or ES. CN-Learn, a machine-learning algorithm designed for identifying CNVs using ES data, consolidates calls from different methods and extracts features from a truth set after training a random forest classifier to recognize true calls [40]. The authors demonstrate the superiority of machine-learning-based methods over Venn-diagram-intersection approaches in identifying high-confidence CNVs, as approximately 50% of the true calls identified were detected by at least one caller. FusorSV [41], a data-mining approach built from short-read WGS, incorporates 8 SV algorithms (BreakDancer [31], BreakSeq2, cnMOPS [42], CNVnator [24], DELLY [34], GenomeSTRiP [43], Hydra [44], and LUMPY [36]) and follows a data-mining approach to characterize the performance of the SV callers against a given truth sequencing set to identify the highest performing ensemble. Cue, a recently developed deep learning-based caller for SV detection, reframes the variant detection approach by transforming sequence alignments into images that capture alignment signals [45]. Subsequently, a trained neural network is employed to generate confidence maps containing the location, type, and genotype of the SVs, ultimately refining and mapping high-confidence SVs to the genome. Employing this strategy, the authors demonstrate Cue's capability to detect deletions, duplications, inversions, and inverted duplications flanked by deletions larger than 5 kb.

ESTABLISHED STRUCTURAL VARIANT BENCHMARKS AND GENERAL POPULATION COHORTS

In recent years, there has been an increasing availability of reference samples for improving accuracy in SV

detection, accompanied by enhancements in sample size, depth, and diversity. However, there is still a notable disparity in the availability of high-quality reference sets for SV detection compared to SNVs. Given the challenges associated with accurately identifying SVs using short-read NGS technologies, useful benchmark reference samples must incorporate multiple orthogonal platforms to adequately describe variation.

Well-characterized reference materials available for the validation of germline SV variants in clinical laboratories include the National Institute of Standards and Technology (NIST) NA12878, the curated sample of a white-ancestry female individual [46,47], which has been extensively studied using PacBio, Oxford Nanopore, and Bionano Optical Genome Mapping. Another high-quality set comprises the Genome in a Bottle (GIAB) Han Chinese trio [48,49] (HG005, HG006, and HG007) and the GIAB Ashkenazi family trio [50] (HG002, HG003, and HG004). These sets have been curated using various orthogonal technologies, including Illumina short-read, Complete Genomics, Ion Proton, Bionano Optical Genome Mapping, and PacBio. The Han Chinese and Ashkenazi family trios sequencing data combine the identification of more than 59,000 deletions and 12,000 insertions. Additionally, the Human Genome Structural Variation Consortium conducted multiplatform curation on trios of Han Chinese, Puerto Rican, and Yoruban Nigerian ancestries, identifying over 100,000 SVs [51].

Including any of the aforementioned reference samples in the validation process of any clinical SV application can aid in estimating sensitivity and specificity calculations. Ideally, laboratories should utilize multiple reference sets in clinical validation of SV identification using WGS [15]. Within the Medical Genome Initiative group, member laboratories reported the use of SV benchmark sample NA12878, along with the variable use of reference samples of Ashkenazi Jewish and Chinese ancestry trios from the Personal Genome Project [52].

The cataloging of SVs from general population cohorts has also significantly increased in recent years. The 1000 Genomes Project [53] was one of the earliest initiatives, in which individuals from European, Han Chinese, Japanese, and Yoruban Nigerian populations were sequenced, with SVs identified using an ensemble of multiple SV detection algorithms. A later release of this project involved the use of short-read WGS data on 2504 individuals from 26 populations and orthogonal techniques (including long-read sequencing data) to identify a wide spectrum of balanced and unbalanced SVs, including deletions, duplications, inversions, multiallelic CNVs, nuclear mitochondrial insertions, and mobile element insertions [4]. This project estimated that on average, an individual harbors approximately 20 million bp affected by SVs per diploid genome.

Subsequent studies have further expanded the number of individuals and the spectrum of SVs identified through WGS technologies. Abel and colleagues [54] interrogated approximately 18,000 human genomes and observed a mean of 4442 high-confidence SVs per human genome. The authors estimated that, on average, individuals carry 2.9 rare coding SVs, which account for 4.0% to 11.2% of rare high-impact coding alleles. They estimated that SVs account for 17.2% of rare alleles in the genome, and approximately 2% of individuals carry ultrarare large SVs, which comprise balanced and complex rearrangements. Collins and colleagues [55], as part of the Genome Aggregation Database (gnomAD v2.1.1), systematically processed data from approximately 15,000 individuals and detected 433,371 SVs using an ensemble of 4 algorithms (Manta [35], DELLY [34], MELT [56], and cnMOPS [57]). They observed an average of 8202 SVs per human genome. The latest release of gnomAD (v4, released November 2023) included 2 SV datasets identified from 63,046 genomes and from 464,297 exomes (CNVs only). Applying the GATK-SV caller to the WGS dataset, the authors identified a total of approximately 1.2 million SVs, with a median of 11,844 SVs per genome [55].

CONSIDERATIONS FOR THE IDENTIFICATION OF STRUCTURAL VARIANTS IN CLINICAL GENOMICS

As of this writing, more than 80 SV callers have been published [58], and the list continues to grow. Multiple studies have assessed the performance of SV callers [59]. For example, Kosugi and colleagues studied the performance of 69 SV algorithms and observed that the combination of algorithms, rather than the combination of read signature methods used in the algorithm, affected the precision and recall of overlapping SV calls [58]. Moreover, the authors observed that different SV detection algorithms perform better toward specific types and/or sizes of SVs. Gabrielaite and colleagues [60] reviewed 50 CNV calling tools and directly evaluated 11 tools to identify the most reliable clinically applicable algorithms for CNV detection by using variants identified by SNP-array as a gold standard. The authors observed that algorithms varied greatly in the number of CNVs identified and exhibited bias toward different CNV lengths. Some tools had high recall of CNVs from arrays for some samples, but poor precision. Both studies observed that no single algorithm could consistently perform with high sensitivity/specificity and across different SV types and sizes. Other sources of variation have been reported across SV algorithms, including mapping methods, sequencing centers, and replicates [61].

The large number of available SV callers underscores the fact that no single method is considered the "best". This is further illustrated by the wide distribution of citations for individual SV callers where the most cited algorithm comprises only 12% of overall citations [19]. Therefore, the question that arises when attempting to implement SV identification using clinical WGS is what is the optimal approach to pursue?

In 2020, Marshall and colleagues, representing the Medical Genome Initiative, outlined best practices for the analytical validation of WGS and recommended that short-read clinical WGS should include the analysis and interpretation of CNVs [52]. Austin-Tse and colleagues, representing the same group, reported best practices for the interpretation and reporting of WGS [62]. They suggested that due to the reduced specificity of SV algorithms and limited understanding of balanced SV variation in the general population, SV methods should be confined to supporting CNV identification and improving breakpoint detection for CNVs identified using read depth-based methods. While balanced SVs could be detected, their recommendation was to limit identification to either established recurrent and pathogenic balanced SVs (eg, the *F8* gene inversion) or known familial balanced SVs.

Marshall and colleagues also summarized the experiences of clinical laboratories in validating WGS for the detection of CNVs [52]. Depending on the laboratory, 7 to 42 positive GMA-derived samples were utilized as positive controls. Among these, a variety of well-described autosomal CNV regions were included, such as 1p, 4p, 9q, 22q terminal regions, and recurrent interstitial CNVs including 7q11.23, 15q13.3, 16p11.2, 16p13.11, 17q21.31, and 22q11.2.

In a recent document from the American College of Medical Genetics and Genomics, Raca and colleagues recommended that NGS-based test validation should encompass a sufficient number of samples, covering every type of SV intended to be reported, and the size range for each type of reportable SV should be defined [63]. For CNV validation, the authors suggested testing at least 30 samples with well-characterized CNVs, representing various genomic regions (including those with differing GC content and complexities), and exhibiting diverse mechanisms (such as segmental duplication mediated recurrent vs nonrecurrent CNVs), sizes, and copy number states. They further recommended that laboratories should focus on achieving high concordance (>95%) between the method selected during validation and the gold standard for clinically significant CNVs. However, they also cautioned that the percentage of reciprocal overlap of CNVs identified by different methods may vary, necessitating stricter filters for genome-to-genome comparisons compared to genome-to-genomic SNP microarray comparisons. Additionally, the authors suggested establishing orthogonal confirmation policies for variant detection, which may involve cytogenetics or molecular methods such as chromosome analysis, fluorescence in situ hybridization, GMA, or MLPA.

As part of the annotation and filtering practices for SVs, multiple groups have agreed upon prioritizing quality metrics, population frequency, overlap with protein-coding genes, overlap with patient's phenotype, and incorporating inheritance information [62,63]. Ideally, allele frequency should be determined using both internal laboratory datasets, where samples were processed using a common SV identification method, and external publicly available datasets derived from WGS (such as gnomAD-SV [55], 1000 Genomes Project [4], or Icelandic SV derived from long-read sequencing [64]), as well as GMA (Database of Genomic Variants [65]). Reciprocal overlap ranges should ideally fall between 50% and 90%. Raca and colleagues posited that SVs observed with an allele frequency of 1% or greater are generally benign and can potentially be eliminated from further consideration. However, due to the high variability of breakpoint detection by different algorithms (even within the same family), recommendations include the use of a 1 kb buffer when filtering for protein-coding regions to ensure the capture of clinically relevant variants [62].

Another consistent recommendation from expert groups is to incorporate visualization of CNV calls using depth-based and B-allele frequency representations. This can be helpful in evaluating large rearrangements and visualizing potential cytogenetic mechanisms [62,63]. Raca and colleagues also recommended that laboratories establish a policy clarifying which variants need confirmation using an orthogonal method and which ones can be reported directly using short-read-based NGS calling [63]. Furthermore, the authors noted that cytogenetic evaluation of certain SVs, such as aneuploidies of acrocentric chromosomes should be performed to determine if a balanced rearrangement such as a Robertsonian translocation is involved, as this impacts recurrence risk counseling. Similarly, other SVs, such as terminal CNVs suggestive of unbalanced translocations, recombinants, or ring chromosomes, and findings suggestive of mosaic chromosomal abnormalities such as 45,X and its variants, isodicentric, ring or marker chromosomes should be cytogenetically characterized for an accurate interpretation and to provide an appropriate guidance for follow-up testing.

DISCUSSION

The identification of SVs has evolved with the incorporation of NGS technologies. This technology has the potential to enable higher resolution and can identify a broader spectrum of variants compared to earlier catalogs solely based on GMA. Multiple algorithms have been described for the identification of SVs using short-read NGS technologies, from single-feature callers to AI-based multicaller methods. Each approach presents distinct strengths and limitations and the translation of SV detection technologies into clinical practice necessitates rigorous validation and standardization protocols to ensure accurate and reliable results.

However, as illustrated by the variety of orthogonal methods used for an accurate identification of SVs in genome assembly benchmark samples, no single technology has been shown to accurately identify all SV in the genome [15]. Emerging approaches are combining multiple platforms, integrating short-read and/or long-read sequencing, and newer methods such as optical genome mapping, to improve SV discovery in constitutional disease and cancer [50].

Best practices outlined by expert groups emphasize the importance of incorporating diverse reference samples and validation sets that encompass the various types and sizes of SVs. Recommendations include defining size ranges for each SV type, achieving high concordance between detection methods and gold standards, and establishing confirmation policies using orthogonal methods. Future studies should address challenges associated with standardization, data visualization, interpretation, and reporting practices. Collaboration among clinical laboratories and ongoing evaluation of SV detection methodologies are essential for advancing the standardization and validation of detection, as well as interpretation of SV in clinical practice.

SUMMARY

SVs, including unbalanced CNVs such as deletions, duplications, and insertions, as well as balanced rearrangements (ie, inversions and translocations) affect more base pairs of the genome than any other variant class. SVs play a crucial role in human genetic conditions, and therefore, their identification in clinical genetics is of significant interest. The advent of NGS has led to improved resolution SV identification, enabling the detection of balanced SVs and novel insertions not previously cataloged. The uniform coverage of PCR-free short-read WGS promises improved resolution of copy-number and potentially balanced SVs along with routine SNV detection in the clinical setting.

The identification of SVs using NGS relies on distinctive read patterns or "signatures" indicative of different SV types. These include changes in read depth, split reads, discordant read pairs, and sequence assembly methods. Hybrid algorithms integrating multiple read signatures have been developed to enhance SV detection precision. Furthermore, emerging AI-based algorithms have improved SV identification using machine learning and data-mining approaches. However, challenges persist in determining the optimal SV detection approach, with more than 80 SV callers published, and no single algorithm or method consistently performing best across different SV types and sizes. Recommendations from expert groups emphasize rigorous validation, standardization protocols, and the incorporation of diverse reference samples to ensure accurate and reliable SV detection in clinical practice. Collaboration among clinical laboratories and ongoing evaluation of SV detection methodologies are essential for advancing standardization and validation efforts.

CLINICS CARE POINTS

- Balanced and unbalanced SVs are associated with a wide variety of human genetic conditions (ie, neurodevelopmental disorders and cancer).
- PCR-free based WGS has the potential to identify a wide range of SVs; however, current recommendations suggest limiting reporting SVs to CNVs or recurrent established pathogenic balanced SVs.
- Best practices outlined by expert groups emphasize the importance of incorporating diverse reference samples and sample sets that encompass various types and sizes of SVs in clinical validation.
- Visualization of large CNVs using B-allele frequency and read-depth plots are useful for evaluating large rearrangements and visualizing potential cytogenetic mechanisms.
- Clinical laboratories should establish policies concerning which SVs require confirmation using orthogonal methods and which ones can be reported directly from short-read-based NGS data.
- Cytogenetic characterization of certain SVs should be performed to accurately define structure, mechanism of origin, and for an accurate interpretation and recurrence risk counseling.

DISCLOSURE

The authors have nothing to disclose.

REFERENCES

[1] Conrad DF, Pinto D, Redon R, et al. Origins and functional impact of copy number variation in the human genome. Nature 2010;464(7289):704–12.

[2] Sudmant PH, Kitzman JO, Antonacci F, et al. Diversity of human copy number variation and multicopy genes. Science 2010;330(6004):641–6.

[3] Alkan C, Coe BP, Eichler EE. Genome structural variation discovery and genotyping. Nat Rev Genet 2011;12(5): 363–76.

[4] Sudmant PH, Rausch T, Gardner EJ, et al. An integrated map of structural variation in 2,504 human genomes. Nature 2015;526(7571):75–81.

[5] Pang AW, MacDonald JR, Pinto D, et al. Towards a comprehensive structural variation map of an individual human genome. Genome Biol 2010;11(5):R52.

[6] Cooper GM, Coe BP, Girirajan S, et al. A copy number variation morbidity map of developmental delay. Nat Genet 2011;43(9):838–46.

[7] Coe BP, Witherspoon K, Rosenfeld JA, et al. Refining analyses of copy number variation identifies specific genes associated with developmental delay. Nat Genet 2014; 46(10):1063–71.

[8] Li Y, Roberts ND, Wala JA, et al. Patterns of somatic structural variation in human cancer genomes. Nature 2020; 578(7793):112–21.

[9] van Belzen I, Schonhuth A, Kemmeren P, et al. Structural variant detection in cancer genomes: computational challenges and perspectives for precision oncology. npj Precis Oncol 2021;5(1):15.

[10] Iafrate AJ, Feuk L, Rivera MN, et al. Detection of large-scale variation in the human genome. Nat Genet 2004; 36(9):949–51.

[11] Sebat J, Lakshmi B, Troge J, et al. Large-scale copy number polymorphism in the human genome. Science 2004; 305(5683):525–8.

[12] Redon R, Ishikawa S, Fitch KR, et al. Global variation in copy number in the human genome. Nature 2006; 444(7118):444–54.

[13] McCarroll SA, Kuruvilla FG, Korn JM, et al. Integrated detection and population-genetic analysis of SNPs and copy number variation. Nat Genet 2008;40(10):1166–74.

[14] Korbel JO, Urban AE, Affourtit JP, et al. Paired-end mapping reveals extensive structural variation in the human genome. Science 2007;318(5849):420–6.

[15] Ho SS, Urban AE, Mills RE. Structural variation in the sequencing era. Nat Rev Genet 2020;21(3):171–89.

[16] Kerkhof J, Schenkel LC, Reilly J, et al. Clinical validation of copy number variant detection from targeted next-generation sequencing panels. J Mol Diagn 2017;19(6):905–20.

[17] Singh AK, Olsen MF, Lavik LAS, et al. Detecting copy number variation in next generation sequencing data from diagnostic gene panels. BMC Med Genom 2021; 14(1):214.

[18] Yao R, Yu T, Qing Y, et al. Evaluation of copy number variant detection from panel-based next-generation sequencing data. Mol Genet Genomic Med 2019;7(1): e00513.

[19] Trost B, Walker S, Wang Z, et al. A comprehensive workflow for read depth-based identification of copy-number variation from whole-genome sequence data. Am J Hum Genet 2018;102(1):142–55.

[20] Campbell PJ, Stephens PJ, Pleasance ED, et al. Identification of somatically acquired rearrangements in cancer using genome-wide massively parallel paired-end sequencing. Nat Genet 2008;40(6):722–9.

[21] Yoon S, Xuan Z, Makarov V, et al. Sensitive and accurate detection of copy number variants using read depth of coverage. Genome Res 2009;19(9):1586–92.

[22] Bentley DR, Balasubramanian S, Swerdlow HP, et al. Accurate whole human genome sequencing using reversible terminator chemistry. Nature 2008;456(7218):53–9.

[23] Magi A, Tattini L, Pippucci T, et al. Read count approach for DNA copy number variants detection. Bioinformatics 2012;28(4):470–8.

[24] Abyzov A, Urban AE, Snyder M, et al. CNVnator: an approach to discover, genotype, and characterize typical and atypical CNVs from family and population genome sequencing. Genome Res 2011;21(6):974–84.

[25] Xie C, Tammi MT. CNV-seq, a new method to detect copy number variation using high-throughput sequencing. BMC Bioinf 2009;10:80.

[26] Krumm N, Sudmant PH, Ko A, et al. Copy number variation detection and genotyping from exome sequence data. Genome Res 2012;22(8):1525–32.

[27] Zhu M, Need AC, Han Y, et al. Using ERDS to infer copy-number variants in high-coverage genomes. Am J Hum Genet 2012;91(3):408–21.

[28] Ye K, Schulz MH, Long Q, et al. Pindel: a pattern growth approach to detect break points of large deletions and medium sized insertions from paired-end short reads. Bioinformatics 2009;25(21):2865–71.

[29] Zhang J, Wang J, Wu Y. An improved approach for accurate and efficient calling of structural variations with low-coverage sequence data. BMC Bioinf 2012;13(Suppl 6):S6.

[30] Tuzun E, Sharp AJ, Bailey JA, et al. Fine-scale structural variation of the human genome. Nat Genet 2005; 37(7):727–32.

[31] Fan X, Abbott TE, Larson D, et al. Break dancer: identification of genomic structural variation from paired-end read mapping. Curr Protoc Bioinformatics 2014; 45(15):6 1–11.

[32] Korbel JO, Abyzov A, Mu XJ, et al. PEMer: a computational framework with simulation-based error models for inferring genomic structural variants from massive paired-end sequencing data. Genome Biol 2009;10(2):R23.

[33] Mahmoud M, Gobet N, Cruz-Davalos DI, et al. Structural variant calling: the long and the short of it. Genome Biol 2019;20(1):246.

[34] Rausch T, Zichner T, Schlattl A, et al. DELLY: structural variant discovery by integrated paired-end and split-read analysis. Bioinformatics 2012;28(18):i333–9.
[35] Chen X, Schulz-Trieglaff O, Shaw R, et al. Manta: rapid detection of structural variants and indels for germline and cancer sequencing applications. Bioinformatics 2016;32(8):1220–2.
[36] Layer RM, Chiang C, Quinlan AR, et al. LUMPY: a probabilistic framework for structural variant discovery. Genome Biol 2014;15(6):R84.
[37] Zarate S, Carroll A, Mahmoud M, et al. Parliament2: accurate structural variant calling at scale. GigaScience 2020;9(12).
[38] Lam HY, Mu XJ, Stutz AM, et al. Nucleotide-resolution analysis of structural variants using BreakSeq and a breakpoint library. Nat Biotechnol 2010;28(1):47–55.
[39] Mohiyuddin M, Mu JC, Li J, et al. MetaSV: an accurate and integrative structural-variant caller for next generation sequencing. Bioinformatics 2015;31(16):2741–4.
[40] Pounraja VK, Jayakar G, Jensen M, et al. A machine-learning approach for accurate detection of copy number variants from exome sequencing. Genome Res 2019; 29(7):1134–43.
[41] Becker T, Lee WP, Leone J, et al. FusorSV: an algorithm for optimally combining data from multiple structural variation detection methods. Genome Biol 2018;19(1): 38.
[42] Klambauer G, Schwarzbauer K, Mayr A, et al. cn.MOPS: mixture of Poissons for discovering copy number variations in next-generation sequencing data with a low false discovery rate. Nucleic Acids Res 2012;40(9):e69.
[43] Handsaker RE, Korn JM, Nemesh J, et al. Discovery and genotyping of genome structural polymorphism by sequencing on a population scale. Nat Genet 2011; 43(3):269–76.
[44] Quinlan AR, Clark RA, Sokolova S, et al. Genome-wide mapping and assembly of structural variant breakpoints in the mouse genome. Genome Res 2010;20(5):623–35.
[45] Popic V, Rohlicek C, Cunial F, et al. Cue: a deep-learning framework for structural variant discovery and genotyping. Nat Methods 2023;20(4):559–68.
[46] Pendleton M, Sebra R, Pang AW, et al. Assembly and diploid architecture of an individual human genome via single-molecule technologies. Nat Methods 2015; 12(8):780–6.
[47] Jain M, Koren S, Miga KH, et al. Nanopore sequencing and assembly of a human genome with ultra-long reads. Nat Biotechnol 2018;36(4):338–45.
[48] Wang YC, Olson ND, Deikus G, et al. High-coverage, long-read sequencing of Han Chinese trio reference samples. Sci Data 2019;6(1):91.
[49] Zook JM, Catoe D, McDaniel J, et al. Extensive sequencing of seven human genomes to characterize benchmark reference materials. Sci Data 2016;3:160025.
[50] Zook JM, Hansen NF, Olson ND, et al. A robust benchmark for detection of germline large deletions and insertions. Nat Biotechnol 2020;38(11):1347–55.
[51] Chaisson MJP, Sanders AD, Zhao X, et al. Multi-platform discovery of haplotype-resolved structural variation in human genomes. Nat Commun 2019;10(1):1784.
[52] Marshall CR, Chowdhury S, Taft RJ, et al. Best practices for the analytical validation of clinical whole-genome sequencing intended for the diagnosis of germline disease. NPJ Genom Med 2020;5:47.
[53] Mills RE, Walter K, Stewart C, et al. Mapping copy number variation by population-scale genome sequencing. Nature 2011;470(7332):59–65.
[54] Abel HJ, Larson DE, Regier AA, et al. Mapping and characterization of structural variation in 17,795 human genomes. Nature 2020;583(7814):83–9.
[55] Collins RL, Brand H, Karczewski KJ, et al. A structural variation reference for medical and population genetics. Nature 2020;581(7809):444–51.
[56] Gardner EJ, Lam VK, Harris DN, et al. The Mobile Element Locator Tool (MELT): population-scale mobile element discovery and biology. Genome Res 2017; 27(11):1916–29.
[57] Tattini L, D'Aurizio R, Magi A. Detection of genomic structural variants from next-generation sequencing data. Front Bioeng Biotechnol 2015;3:92.
[58] Kosugi S, Momozawa Y, Liu X, et al. Comprehensive evaluation of structural variation detection algorithms for whole genome sequencing. Genome Biol 2019; 20(1):117.
[59] Cameron DL, Di Stefano L, Papenfuss AT. Comprehensive evaluation and characterisation of short read general-purpose structural variant calling software. Nat Commun 2019;10(1):3240.
[60] Gabrielaite M, Torp MH, Rasmussen MS, et al. A comparison of tools for copy-number variation detection in germline whole exome and whole genome sequencing data. Cancers 2021;(24):13.
[61] Khayat MM, Sahraeian SME, Zarate S, et al. Hidden biases in germline structural variant detection. Genome Biol 2021;22(1):347.
[62] Austin-Tse CA, Jobanputra V, Perry DL, et al. Best practices for the interpretation and reporting of clinical whole genome sequencing. NPJ Genom Med 2022; 7(1):27.
[63] Raca G, Astbury C, Behlmann A, et al. Points to consider in the detection of germline structural variants using next-generation sequencing: A statement of the American College of Medical Genetics and Genomics (ACMG). Genet Med 2023;25(2):100316.
[64] Beyter D, Ingimundardottir H, Oddsson A, et al. Long-read sequencing of 3,622 Icelanders provides insight into the role of structural variants in human diseases and other traits. Nat Genet 2021;53(6):779–86.
[65] MacDonald JR, Ziman R, Yuen RK, et al. The database of genomic variants: a curated collection of structural variation in the human genome. Nucleic Acids Res 2014; 42(Database issue):D986–92.

Advances in Molecular Pathology 7 (2024) 175–183
ADVANCES IN MOLECULAR PATHOLOGY

Sequencing Platforms

John M. O'Shea, PhD[a,b], Hunter Best, PhD[a,b], Makenzie L. Fulmer, PhD[a,b,*]
[a]Department of Pathology, University of Utah School of Medicine, Salt Lake City, UT, USA; [b]ARUP Laboratories, 500 Chipeta Way, Salt Lake City, UT 84108, USA

KEYWORDS
• Next-generation sequencing platforms • NGS • Short-read sequencing • Long-read sequencing • Genome

KEY POINTS

- Next-generation sequencing has revolutionized the diagnosis of genetic disorders and the ability to interrogate the human genome.
- Short-read sequencing offers high throughput and read accuracy, with diminished capacity to detect structural variation and interrogate highly complex regions of the genome.
- Long-read sequencing has an improved ability to identify structural variation and complex, repetitive regions in the genome.
- Currently, short-read sequencing technologies are more widely used in clinical testing compared to long-read sequencing.

INTRODUCTION

The rapid evolution of sequencing technologies continues to have a colossal impact on the life sciences. Traditional Sanger sequencing, which first debuted in 1977, has been a front-runner in clinical genetic testing and continues to be a gold standard [1]. However, with its low throughput and considerable cost, implementation of testing for diseases with genetic heterogeneity using multigene panels has been limited. Next-generation sequencing (NGS), a high-throughput methodology that allows for rapid sequencing of DNA and RNA at a reduced cost, has therefore become a preferred sequencing methodology and has revolutionized the field of genetics and genomics. With the initiation of this massively parallel sequencing method, substantial progress has been made in the discovery of new genes implicated in human disease in the last decade, allowing for more accurate diagnoses and more directed treatment options for patients. A brief comparison of Sanger sequencing and NGS is described in Fig. 1.

NGS offers the ability to sequence all genes associated with a disorder at a price and turnaround time that is far superior to traditional Sanger sequencing. The current scope of NGS is broad, and testing is appropriate in all stages of life: from preconception or fetal screening to adult-onset disorders. Therefore, laboratories in both commercial and academic settings have quickly employed NGS technology for clinical diagnostics, especially for clinical indications where panel-based testing is the proper approach. To put things into perspective, we compare the time and cost of genome sequencing between the 2 methodologies. The genome of J. D. Watson was sequenced using NGS in under 2 months, costing less than US$1 million. In comparison, as part of the Human Genome Project, sequencing of J. C. Venter's genome using Sanger sequencing technology took almost 15 years to complete and cost over US$100 million [2,3]. More recently, the NGS technology has significantly improved whereby a full human genome can be sequenced with a few days for less than US$1000.

*Corresponding author, *E-mail address:* makenzie.fulmer@aruplab.com

https://doi.org/10.1016/j.yamp.2024.06.007 www.advancesinmolecularpathology.com
2589-4080/24/

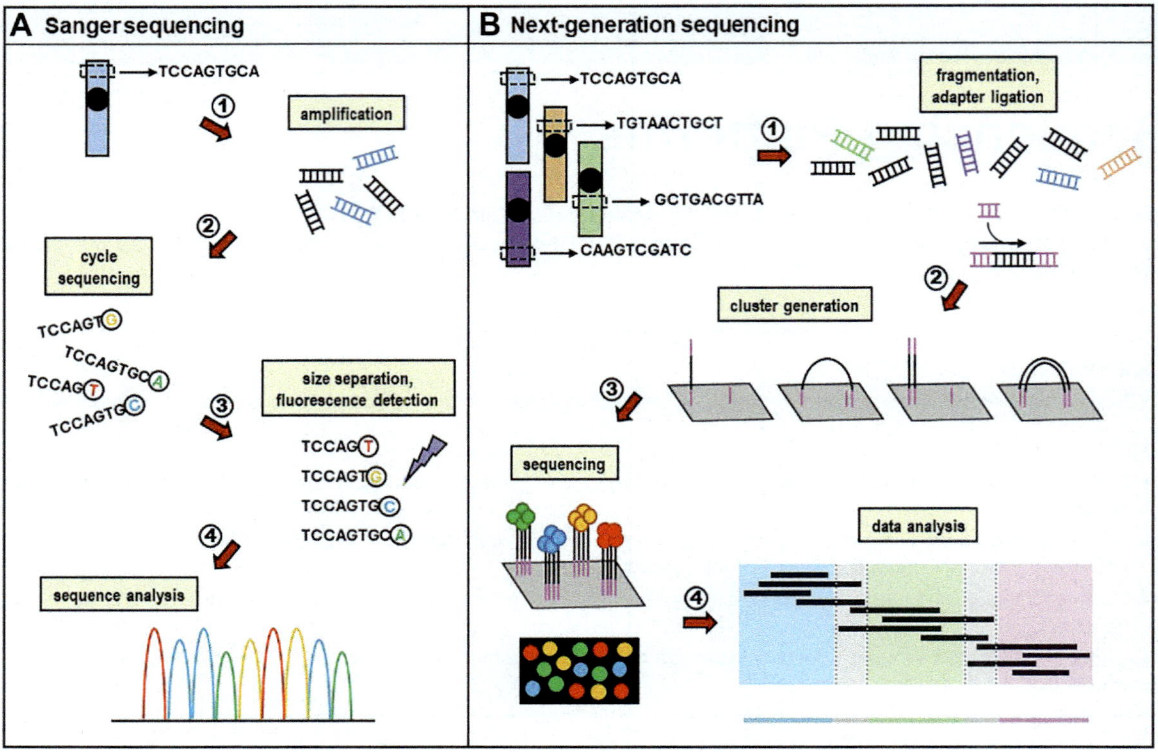

FIG. 1 Comparison of Sanger and NGS. (**A**) Sanger sequencing: (1) A region of interest is exponentially amplified using PCR. (2) Cycle sequencing is performed using chain termination PCR, with incorporation of fluorescently labeled nucleotides. (3) Size separation of the fragments is performed, generally using capillary electrophoresis. A laser is used to detect the specific nucleotide fluorophore on each fragment. (4) Raw data are converted to an electropherogram and aligned to a known sequence for data analysis. (**B**) NGS: (1) Genomic DNA from multiple regions of interest is fragmented and adapters are ligated to the sheared strands, creating a library. (2) The library is loaded onto a flow cell, where the fragments bind to complementary library adapters. Generation of clustered DNA strands generally occurs through bridge amplification. (3) Sequencing is performed using a terminator-based method, and cameras record the fluorescently labeled nucleotides during each sequencing cycle to create a digital image. (4) Sequence reads are aligned utilizing de novo assembly or mapped back to a known genome. The assembled genome sequence can then be analyzed.

Variation of the human genome is not limited to just single base changes in our DNA. There are also insertions and deletions of single or multiple bases, large genomic duplications and deletions of exons or whole gene(s), and complex rearrangements such as translocations or inversions. While Sanger sequencing provides the capability of discovering substitutions or small insertions or deletions, it lacks the ability to capture copy number variants (CNVs) or rearrangements and, therefore, must be supplemented with additional technologies. For instance, exon-level deletions and duplications account for around 15% of *BRCA1* and *BRCA2* mutations identified in hereditary breast and ovarian cancers [4]. Clinical testing for these genes using Sanger sequencing alone would miss a considerable number of pathogenic aberrations in *BRCA1* and *BRCA2*; therefore, a secondary method, which can detect large deletions and duplication events, such as multiplex-ligation probe amplification, would be necessary in order to increase the clinical sensitivity of the assay. The need for additional assays increases the amount of DNA needed from the patient, cost for the patient and laboratory, and turnaround time. Any delay in testing is a detriment to the patient and may have a negative impact on treatment decisions by the physician. NGS technology has the capacity to capture a broader spectrum of variants than traditional Sanger sequencing, so that only one assay needs to be performed in order to assess both small and large genetic changes.

Genetic conditions with considerable genetic heterogeneity, such as cardiomyopathies and RASopathies, are typically prioritized for panel testing as these generally include numerous different genes. Other disorders that are implicated by a single gene may have a cascade testing strategy based on severity of phenotype. Hemophilia A, which is caused by pathogenic variants in *F8*, is a heritable bleeding disorder in which the blood does not clot effectively, and affected persons are subjected to prolonged bleeding after trauma [5]. The phenotypic spectrum of this disorder ranges from mild to severe, and tiered testing is generally utilized in determining the causative genetic change. Clinical information, such as FVIII levels in the patient, is important in determining the best testing approach. For example, an individual who is severely affected would begin with testing to detect the most common pathogenic aberrations implicated in severe hemophilia A, inversion of intron 22 or intron 1. If negative, then testing would be reflexed to sequencing to look for small changes in the coding regions and exon/intron boundaries. Finally, if this testing is negative, the patient sample would be reflexed to deletion/duplication analysis. This tiered approach is very costly and time consuming, and with the advancements in NGS technology, could be consolidated into a single testing platform at a reduced cost and turnaround time. For patients with a complex clinical presentation that does not fit into a specific diagnostic category, use of whole exome or whole genome sequencing (WGS) may be implemented in order to target a broader set of genes in an attempt to end a diagnostic odyssey. Rapid WGS has also been brought to the forefront for use in the neonatal intensive care unit for critically ill newborns [6].

Individuals can have multiple cell lines that are derived from a single zygote but are genotypically different from one another. This phenomenon, termed mosaicism, can be present in both germline and somatic cells. Mosaicism occurs as a result of single nucleotide variants (SNVs), CNVs, and simple or complex chromosomal rearrangements, and the ratio of these changes compared to normal cells may differ between tissue type and location within the body [7]. While there are several molecular and cytogenetics techniques that allow for the detection of mosaic aberrations within the body, such as Giemsa staining, fluorescent in situ hybridization, chromosomal microarray (CMA), and various polymerase chain reaction (PCR) techniques including Sanger, each assay may only detect a single type of change within the genome, with variable limits of detection. For instance, CMA will detect large deletions and duplications, but it is not designed to detect small copy number changes or SNVs. Implementation of NGS technologies has provided the opportunity to assess low-level mosaic changes that include not only SNVs and CNVs but also other complex chromosomal rearrangements such as translocations. The advantage of employing NGS methods over other molecular and cytogenetic methods has clear utility for disorders such as tuberous sclerosis, which is commonly associated with somatic mosaicism [8]. Additionally, an implication for somatic mosaicism in diseases, not commonly associated with mosaicism, has recently become known. For example, pathogenic germline variants in *PTEN* are associated with Cowden syndrome, a disorder characterized by the presence of hamartomas and an increased risk of developing certain cancers. One study highlighted a patient with Cowden syndrome who tested negative for *PTEN* variants by Sanger sequencing of peripheral blood, but NGS testing was able to identify a frameshift variant in *PTEN* at a low frequency in the same sample [9]. Fibroblasts from this individual were then tested, and this frameshift variant was detected at a heterozygous level, confirming mosaicism in this individual. Other large studies have shown that apparent somatic mosaicism may be relatively common in individuals with epilepsy, autism, or intellectual disability [10–12].

Advancements in NGS technology have been crucial to our understanding of the human genome. For instance, when the sequencing of the human genome was originally announced using chain-terminating methods, it still lacked a considerable percentage of genomic DNA. In 2013, new data became available that covered more of the human genome using short-read NGS, but approximately 8% was still lacking [13]. Short-read NGS technologies, which are referred to as second-generation sequencing, lack the ability to sequence long stretches of DNA. As a result, preferential amplification of repetitive DNA can occur during PCR, and the generation of sufficient overlap sequences from the DNA fragments may fail to occur [14,15]. While a useful tool for clinical diagnostics, the downfalls of short-read technologies do pose a major challenge for de novo assembly of the human genome due to repetitive and/or highly complex regions [16]. The missing regions of the genome have typically included repetitive regions of DNA, and it was not until 2022 that a large majority of these gaps could be resolved by the implementation of long-read sequencing [17]. Referred to as third-generation sequencing, long-read sequencing can address some of the shortcomings of Sanger and short-read NGS by sequencing a single molecule at read lengths of 5 to 30 kilobases, eliminating the potential for amplification bias and producing better sequence assembly with sufficient overlap [15,18]. Despite its suitability for de novo assembly in terms of repeat region resolution, detection of structural variants, and the ability to target the epigenome and transcriptome, the per read accuracy and throughput of long-read sequencing still remains poor compared to short-read technologies [14,19,20].

LIBRARY PREPARATION METHODS

To facilitate the pooling of multiple samples onto a single sequencing flow cell and to improve error rates, some approaches to library preparation protocols are now commonly implemented. Pooling of samples is made possible using sample-specific indexes, incorporated into the adapter sequences prior to library amplification. When each sample to be loaded on to the same flow cell is given a unique index, it allows the reads to be assigned to the correct sample during the demultiplexing step in the analysis pipeline [21–23]. Unique molecular identifiers (UMIs) can also be incorporated into the adapter sequence to aid in the reduction of errors introduced during PCR steps in the library preparation and sequencing processes [24,25]. These UMI sequences are composed of a combination of random nucleotides, typically 3 to 8 bp in length. Once adapters are ligated onto the fragmented DNA, there will be an almost unique combination of barcode sequences, split across both adapters. This allows for the identification of variants present in all copies of the molecular family, and the disregarding of errors that occur during library amplification or sequencing [26,27]. Additional improvements in library preparation efficiency can also be achieved using Tn5 transposase-based, or tagmentation method, which combines DNA cleavage and adapter ligation into a single reaction. This helps with process automation and throughput [28]. Almost all of the short-read platforms we will discuss next can incorporate some or all of these methods to improve accuracy of the data obtained from the sequencing run.

SHORT-READ SEQUENCING PLATFORMS

Illumina

Sequencing by synthesis (SBS) technology was developed and commercialized by Solexa Sequencing in the 1990s, culminating in the release of the first high-throughput sequencing platform, the Genome Analyzer in 2006 [29]. SBS allowed researchers to generate up to 1 gigabase (Gb) of data from a single run, dramatically increasing the throughput over previous technologies. By incorporating fluorescently labeled reversible terminator nucleotides and clustering amplified fragments of DNA onto flow cells, the sequencing speed, fidelity, and cost were all improved. Illumina acquired Solexa in 2007, and it formed the basis for the current sequencing methodology utilized in Illumina sequencers [30,31]. This is the most commonly used method in clinical molecular laboratories.

In the Illumina short-read method, DNA is fragmented and Illumina-specific adapters are ligated onto these DNA fragments. Adapter-ligated libraries can either be PCR amplified or be loaded on the sequencer without an amplification step (PCR-free sequencing) [32]. Clusters are generated on the flow cell, through bridge amplification, which helps increase the signal and the fidelity of base calling, although this can also lead to template error expansion [33]. The libraries are then able to undergo sequencing.

Initially, 4 different fluorescent colors were used, one for each nucleotide. Each sequencing cycle leads to the incorporation of a single nucleotide, which can be deciphered based on the fluorescent signal of the cluster. More recent instruments are using 2 fluorescent colors, with the additional nucleotides using either a mixture of both colors, and a nonfluorescently labeled nucleotide, which is read by an absence of fluorescence signal. This simplifies the optics systems used in these 2 color sequencing instruments.

The reversible terminator chemistry allows for only a single nucleotide to be incorporated into the extending DNA chain in each sequencing cycle. After the fluorescent signals are imaged, the fluorescent dyes are washed away, leaving the 3′ hydroxyl group available for the next nucleotide to be incorporated in the next cycle.

Ion Torrent

Ion semiconductor sequencing was developed by Ion Torrent Systems, with the first sequencing instrument, the Personal Genome Machine, being released in 2010. Rather than using fluorescently labeled nucleotides, which requires more complex and expensive optics and imaging capacity, this technology sought to simplify the sequencing process by measuring the release of hydrogen ions during nucleotide incorporation into the extending DNA strand [34]. The ions are detected via an ion-sensitive field effect transistor [35]. Individual DNA molecules are incorporated into separate microwells enabling the sequence of the specific DNA strand to be determined.

At each cycle, standard deoxynucleotide triphosphates are introduced individually onto the sequencing chip in sequential manner, with the remaining nucleotides being washed away prior to the addition of the next nucleotide. If a nucleotide is successfully incorporated into the extending DNA strand, a change in pH will occur due to the release of hydrogen ions from the extension reaction, allowing the instrument to determine the sequence.

Ultima Genomics

Ultima Genomics UG 100 Sequencer utilizes an open flow cell design on a circular 200 mm silicon wafer, which is a standard low-cost substrate commonly used in the semiconductor industry. By additionally incorporating contactless spin coating, a technique that was developed for and is commonly used in the computer chip industry, they have also eliminated more complex microfluidics systems from the platform. They also use what they describe as "mostly natural sequencing by synthesis chemistry," with fluorescently labeled sequencing nucleotides that do not incorporate reversible terminator chemistry, a common approach used in other sequencing platforms, another mechanism that lowers reagent cost. Finally, Ultima uses neural network-enabled base calling to improve accuracy [36]. This results in an innovative and cost-effective sequencing solution, with an advertised cost of WGS of approximately US$100.

Element Biosciences

Avidity base chemistry (ABC) was a process developed by Element Biosciences. Rather than a PCR-based amplification process, clusters of the same DNA strand are generated via rolling circle amplification (RCA), helping to reduce template error expansion, which can occur with PCR bases amplification processes [33]. The RCA-generated DNA copies form tightly bound structures, termed polonies, and these structures form the backbone for the binding of an avidite, a dye-labeled polymer with the same nucleotide [37,38]. The avidites detect bases in the polony in a sequential manner and amplify the signal for optical detection. A low-binding surface chemistry was also developed, improving the contrast to noise ratio and reducing the number of fluorescent molecules required for optical detection. Scores, or the probability of the sequencer incorrectly calling a base at any given position 1 in 10,000 (1:10,000) times, are frequently obtained, with some libraries even reaching a score (1:100,000 times) [39–41]. This makes this platform particularly suited to sequencing to a low depth of coverage while calling variants with confidence.

Complete Genomics

Complete Genomics utilizes rolling circle replication (RCR) to amplify DNA molecules into self-assembling DNA nanoballs (DNBs), a process also based on the multiplexed polony technique [38,42]. The nanoballs are loaded onto flow cells with etched patterns of approximately 200 nm uniformly spaced binding sites. Combinatorial probe-anchor synthesis (cPAS) chemistry then incorporates fluorescently labeled reversibly terminating probes, which allows the optical system to determine the sequence of the DNB [43]. The combined benefits of the PCR-free amplification and the high occupancy of DNBs on flow cell enable accurate and cost-effective sequencing.

LONG-READ SEQUENCING PLATFORMS

Most sequencing data generated to date has focused on read lengths of between 50 and 300 nucleotides. After these sequences are aligned to a reference genome, differences from the reference can be detected. The short length of the fragments works well for many different types of variants, particularly SNVs and small insertions and deletions. It is also possible to detect more complex structural variants, such as CNVs and inversions (INVs), through bioinformatic approaches developed specifically for this purpose, including read depth, read pair, and split read techniques [44]. However, short-read sequencing continues to struggle with certain regions of the genome, such as repetitive and high GC content regions, making some differences difficult to detect, repeat expansions being a very important example [45–47]. Additionally, phasing of variants to the same or different chromosomes can be important in determining whether the variant pair can lead to disease. Many of these shortcomings are addressed by long-read sequencing technologies [48,49]. In addition, long-read platforms can detect epigenetic changes to DNA, adding an additional layer of information that can be generated from long-read sequencing technologies [50,51]. One drawback to long-read sequencing has historically been an increased error rate in base calling. More recent improvements have reduced these concerns, and it is now possible to generate data with error rates comparable to short-read sequencing platforms. Next, we will discuss the 2 most common long-read platforms and a modification to short-read sequencing methods that allow for longer reads to be assembled from short-read data (Table 1).

TABLE 1
Comparison of Short-Read and Long-Read Sequencing Platforms

	Platform	Sequencing Method	Detection	Amplification	Single or Paired End	Read Length	Q30
Short Read	Illumina (San Diego, CA)	SBS	Optical	Bridge	P	2 × 50 – 2 × 300	≥85 – 90%
	Ion Torrent (Waltham, MA)	SBS	Ion	Emulsion PCR (emPCR)	—	—	—
	Ultima Genomics (Newark, CA)	SBS	Optical	emPCR	S	1 × 225 – 300+	>85%
	Element Biosciences (San Diego, CA)	Avidites	Optical	RCA	P	2 × 75 – 2 × 300	>85 – 90%
	Complete Genomics (San Jose, CA)	cPAS	Optical	RCR	P	2 × 50 – 2 × 300	>85%
Long Read	PacBio (Menlo Park, CA)	—	Optical	Na	S	10 – 20 kbp	>90
	Oxford Nanopore Technologies (Oxford Science Park, OX)	—	Current	Na	S	20 bp – 4 Mbp	—

Pacific Biosciences

Pacific Biosciences (PacBio) developed a sequencing methodology that immobilizes a single circularized DNA fragment onto the bottom of a cylindrically shaped well, known as zero-mode waveguides (ZMWs), on the surface of a nanofluidic chip, known as a single molecule, real-time (SMRT) cell [52,53]. SMRT cells can contain millions of ZMWs, and multiple SMRT cells can be run in parallel on a single instrument, allowing for a large number of long DNA molecules to be sequenced simultaneously. Long double-stranded DNA fragments are converted into circular DNA molecules through the ligation of SMRTbell adapters to both ends. A DNA polymerase is attached to the SMRTbell circular DNA, and as individual nucleotides are incorporated into the expanding DNA strand, light is released corresponding to the specific nucleotide, which can be detected via an optical system. Differences in the kinetics of the nucleotide incorporation also allow for epigenetic modifications to be detected, without any additional processing steps such as bisulfite or enzymatic conversion [50]. Improvements in the platform and in sequencing methods, including PacBio HiFi sequencing, have dramatically reduced error rates, which was one of the major downsides to earlier long-read sequencing methodologies, while still maintaining average read lengths of 10 to 25 kbp [54].

Oxford Nanopore Technologies

Oxford Nanopore Technologies approach to sequencing long strands of DNA utilizes an array of tiny holes, known as nanopores, embedded in an electro-resistant membrane. The flow of current through these nanopores can be disrupted by any molecules passing through, such as single-stranded DNA, and each molecule has a specific disruption pattern, allowing for the sequencing of native DNA strands [55,56]. This can also be applied to RNA and other biomolecules such as proteins [57,58]. Sample preparation consists of the addition of an adaptor and motor protein, which controls the translocation of the single-stranded DNA molecule through the nanopore. Since modified nucleotides will also have a specific disruption pattern, epigenetic modifications can also be captured with this technology. DNA molecules from as short as 20 bp and as long as 4 Mbp have been sequenced on this platform, with 10 to 300 kbp being more typical [59]. Real-time availability of the data allows for adaptive sequencing to be utilized, which allows the instrument to focus on specific user-defined regions or improve coverage uniformity by focusing later sequencing on low coverage regions [60].

Illumina Complete Long-Read

Illumina has developed a method allowing sequencing information from their short-read platforms to generate long-read data. This is achieved by creating "land marked" DNA from long DNA strands prior to processing in a short-read sequencing protocol. The "land marked" DNA can then be assembled informatically into long-read sequences of up to 5 to 7 kbp. Other groups have developed alternative approaches, such as transposase enzyme-linked long-read sequencing, which can generate phased reads of DNA sequences up to 20 to 110 kbp [61]. These approaches can be incorporated into standard WGS workflows allowing for both short-read and long-read data to be obtained simultaneously, resulting in a more complete genome. However, the lengths obtained via this method can be less than those obtained from dedicated long-read platforms and have the other disadvantages seen with short-read platforms discussed earlier.

SUMMARY

Improvements to NGS platforms and techniques are rapidly allowing for increasingly more complex and comprehensive clinical questions to be answered. Additionally, increased competition among platforms should result in reduced costs, leading to improved access to these testing options for a broader population. Many clinical questions can be resolved using current approaches, but for a subset of patients, these approaches are not sufficient. Utilizing long-read sequencing and incorporating epigenetic analysis should increase diagnostic yields above what current practices allow. It is also possible that one clinical test will provide the same diagnostic information as the multiple approaches currently routinely used (ie, genomic microarray, chromosome analysis—karyotype, exome sequencing/WGS). This would provide the opportunity to reduce the time to diagnosis for many patients, allowing for targeted treatments and planning to be implemented in a much timelier manner.

CLINICS CARE POINTS

- Advances in next generation sequencing technologies have facilitated accurate diagnoses for a wide variety of genetic conditions, at a relatively low cost and acceptable turnaround time.
- Panel testing provides a convenient and cost-effective method of obtaining a diagnosis, when the clinical team has strong suspicion for a specific genetic condition.
- Long read sequencing platforms have the potential to combine many diagnostic questions into a single unified platform, leading to simplified test selection for clinical teams and quicker diagnoses for patients and their families.
- Exome and whole genome short read sequencing is being utilized more frequently as a first-tier test due to its ability to interrogate a wide range of abnormalities and a continued decrease in sequencing costs.
- Ongoing improvements to sequencing methods and bioinformatic analysis pipelines will allow for increasingly more complex genetic questions to be answered.

DISCLOSURE

The authors have nthing to disclose.

REFERENCES

[1] Sanger F, Nicklen S, Coulson AR. DNA Sequencing with Chain-Terminating Inhibitors. Proc Natl Acad Sci U S A 1977;74(12):5463–7, (DNA Polymerase/Nucleotide Sequences/Bacteriophage 4X174).

[2] Levy S, Sutton G, Ng PC, et al. The Diploid Genome Sequence of an Individual Human. PLoS Biol 2017; 5(10):e254. https://doi.org/10.1371/journal.pbio.

[3] Wheeler DA, Srinivasan M, Egholm M, et al. The complete genome of an individual by massively parallel DNA sequencing. Nature 2008;452(7189):872–6. https://doi.org/10.1038/nature06884.

[4] Petrucelli N, Daly MB, Pal T. BRCA1- and BRCA2-Associated Hereditary Breast and Ovarian Cancer. 1993. Available at: https://www.ncbi.nlm.nih.gov/books/NBK1247/. [Accessed 27 March 2024].

[5] Konkle BA, Nakaya Fletcher S. Hemophilia A. 1993. Available at: https://www.ncbi.nlm.nih.gov/books/NBK1404/. [Accessed 27 March 2024].

[6] Lewis R, O'Shea J, Best D, et al. Rapid whole genome sequencing in critically ill newborns. In: Tsongalis G, editor. Advances in molecular pathology6. 2023. 2023. p. 175–86.

[7] Spinner NB, Conlin LK. Mosaicism and clinical genetics. Am J Med Genet C Semin Med Genet 2014;166C(4): 397–405. https://doi.org/10.1002/ajmg.c.31421.

[8] Verhoef S, Bakker L, Tempelaars AM, et al. High rate of mosaicism in tuberous sclerosis complex. Am J Hum Genet 1999;64(6):1632–7. https://doi.org/10.1086/302412.

[9] Pritchard CC, Smith C, Marushchak T, et al. A mosaic PTEN mutation causing Cowden syndrome identified by deep sequencing. Genet Med 2013;15(12):1004–7. https://doi.org/10.1038/gim.2013.51.

[10] Acuna-Hidalgo R, Bo T, Kwint MP, et al. Post-zygotic Point Mutations Are an Underrecognized Source of De Novo Genomic Variation. Am J Hum Genet 2015;97(1):67–74. https://doi.org/10.1016/j.ajhg.2015.05.008.

[11] Freed D, Pevsner J. The Contribution of Mosaic Variants to Autism Spectrum Disorder. PLoS Genet 2016;12(9): e1006245. https://doi.org/10.1371/journal.pgen.1006245.

[12] Stosser MB, Lindy AS, Butler E, et al. High frequency of mosaic pathogenic variants in genes causing epilepsy-related neurodevelopmental disorders. Genet Med 2018;20(4):403–10. https://doi.org/10.1038/gim.2017.114.

[13] Nurk S, Koren S, Rhie A, et al. The complete sequence of a human genome. Science 2022;376(6588):44–53. https://doi.org/10.1126/science.abj6987.

[14] Adewale BA. Will long-read sequencing technologies replace short-read sequencing technologies in the next 10 years? Afr J Lab Med 2020;9(1):1340. https://doi.org/10.4102/ajlm.v9i1.1340.

[15] Olivucci G, Iovino E, Innella G, et al. Long read sequencing on its way to the routine diagnostics of genetic diseases. Front Genet 2024;15:1374860. https://doi.org/10.3389/fgene.2024.1374860.

[16] Neerman N, Faust G, Meeks N, et al. A clinically validated whole genome pipeline for structural variant detection and analysis. BMC Genom 2019;20(Suppl 8):545. https://doi.org/10.1186/s12864-019-5866-z.

[17] Marx V. Method of the year: long-read sequencing. Nat Methods 2023;20(1):6–11. https://doi.org/10.1038/s41592-022-01730-w.

[18] Mastrorosa FK, Miller DE, Eichler EE. Applications of long-read sequencing to Mendelian genetics. Genome Med 2023;15(1):42. https://doi.org/10.1186/s13073-023-01194-3.

[19] Amarasinghe SL, Su S, Dong X, et al. Opportunities and challenges in long-read sequencing data analysis. Genome Biol 2020;21(1):30. https://doi.org/10.1186/s13059-020-1935-5.

[20] Lin B, Hui J, Mao H. Nanopore Technology and Its Applications in Gene Sequencing. Biosensors (Basel) 2021; 11(7). https://doi.org/10.3390/bios11070214.

[21] Kircher M, Sawyer S, Meyer M. Double indexing overcomes inaccuracies in multiplex sequencing on the Illumina platform. Nucleic Acids Res 2012;40(1). https://doi.org/10.1093/nar/gkr771.

[22] Rohland N, Reich D. Cost-effective, high-throughput DNA sequencing libraries for multiplexed target capture. Genome Res 2012;22(5). https://doi.org/10.1101/gr.128124.111.

[23] Meyer M, Kircher M. Illumina sequencing library preparation for highly multiplexed target capture and sequencing. Cold Spring Harb Protoc 2010;5(6). https://doi.org/10.1101/pdb.prot5448.

[24] Jabara CB, Jones CD, Roach J, et al. Accurate sampling and deep sequencing of the HIV-1 protease gene using a Primer ID. Proc Natl Acad Sci U S A 2011;108(50). https://doi.org/10.1073/pnas.1110064108.

[25] Kinde I, Wu J, Papadopoulos N, et al. Detection and quantification of rare mutations with massively parallel sequencing. Proc Natl Acad Sci U S A 2011;108(23). https://doi.org/10.1073/pnas.1105422108.

[26] Schmitt MW, Kennedy SR, Salk JJ, et al. Detection of ultra-rare mutations by next-generation sequencing. Proc Natl Acad Sci U S A 2012;109(36). https://doi.org/10.1073/pnas.1208715109.

[27] Kukita Y, Matoba R, Uchida J, et al. High-fidelity target sequencing of individual molecules identified using barcode sequences: De novo detection and absolute quantitation of mutations in plasma cell-free DNA from cancer patients. DNA Research 2015;22(4). https://doi.org/10.1093/dnares/dsv010.

[28] Adey AC. Tagmentation-based single-cell genomics. Genome Res 2021;31(10):1693–705. https://doi.org/10.1101/gr.275223.121.

[29] Rodriguez R, Krishnan Y. The chemistry of next-generation sequencing. Nat Biotechnol 2023;41(12). https://doi.org/10.1038/s41587-023-01986-3.

[30] Bentley DR, Balasubramanian S, Swerdlow HP, et al. Accurate whole human genome sequencing using reversible terminator chemistry. Nature 2008;456(7218). https://doi.org/10.1038/nature07517.

[31] Chen F, Dong M, Ge M, et al. The History and Advances of Reversible Terminators Used in New Generations of Sequencing Technology. Dev Reprod Biol 2013;11(1). https://doi.org/10.1016/j.gpb.2013.01.003.

[32] Zhou G, Zhou M, Zeng F, et al. Performance characterization of PCR-free whole genome sequencing for clinical diagnosis. Medicine (United States) 2022;101(10). https://doi.org/10.1097/MD.0000000000028972.

[33] Nix DA, Hellwig S, Conley C, et al. The stochastic nature of errors in next-generation sequencing of circulating cell-free DNA. PLoS One 2020;15(2). https://doi.org/10.1371/journal.pone.0229063.

[34] Slatko BE, Gardner AF, Ausubel FM. Overview of Next-Generation Sequencing Technologies. Curr Protoc Mol Biol 2018;122(1). https://doi.org/10.1002/cpmb.59.

[35] Lee CS, Kyu Kim S, Kim M. Ion-sensitive field-effect transistor for biological sensing. Sensors 2009;9(9). https://doi.org/10.3390/s90907111.

[36] Almogy G, Pratt M, Oberstrass F, et al. Cost-efficient whole genome-sequencing using novel mostly natural sequencing-by-synthesis chemistry and open fluidics platform. bioRxiv 2022. https://doi.org/10.1101/2022.05.29.493900.

[37] Arslan S, Garcia FJ, Guo M, et al. Sequencing by avidity enables high accuracy with low reagent consumption. Nat Biotechnol 2024;42(1):132–8. https://doi.org/10.1038/s41587-023-01750-7.

[38] Shendure J, Porreca GJ, Reppas NB, et al. Accurate multiplex polony sequencing of an evolved bacterial genome. Science (1979) 2005;309(5741). https://doi.org/10.1126/science.1117389.

[39] Sprang M, Kruger M, Andrade-Navarro MA, et al. Statistical guidelines for quality control of next-generation sequencing techniques. Life Sci Alliance 2021;4(11). https://doi.org/10.26508/LSA.202101113.

[40] Cock PJA, Fields CJ, Goto N, et al. The Sanger FASTQ file format for sequences with quality scores, and the Solexa/Illumina FASTQ variants. Nucleic Acids Res 2009;38(6). https://doi.org/10.1093/nar/gkp1137.

[41] Ewing B, Green P. Base-calling of automated sequencer traces using phred. II. Error probabilities. Genome Res 1998;8(3). https://doi.org/10.1101/gr.8.3.186.

[42] Drmanac R, Sparks AB, Callow MJ, et al. Human genome sequencing using unchained base reads on self-assembling DNA nanoarrays. Science (1979) 2010; 327(5961). https://doi.org/10.1126/science.1181498.

[43] Fehlmann T, Reinheimer S, Geng C, et al. cPAS-based sequencing on the BGISEQ-500 to explore small non-coding RNAs. Clin Epigenet 2016;8(1). https://doi.org/10.1186/s13148-016-0287-1.

[44] Minoche AE, Lundie B, Peters GB, et al. ClinSV: clinical grade structural and copy number variant detection from whole genome sequencing data. Genome Med 2021; 13(1). https://doi.org/10.1186/s13073-021-00841-x.

[45] Benjamini Y, Speed TP. Summarizing and correcting the GC content bias in high-throughput sequencing. Nucleic Acids Res 2012;40(10). https://doi.org/10.1093/nar/gks001.

[46] Treangen TJ, Salzberg SL. Repetitive DNA and next-generation sequencing: Computational challenges and solutions. Nat Rev Genet 2012;13(1). https://doi.org/10.1038/nrg3117.

[47] Tilak MK, Botero-Castro F, Galtier N, et al. Illumina Library Preparation for Sequencing the GC-Rich Fraction of Heterogeneous Genomic DNA. Genome Biol Evol 2018;10(2). https://doi.org/10.1093/gbe/evy022.

[48] Logsdon GA, Vollger MR, Eichler EE. Long-read human genome sequencing and its applications. Nat Rev Genet 2020;21(10). https://doi.org/10.1038/s41576-020-0236-x.

[49] Feng Z, Clemente JC, Wong B, et al. Detecting and phasing minor single-nucleotide variants from long-read sequencing data. Nat Commun 2021;12(1). https://doi.org/10.1038/s41467-021-23289-4.

[50] Ni P, Nie F, Zhong Z, et al. DNA 5-methylcytosine detection and methylation phasing using PacBio circular consensus sequencing. Nat Commun 2023;14(1). https://doi.org/10.1038/s41467-023-39784-9.

[51] Simpson JT, Workman RE, Zuzarte PC, et al. Detecting DNA cytosine methylation using nanopore sequencing. Nat Methods 2017;14(4). https://doi.org/10.1038/nmeth.4184.

[52] Koren S, Schatz MC, Walenz BP, et al. Hybrid error correction and de novo assembly of single-molecule sequencing reads. Nat Biotechnol 2012;30(7). https://doi.org/10.1038/nbt.2280.

[53] Eid J, Fehr A, Gray J, et al. Real-time DNA sequencing from single polymerase molecules. Science (1979) 2009; 323(5910). https://doi.org/10.1126/science.1162986.

[54] Hon T, Mars K, Young G, et al. Highly accurate long-read HiFi sequencing data for five complex genomes. Sci Data 2020;7(1). https://doi.org/10.1038/s41597-020-00743-4.

[55] Howorka S, Cheley S, Bayley H. Sequence-specific detection of individual DNA strands using engineered nanopores. Nat Biotechnol 2001;19(7). https://doi.org/10.1038/90236.

[56] Kasianowicz JJ, Brandin E, Branton D, et al. Characterization of individual polynucleotide molecules using a membrane channel. Proc Natl Acad Sci USA 1996;93. https://doi.org/10.1073/pnas.93.24.13770.

[57] Dorey A, Howorka S. Nanopore DNA sequencing technologies and their applications towards single-molecule proteomics. Nat Chem 2024;16(3). https://doi.org/10.1038/s41557-023-01322-x.

[58] Martin-Baniandres P, Lan WH, Board S, et al. Enzyme-less nanopore detection of post-translational modifications within long polypeptides. Nat Nanotechnol 2023; 18(11). https://doi.org/10.1038/s41565-023-01462-8.

[59] Anukul N, Jenjaroenpun P, Sirikul C, et al. Ultrarapid and high-resolution HLA class I typing using transposase-based nanopore sequencing applied in pharmacogenetic testing. Front Genet 2023;14. https://doi.org/10.3389/fgene.2023.1213457.

[60] Loose M, Malla S, Stout M. Real-time selective sequencing using nanopore technology. Nat Methods 2016;13(9). https://doi.org/10.1038/nmeth.3930.

[61] Chen Z, Pham L, Wu TC, et al. Ultralow-input single-tube linked-read library method enables short-read second-generation sequencing systems to routinely generate highly accurate and economical long-range sequencing information. Genome Res 2020;30(6). https://doi.org/10.1101/gr.260380.119.